—What causes baldness?
—How much sleep should you get?
—What special care should you give your skin?
—Has the link between cancer and cigarettes been proven?
—What is your optimal weight?
—What foods should you avoid to maintain your heart in a healthy condition?
—How do you deal with a child who is a picky eater?
—What is the best exercise to relieve stress?
—Are there effective treatments for sexual frigidity and impotence?
—What are the facts and myths about old age?
—What are the special nutritional needs of a pregnant woman?

THE HEALTHY BODY

A Maintenance Manual

Thousands of such questions are answered for you in this complete and practical guide that speaks to you directly in words and pictures you can instantly understand and benefit from.

THE DIAGRAM GROUP is the creator of this unique format for conveying the most up-to-date health information and advice to the reading public. Previous books by The Diagram Group, such as *Man's Body*, *Woman's Body*, and *Child's Body*, have appeared in 17 languages and sold over 5 million copies in 20 countries.

THE HEALTHY BODY

A Maintenance Manual

BY THE DIAGRAM GROUP

A PLUME BOOK
NEW AMERICAN LIBRARY
MOSBY
TIMES MIRROR
NEW YORK AND SCARBOROUGH, ONTARIO

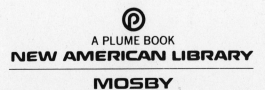

MOSBY MEDICAL LIBRARY

Publisher's note:
The ideas, procedures, and suggestions contained in this book are not intended as a substitute for consulting with your physician. All matters regarding your health require medical supervision.

NAL books are available at quantity discounts when used to promote products or services. For information please write to:
Premium Marketing Division,
The New American Library, Inc., 1633 Broadway,
New York, New York 10019

Library of Congress Catalog Card Number: 81-82816

PLUME TRADEMARK REG. U.S. PAT. OFF. AND FOREIGN COUNTRIES
REGISTERED TRADEMARK—MARCA REGISTRADA
HECHO EN WESTFORD, MASS., U.S.A.

SIGNET, SIGNET CLASSICS, MENTOR, PLUME, MERIDIAN and NAL BOOKS are published *in the United States* by The New American Library Inc., 1633 Broadway, New York, New York 10019, *in Canada* by The New American Library of Canada Limited, 81 Mack Avenue, Scarborough, Ontario M1L 1M8.

Mosby Books are published by
The Mosby Press, The C. V. Mosby Company,
11830 Westline Industrial Drive, St. Louis, Missouri 63141

First Printing, November, 1981

First Mosby Medical Library Printing, April, 1982

1 2 3 4 5 6 7 8 9

PRINTED IN THE UNITED STATES OF AMERICA

Consultants

Cyril J Jones, MD
Clinical Professor of Surgery, State University of New York; Chief Medical Officer, New York Fire Service

Dr Ian Anderson
Consultant cardiologist, Harley Street

Dr Paul Basset and Dr Keith Langley
Centre de Neurochemie, Strasbourg

Mrs A Borrill
Inner London Education Authority Tutor for Physical Fitness in Retirement

Camden Borough Council Homes for the Elderly

Family Planning Association

Dr D B Garrioch
Consultant in Obstetrics and Gynaecology, Pembury Hospital

Dr H Gough-Thomas
Executive Director, National Council on Alcoholism

Frances Haste
Research Associate, St George's Hospital Medical School

Mr R A C Hoppenbrouwers
University College Dental Hospital

Sally Humphreys
Psychologist

Professor P J Lawther
Professor of Environmental and Preventive Medicine, University of London and St Bartholomew's Hospital

Dr Gwyneth Lewis
Medical Officer, Sussex University

Dr M Modell
The James Wigg Practice

Shirley Norman
Tutor of Physical Fitness for Inner London Education Authority

Janet Pilkington
Sector Chiropodist (Windsor/Maidenhead), East Berkshire Health District

Dr C Ray
Lecturer in Psychology, Brunel University

Robert Royston
Psychotherapist

Dr M K Thompson
General Practitioner in Croydon, Surrey

Michael Tristram
Director, RELEASE

THE DIAGRAM GROUP

Editor Gail Lawther

Contributors Maureen Cartwright, David Lambert, Ruth Midgley, Caroline Tomalin

Indexer Mary Ling

Art editors Mark Evans, Richard Hummerstone

Artists Stephen Clark, Sean Gilbert, Brian Hewson, Kathleen McDougall, Janos Marffy, Graham Rosewarne

Foreword

The inner workings of our bodies are probably a mystery to most of us. Chances are that we know more about the functioning of our automobiles or our plumbing than we do about our heart or our digestive system.

The editors of THE HEALTHY BODY believe that it is through an understanding of our own body and an awareness of its capabilities that we can gain better control of our health. The proverb "An ounce of prevention is worth a pound of cure" is particularly relevant. Each individual should assume personal responsibility for his or her own health. It is interesting to note that the words "healthy body" can be divided up into "heal thy body."

Medical science and its language are frequently complex, but our goal in THE HEALTHY BODY has been to express this information in terms that the general reader can easily understand. By the frequent use of anatomical illustrations, the unseen workings of our bodies are made clear, and by the use of charts, medical statistics are displayed in a way that is immediately comprehensible.

During the creation of the book, all text and drawings were submitted to a panel of medical specialists, who have carefully checked and approved the material. It is the job of these men and women of the medical profession to examine daily the defects of our bodies – defects that are all too often the result of ignorance or malpractice. We of the Diagram Group hope that THE HEALTHY BODY will provide you with an enjoyable means of discovering knowledge about your body, and that it will encourage the maintenance of the healthy and vital life that is your natural birthright.

Contents

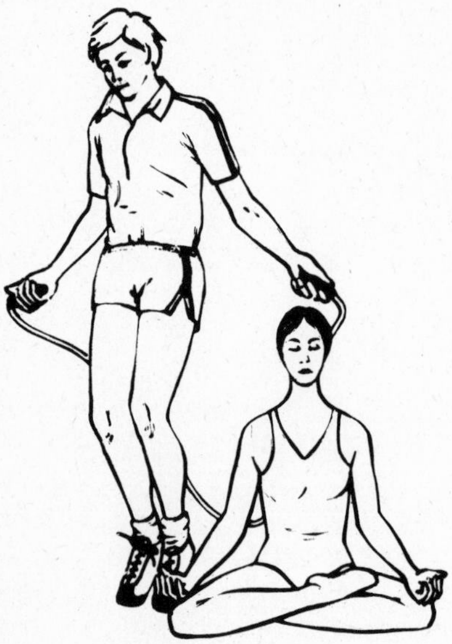

Chapter 1

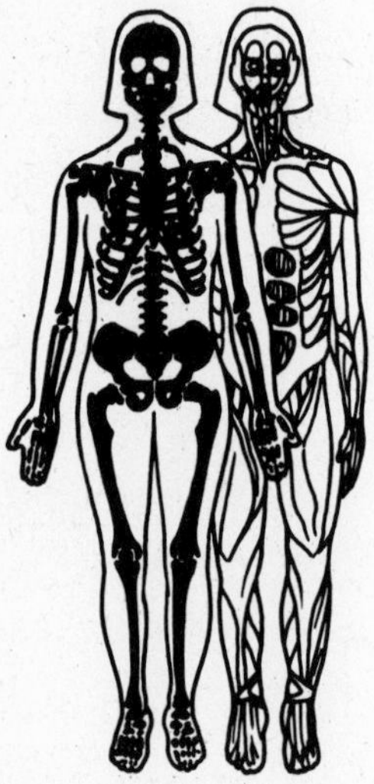

Chapter 2

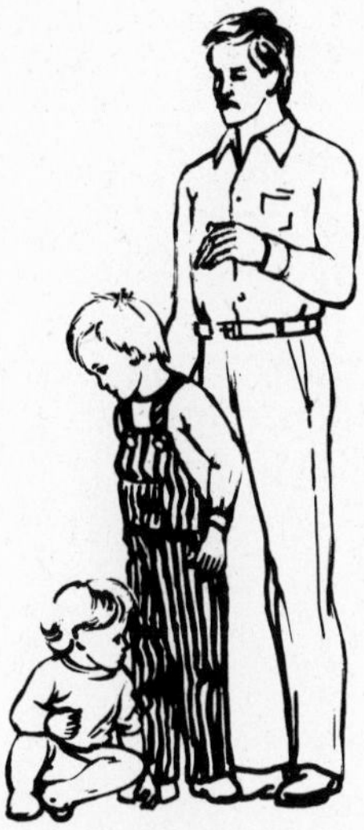

Chapter 3

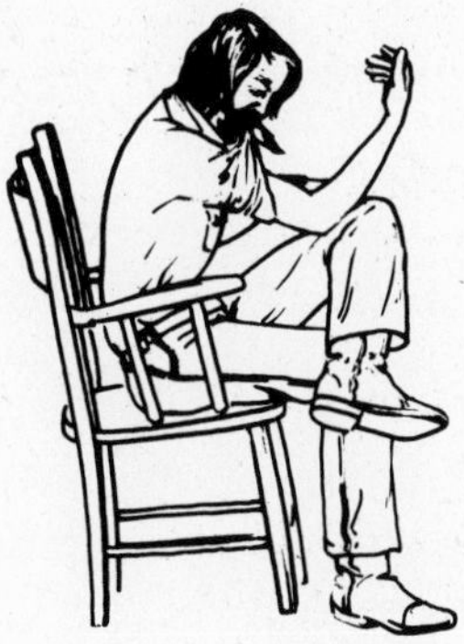

Chapter 4

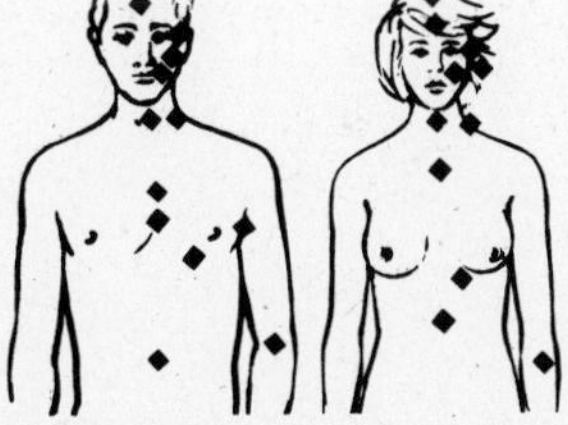

Chapter 5

CHAPTER 1

A HEALTHY ENVIRONMENT

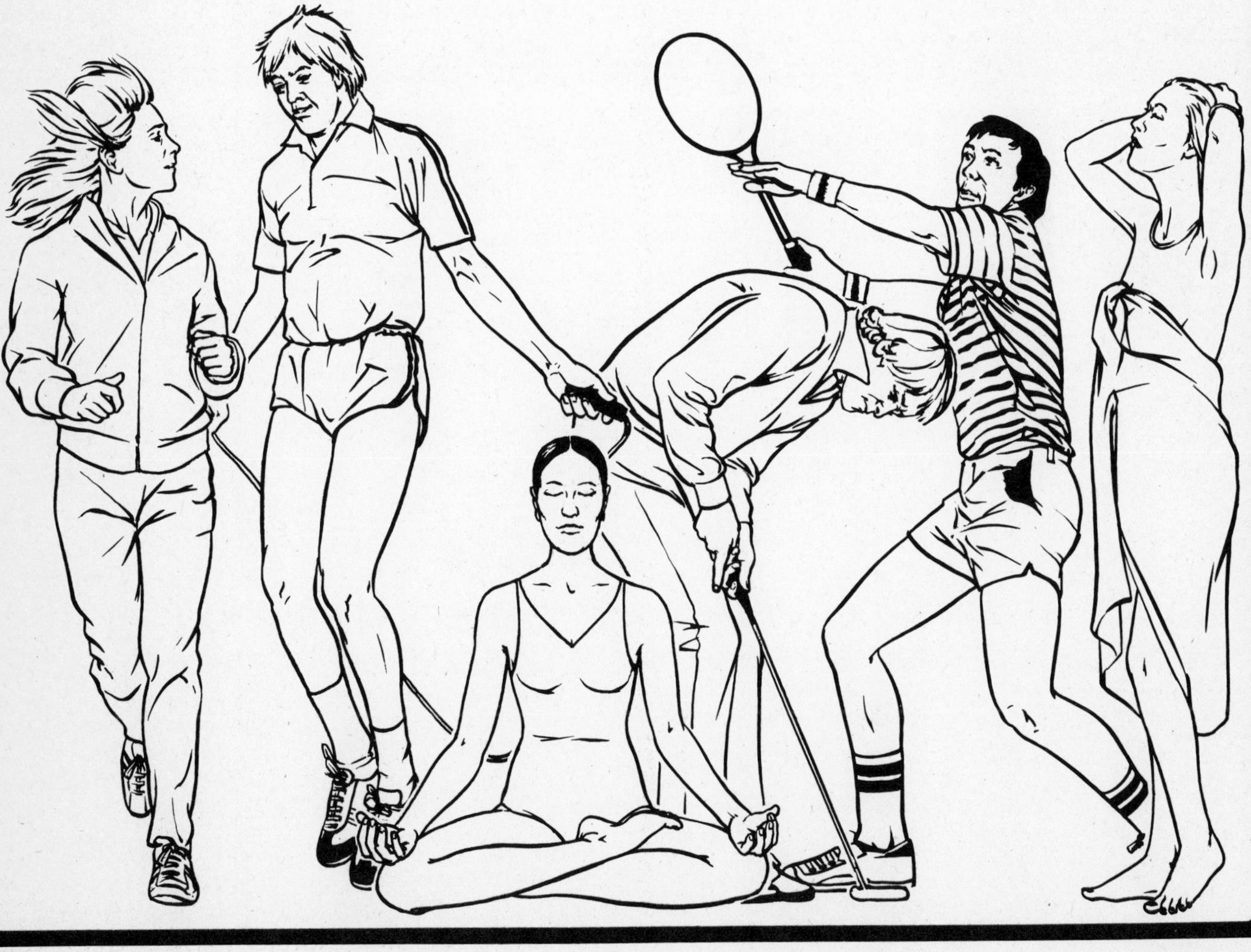

Introduction

A healthy environment is a prerequisite for helping you to maintain a healthy body. This chapter covers various matters concerning your physical and mental wellbeing, and provides information you can use in order to get to know your own body better and to provide for its needs. Some of these hints and guidelines are very easy to put into practice; others, such as providing a safe environment and a nutritious diet, may require a rethinking of your lifestyle. All of them, however, will help you toward a healthier body. On these pages we summarize the topics covered in this chapter.

Sources of help
This section deals with some of the individuals and organizations that can be incorporated into your personal health plan. Don't be ashamed to take full advantage of the services available from outside resources; you should never need to feel embarrassed, as your pursuit of a healthy body is entirely praiseworthy. Some of the sources of help available are orthodox, such as doctors, social workers, and gymnasiums; others are less so – acupuncturists, masseurs etc. Choose carefully the sources of help that best fit your needs and wishes.

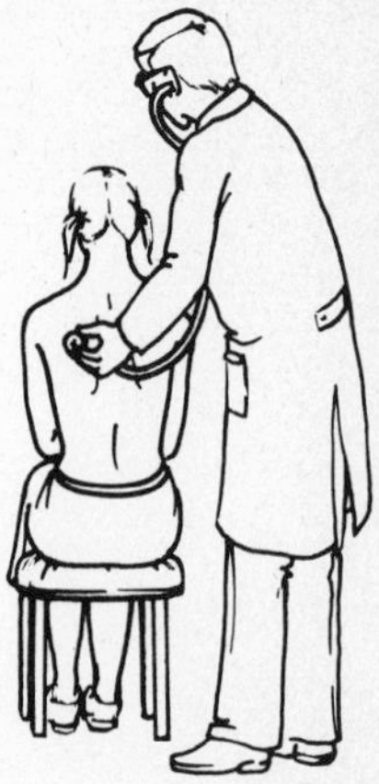

Body and environment
Knowledge of your body and its functions, its likes and dislikes, its habits and characteristics, can be a great ally in health matters. If you are familiar with the normal functioning of your body, you will be quickly aware of anything that is changed or disturbed in its pattern. This section suggests some of the things you ought to know about your body, and also certain precautions you can take against emergencies. Learn to know and understand your body and you will certainly reap benefits in your health.

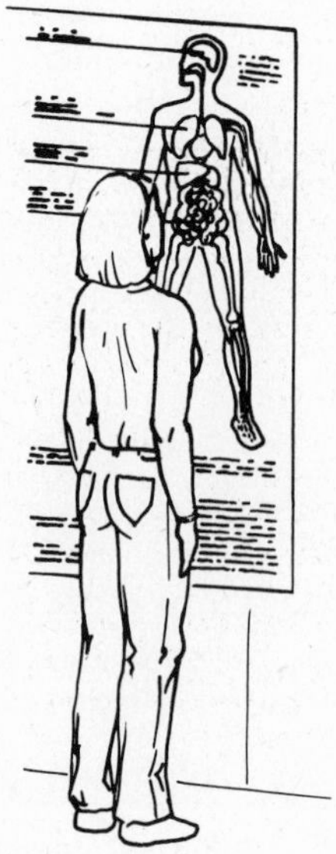

Hygiene
Hygiene is mainly concerned with preventing the spread of disease. Cleanliness and certain hygiene precautions drastically reduce the number of germs on your body, in your household, in your food and on your pets. Some diseases travel very slowly and affect only a few people; others travel very rapidly from one person to another; both kinds can be hampered in their progress by sensible hygiene. Careful food preparation can eliminate numerous potential health hazards; the section deals also with hygiene during illness, with pets, and when traveling.

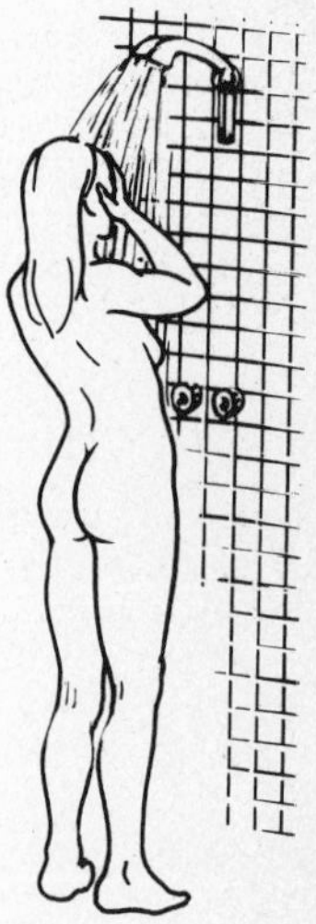

Safety
The tragedy of accidental deaths and injuries is that most of them could have been prevented with a little care, forethought or organization. Safety hazards include fire, gas, electricity, poisons, falls, drowning, dangerous or misused tools and equipment, firearms and traffic dangers. This section looks at many aspects of safety and provides a basic code that could save lives. Make your home as safe as possible, not only for children and the elderly but for everyone.

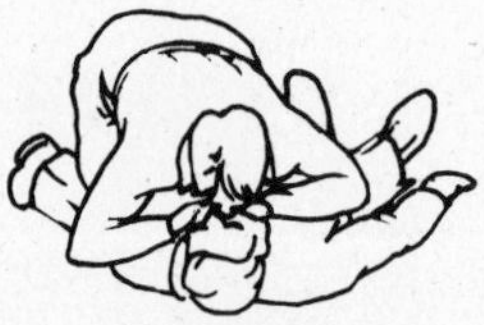

Nutrition
Eating a well-balanced diet benefits your body in many ways. It enables the various parts of your body to function efficiently: for instance certain organs need small amounts of particular trace elements or minerals. It encourages healthy growth and development: for example the calcium that is so important in the diets of babies and young children enables their bones to form properly. It also helps to protect your body from disease: adequate vitamins increase your body's resistance and make it more capable of fighting infections. In this section we look at the components of a good diet.

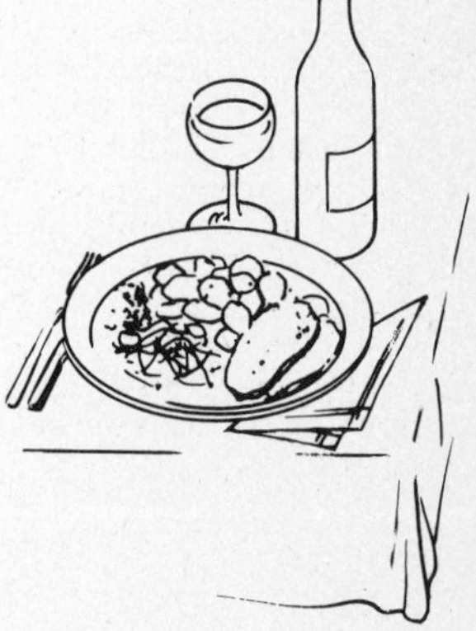

Energy and calories
Energy is supplied to the body by the calories in the food we eat. In order to function to their full capabilities, our bodies need to receive sufficient calories for conversion into energy that can be used by the muscles. In this section we examine the energy output of males and females of various ages and look at their calorie requirements. We also look at the calorie contents of a selection of common foods.

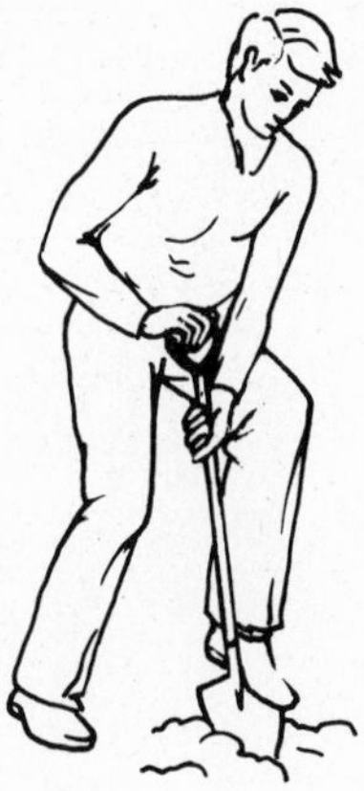

Eating problems
Eating problems can take many forms. Some are physiological, such as the enormous appetite caused in a body infested with tapeworms, or the cravings for particular foods that are often associated with pregnancy. In this section we look at two of the most common eating disorders: overeating and undereating. In both types of disorder the body no longer responds to its physical needs; instead, the pattern of eating is dictated by psychological factors. We examine some of the health problems associated with overeating and undereating and suggest some ways of changing the appetite patterns.

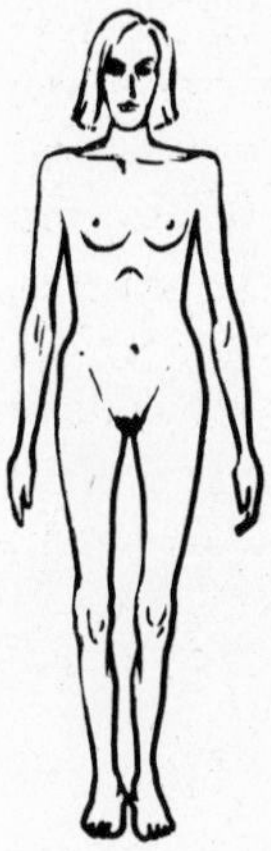

Reducing
Reducing, or dieting, is the removal of excess body weight in the form of fat. Excess stores of fat provide no benefit to the body, in fact they increase its risk of developing numerous diseases and medical conditions, so the pursuit of a healthy body includes ridding it of any excess weight. We give tables of suggested weights for both sexes, and also give practical advice on how to reduce the excess fat, including dietary guidelines and exercises.

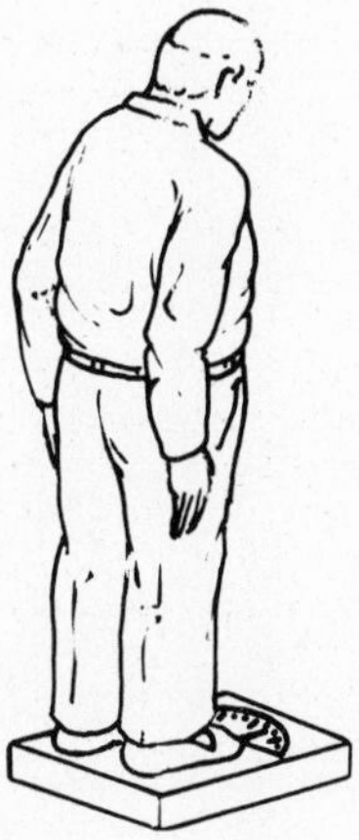

Exercise
Exercise is a fundamental bodily need. It pumps the blood faster around the body, speeds up the metabolism, and makes the internal organs work more efficiently; it also helps to keep the muscles toned up so that the body looks in good shape. Different occupations provide different amounts of exercise: dancers exercise rigorously as part of their training, but office workers seldom move from their desks during the day. In this section we show you ways of organizing your own exercise program to suit your needs, and give many examples of different types of exercise.

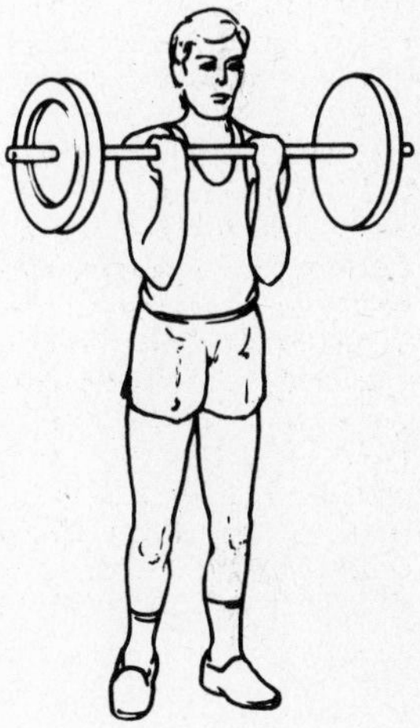

Sleep
Sleep is an enigmatic state that scientists find very difficult to examine. However it is known that satisfactory sleep is necessary for both life and sanity; a person deprived of sleep for several days suffers severe personality disturbances, and longer deprivation will lead eventually to death. In this section we look at some of the requirements for healthy sleep and examine ways in which these needs can be met.

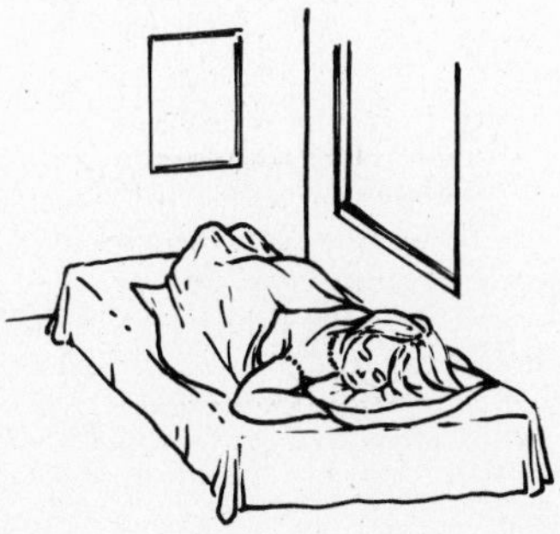

Relaxation
Relaxation can be physical or mental, and the best kind of relaxing activity is one that combines the two elements. Relaxation provides a peaceful oasis in the middle of a busy and hectic life, and provides a time when body and mind can renew themselves without pressure. It will probably be hard to find a time each day when you can relax completely, ideally alone and without interruption, but it is worth making the effort as you will work more efficiently the rest of the time if your body and brain have been refreshed.

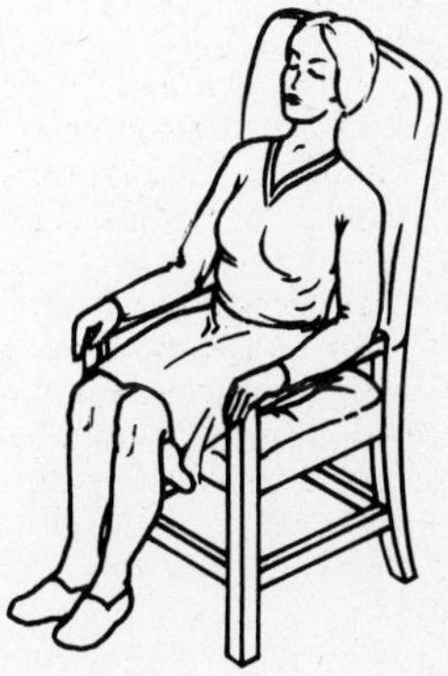

Sources of help

Good health care begins in the home, in the way you run your life and treat your body, but outside the home there are many individuals and organizations that can be used to give advice and support, and provide diagnoses, back-up care and treatment for medical problems that are beyond the scope of home care. Unfortunately some so-called health treatments may be misrepresented or even devoid of any real benefit, encouraging you to part with money by promising spectacular results, and they should be examined carefully. On these pages we look at some of the health services and activities that you could beneficially include in your health program, showing the advantages and drawbacks of each; find a combination that suits your own character and health situation.

Doctors and specialists
Your family doctor can be a tremendous help in encouraging you to maintain your body in a healthy condition. He can provide encouragement and support as well as specific advice on your medical condition and treatment of diseases, and will be able to work even more effectively if he knows your family and work situation as well as your medical history. Specialists work in a specific area of medicine such as gynecology, gastroenterology, pediatrics etc; your doctor may refer you to a specialist for a particular problem, or it may be possible to consult one on your own initiative.

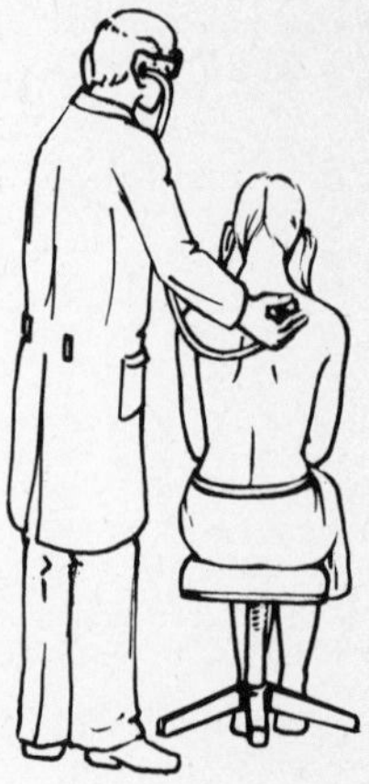

Exercises
Exercises may be designed to improve your general health, or they may be specifically worked out to exercise a particular part of your body, for instance if you wish to lose inches from your hips or firm up your bustline. Physiotherapy exercises are designed to exercise a limb or muscle that has been weakened through accident, disease or disuse. Exercises may be done at home, so that they are fitted into your daily routine, or you may prefer to join a gymnasium where you can work out under supervision and make use of their exercise machines and gymnasium equipment.

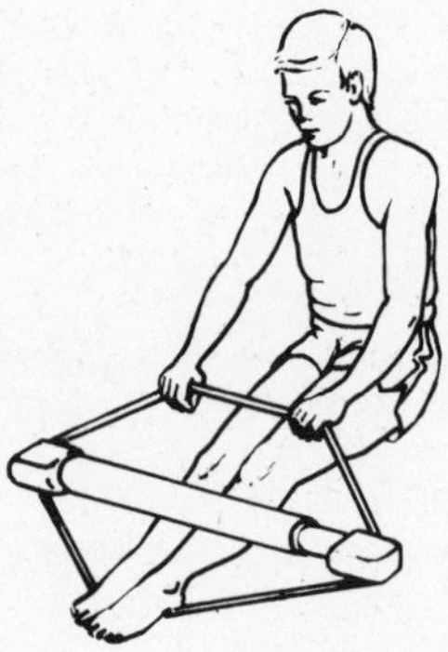

Sport and recreation
Relaxation is an important part of maintaining a healthy body, and there are many activities that will help you to relax. These may be as gentle as sport spectatorship or cooking, or as strenuous as rock climbing or parachuting. Some sports provide excellent exercise as well as the enjoyment of participating in them; any sport that causes you to exercise your heart and lungs will have a beneficial effect on your body if you do not overdo it. Sports range from those that do not require much movement, such as archery or darts, to those that use the whole body, such as football, hockey or skating.

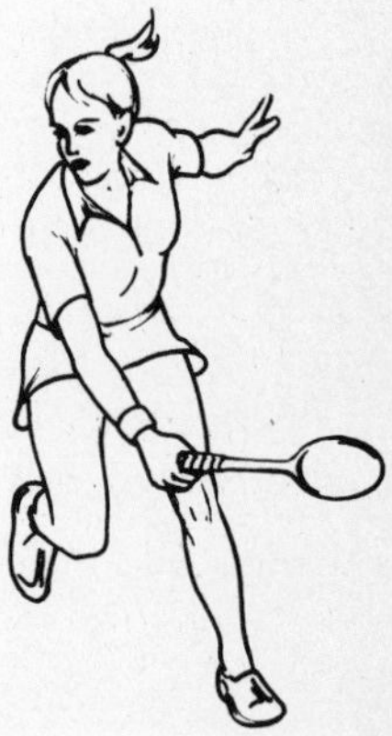

Individual and group therapy
Psychotherapy is intended to help individuals to talk out their psychological problems in order to come to terms with them and overcome their effects. This may be done under the leadership of a specialist psychotherapist, who may be recommended by your doctor or approached privately, or you may choose to join a therapy group. These groups are usually guided by a psychiatrist or therapist, who aims to help the members of the group to discover some of their own problems and ways of overcoming them. Frank discussion and physical "encounter therapy" may be encouraged to help remove inhibitions.

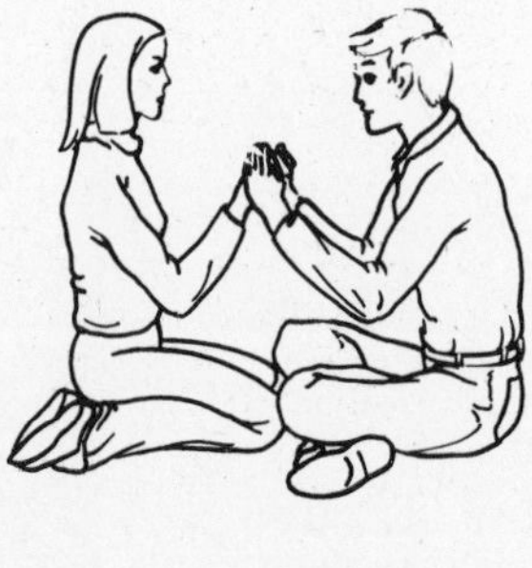

Self-help groups
Self-help groups are usually set up by people who have a problem in common, for mutual aid and support and for finding out new information and perhaps forming action groups. The members of the group may be alcoholics, parents of handicapped children, dieters, gamblers, single parents, families of the mentally disturbed etc. This kind of organization can provide invaluable help for individuals facing seemingly insurmountable problems not specifically provided for by the health services. If there is no self-help group near you, you could consider forming your own.

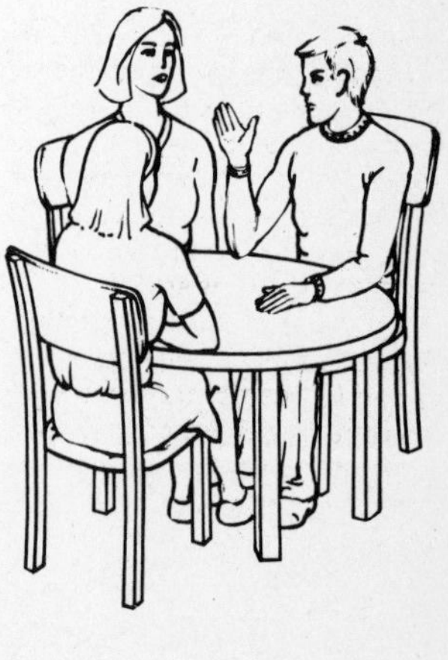

Steam treatments
Saunas and steam baths provide heat in a high humidity that can help to relax the muscles and tone up the skin over the entire body. They tend to cause a temporary loss of weight because of the water lost through perspiration, but this weight is regained as soon as you drink a glass of water after the sauna. Steam treatments do not help in improving the fitness or flexibility of the body, but they can be an aid to relaxation. Rubberized sweatsuits, designed to be worn while exercising, also cause a temporary loss of weight by making the body perspire.

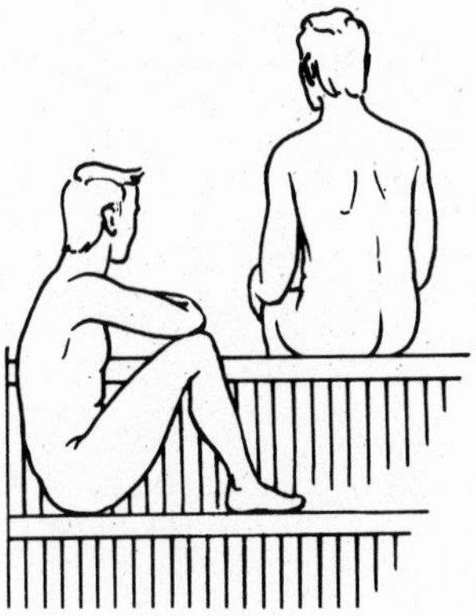

Baths
The therapeutic properties of particular sources of water have been claimed for hundreds of years. The springs or spa waters may be hot or cold, and they may be intended for bathing, drinking or both. Many of these waters contain large proportions of certain minerals or salts, and there are a few cases where these may be truly beneficial, but in many other cases no particular result will be noticed; relaxation may be a pleasant side effect of warm baths, but this is equally true in your own bathtub at home. Mud baths may help to tone up the skin but will have no effect on general health.

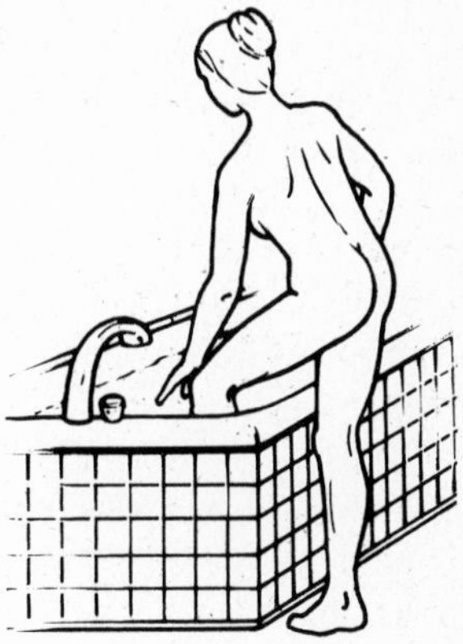

Massage
Massage is the manipulation of body tissues in order to release tension. The massage may take the form of gentle rubbing with the fingertips or palms, kneading of folds of skin, or pummeling the body tissue with the edges of the hands or with clenched fists. Massage improves the blood supply to the part massaged and so can help to disperse the waste products collected in stiff muscles; it can also help to relax and un-knot overworked muscles and tendons. Massage does not have any real effect on fitness; it is more a form of therapy than exercise.

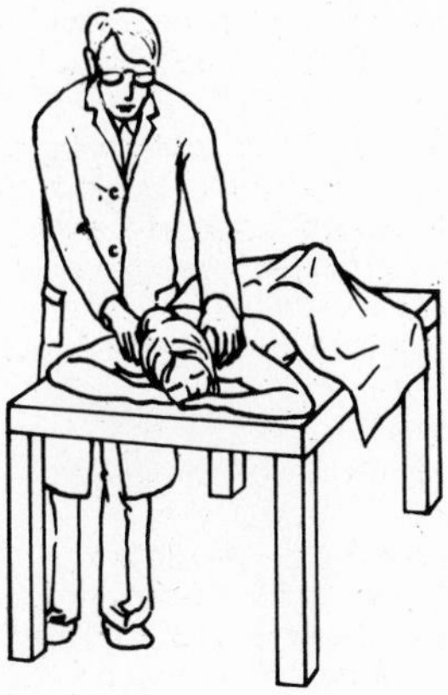

Meditation
Meditation techniques are not really forms of exercise, but may improve your wellbeing by helping the mind and body to relax; this can be particularly important in medical conditions that are aggravated by stress, such as heart disease, high blood pressure, migraine etc. Meditation may take the form of simply sitting or lying in one position and consciously removing all subjects of tension from the mind, or it can be part of a series of gentle movements, as in yoga sequences, K'ai Men and T'ai Chi, which may also aid flexibility and muscle tone.

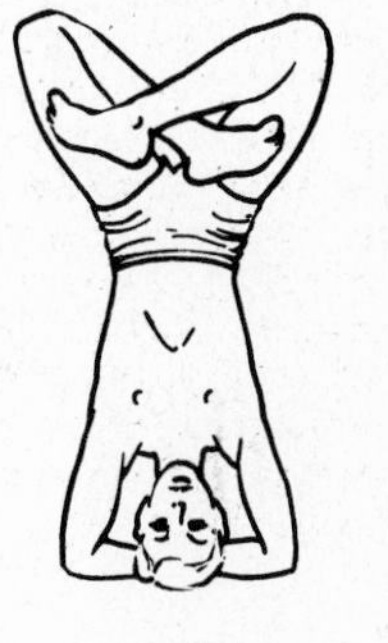

Acupuncture and hypnotism
Acupuncture is based on the blocking or stimulation of various nerve points around the body. The technique is used as an anesthetic in many Oriental countries, but it may also be used, enthusiasts claim, to help an individual to diet or to alter his behavior in other ways. Hypnotism is also becoming popular as a means of altering behavior patterns such as overeating or smoking, partly by suggestion to the person under hypnosis and partly by encouraging the subject to talk through psychological problems that may not be evident to him when not under hypnosis.

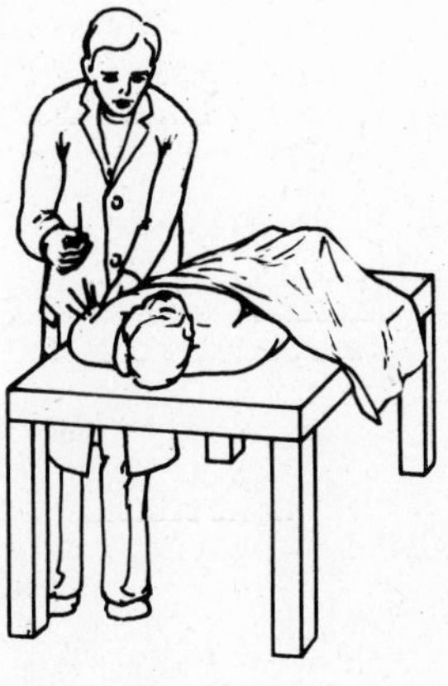

Health farms
Health farms often combine aspects of many types of health treatment. People may use health farms for reducing, for getting back into shape, or simply for escaping from the pressures of everyday life. The farms usually offer the opportunity to exercise, swim, learn new sports, dance etc as well as providing massage, saunas, individual diets and beauty therapy, often in luxurious surroundings. Health farms may be useful for people who lack the self-discipline to exercise or diet on their own, but they are usually very expensive.

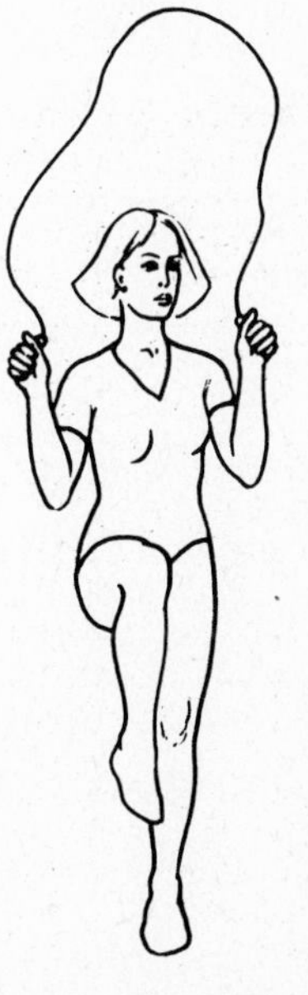

Body and environment

The physical aspects of your environment can have very direct results on the wellbeing of your body, and with a little care you will be able to alter many of these circumstances to suit your own body and lifestyle. Your clothes can be chosen to help your body toward better health, and a knowledge of the characteristics and responses of your own body is invaluable in recognizing any changes, problem areas, warning signs or illnesses and helping you to avoid their complications. On these pages we show you some of the things that you can do in your daily routine to make life healthier for your body.

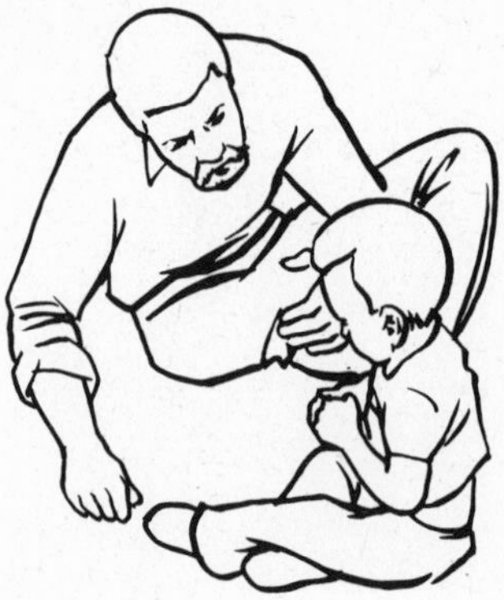

Personal care and age
The care a person requires depends very much on his or her age; even environmental factors of care alter with age. Babies and old people are particularly susceptible to cold, and will usually require higher room temperatures than older children or adults. Babies are totally dependent on others, and parents should be aware of the potentially damaging effects of restricting a baby's movements with tight clothing or damaging its developing bones with ill-fitting footwear. Growing children should be taught an increasing awareness of the factors that help or hinder a healthy body.

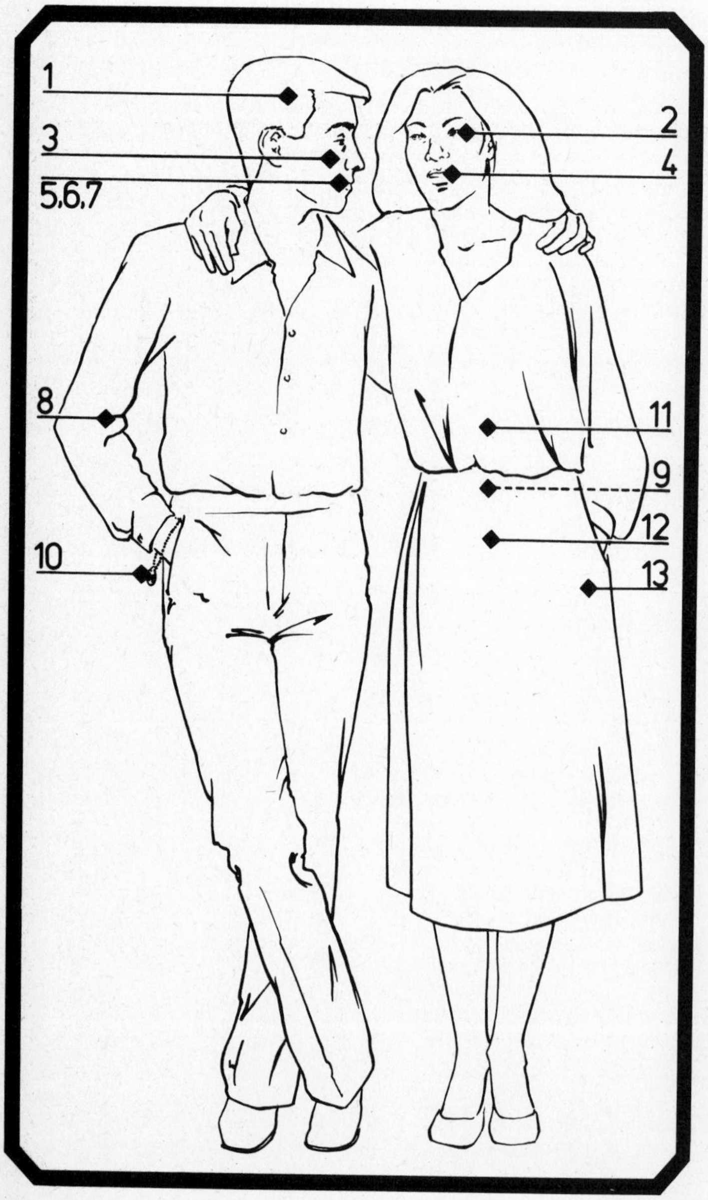

Personal check list
Listed here are some of the facts that you should know about your own body and ways in which you can help to keep it in optimum health.

1 Be aware of your hair type – whether it is dry, brittle, greasy, fine, prone to dandruff etc – and give it the appropriate shampoo or medication.
2 Have your vision checked regularly by an ophthalmologist.
3 Know any allergies you have to such things as pollen, household dust, animal fur etc, and avoid the allergens as much as possible. Know how to treat an allergic reaction if you are prone to them.
4 Understand your own skin type and complexion. If you have greasy skin, don't use a greasy moisturizer; if you have sensitive skin, don't sunbathe for long periods.
5 Practice good dental hygiene, and visit your dentist regularly so that he can forestall decay as much as possible. Avoid a diet high in sugar.
6 Know the name and the purpose of any medication you are taking, and make sure that you are aware of any side-effects.
7 Know how to take your own temperature, and be aware of the physical symptoms of high temperature or fever.
8 Know your own blood group, and those of your immediate family; this could save valuable time in an emergency.
9 Practice good posture when walking, sitting or lying down; make alterations in the furniture you use at home and at work if necessary.
10 Wear a clearly seen identification tag or bracelet if you have any condition or are taking any medication that would affect emergency medical treatment (eg diabetes, hemophilia) and carry written confirmation of your condition if you are pregnant.
11 Be aware of the normal working of your digestive system, as many illnesses and diseases first show themselves in digestive abnormalities.
12 Maintain good menstrual and sexual hygiene.
13 Be aware of your weight and general physique, so that you will recognize any dangerous weight gain or loss or any unusual change in body shape.

Home environment
The home environment can be used in many ways to help you to maintain a healthy body. The rooms should be protected from extremes of temperature; the ideal temperature is around 65–70°F, although individual needs and preferences vary. Adequate ventilation is necessary to circulate the air and remove cigarette smoke and carbon dioxide, but the house should be free from direct drafts. Humidity is also important: a high humidity is uncomfortable and tiring, but a low humidity dries up the mucous membranes of the nose and mouth and contributes to respiratory problems. All rooms should be well lit.

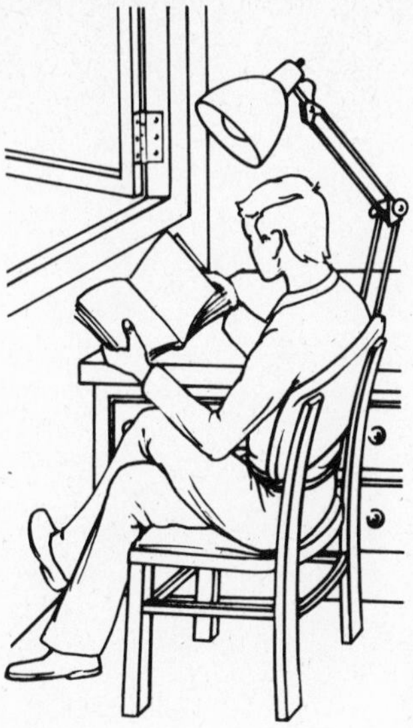

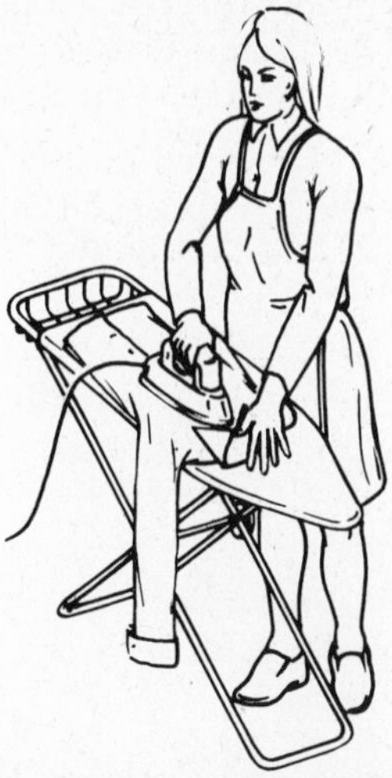

Furniture
Your body assumes different shapes depending on the furniture it is using; if it is repeatedly bent into poor positions, permanent damage may result. Work chairs should be fairly upright and should allow the spine to rest in as natural a position as possible; workbenches should be neither too high nor too low. Beds should be comfortable but firm; soft beds allow the body to sink into the mattress and do not support the spine adequately. Sinks, stoves, ironing boards etc should all be placed at the correct height so that you do not have to stoop over them or reach uncomfortably high.

Clothing
Clothing and related accessories should be comfortable, safe, clean and easily cared for.
1 Hats or wigs should not be worn all the time, as they prevent air from getting to the scalp. If you wear a wig for cosmetic reasons, take it off at night.
2 Glasses or contact lenses should be checked frequently by your ophthalmologist to make sure that they still meet your requirements. Contact lenses should always be cleaned before they are inserted.
3 Jewelry should be made of hypoallergenic metal (this is especially true of earrings) or a material such as wood or plastic, and should have no sharp or hard edges. If you wear a bracelet or necklace all the time, take it off occasionally and clean it so that it does not harbor bacteria.
4 The fibers your clothes are made of should suit their function and your lifestyle. Wear natural fibers if you are prone to perspiration, and check clothes before you buy them to make sure that they do not contain any fibers that you know you are allergic to.
5 Do not wear clothes that are uncomfortably tight around the chest, as these can restrict your breathing and affect your posture adversely.
6 If you have heavy breasts, wear a good supporting brassiere so that the muscles are not stretched. During pregnancy, avoid clothes with tight yokes as these restrict the breasts.
7 Do not wear clothes with a very tight waistband as this can cause great discomfort and affect the digestion adversely.
8 Underwear should be clean daily, and should not be too tight. Natural fibers are often preferable to synthetic ones as they keep the genitals cooler.
9 If you wear stockings, do not keep them up with elastic garters as these can aggravate varicose veins.
10 Socks should be clean every day, and should be long enough to fit the foot when they are unstretched; this will prevent them from restricting the toes.
11 Shoes should be well-fitting, with a low, wide heel and good support for the arch and instep. Wear fashion shoes only occasionally, and certainly not all day at work.

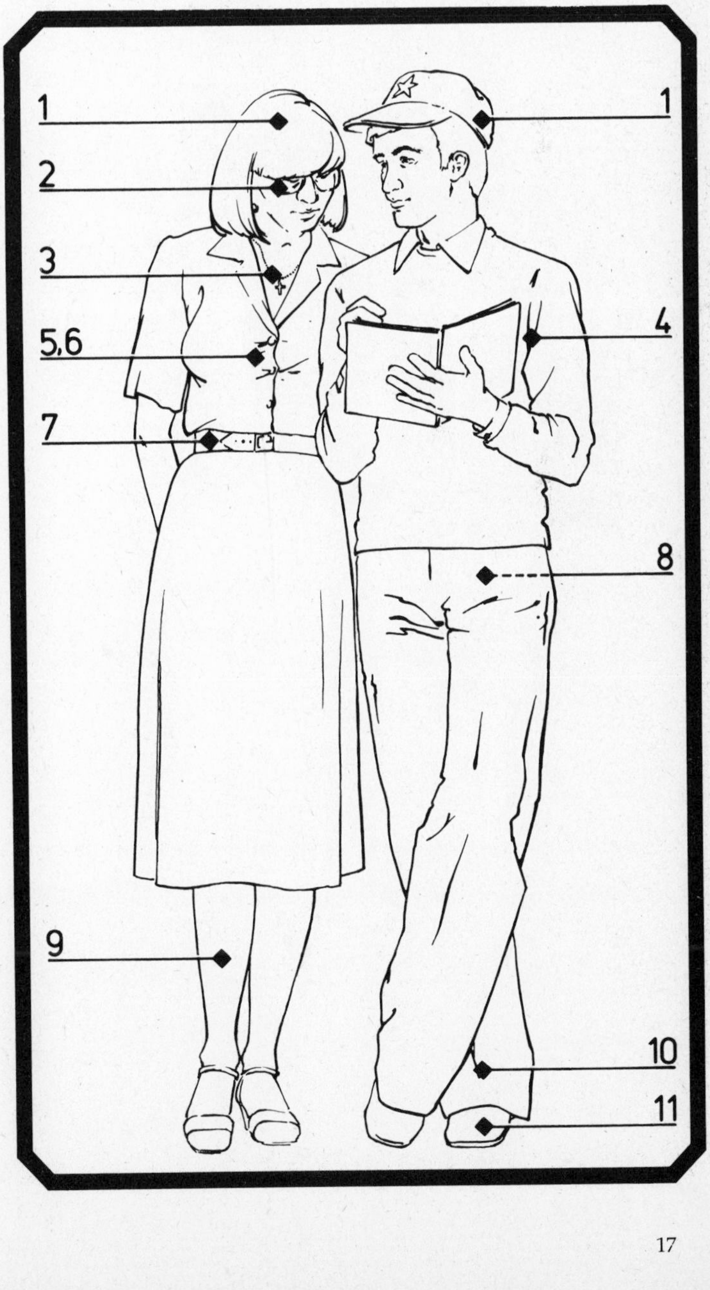

Hygiene

Good hygiene is a vitally important requirement in preventing the spread of infectious diseases. Diseases can reach epidemic proportions if a water supply is contaminated or if the organisms reach a widespread vector (carrying) population such as flies, rats or mosquitoes. Widespread outbreaks of disease can also occur through contaminated food — for instance when many people have eaten at a restaurant where the food has borne germs, or when one contaminated animal has been among many prepared in the same batch in a foodstuffs factory. On these pages, however, we talk mainly about personal hygiene. Following these guidelines should help you avoid disease yourself, and also prevent you from transmitting germs to others.

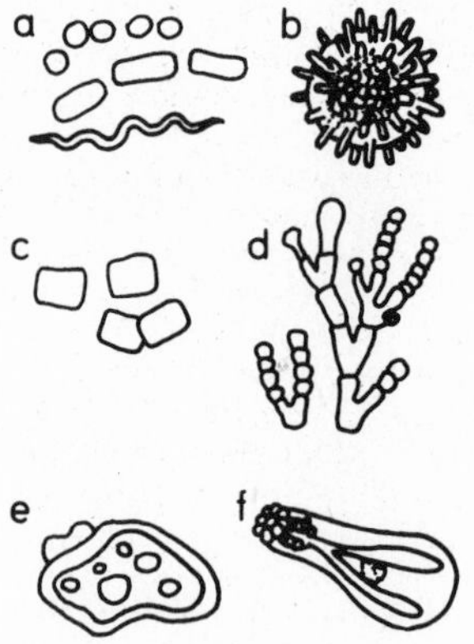

Disease organisms
Most diseases are transmitted by one of the following types of organism.
a Bacteria are microscopic one-celled carriers of infections such as diphtheria and tuberculosis.
b Viruses are tiny parasites carrying diseases such as the common cold and influenza.
c Rickettsias are germs found in fleas and lice; they cause various uncommon diseases.
d Fungi are non-green plants, and cause ringworm, athlete's foot, thrush etc.
e Protozoan (one-celled) parasites cause diseases, including malaria.
f Metazoan (many-celled) parasites include tapeworms, lice and fleas.

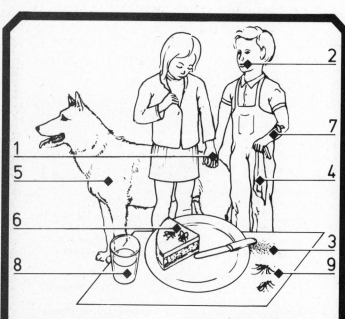

The spread of disease
The illustration *above* shows some of the ways in which disease is commonly spread.
1 Direct contact, such as kissing, sexual intercourse, holding hands etc, is responsible for spreading many germs.
2 Droplets are frequent carriers of bacteria and viruses; the droplets may be coughed, sneezed or breathed out, and then inhaled by other people.
3 Dust may harbor airborne particles, which are later inhaled by others.
4 Objects such as washcloths, handkerchiefs and tissues that have been used by an infected person are an ideal breeding ground for bacteria.
5 Pets and farm animals may be carriers of diseases or parasites.
6 Insects, especially flies, are frequently carriers of disease, and are particularly drawn to uncovered food, which they then contaminate.
7 Dirt entering a break in the skin often harbors disease.
8 Contaminated food or water, or dirty utensils, can harbor and transmit germs to many people.
9 Parasitic animals such as mosquitoes, ticks and fleas can transmit disease to the host.

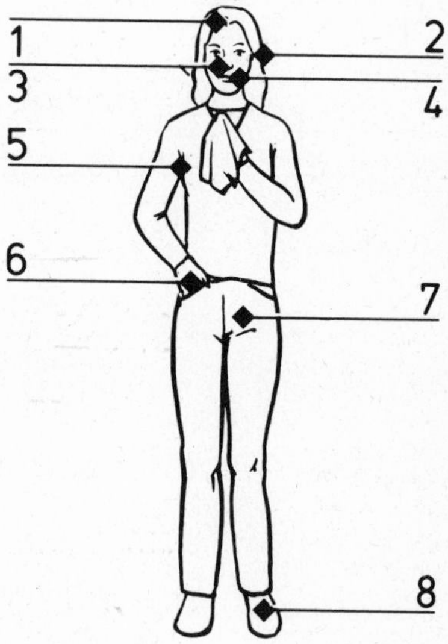

Personal hygiene
The diagram *above* shows the areas of the body to which you should pay particular attention in order to maintain a high standard of personal hygiene.
1 Wash your hair regularly, and inspect it for lice and nits if there is an epidemic in your neighborhood.
2 Clean your ears daily with a damp washcloth.
3 Blow your nose into a clean handkerchief or tissue when necessary.
4 Clean your teeth frequently, ideally after every meal, and use antiseptic gargles if you have a mouth or throat infection. Cover your mouth and nose with a clean handkerchief whenever you cough or sneeze, so as few infected droplets as possible transfer to the air around you.
5 Take a thorough, allover wash, shower or bath each day, paying particular attention to your underarms, groin and feet.
6 Wash your hands after visiting the toilet, and before preparing food.
7 Wear a clean set of underwear each day.
8 Change your socks or stockings every day, and keep your feet clean so that they do not perspire too much.

Children
Children need to be taught good hygiene habits as early as possible, since they are not naturally clean beings! Make sure that your child washes his hands after visiting the toilet, and also before every meal; dirt of all sorts accumulates on the hands. Keep children's fingernails short so that they are easy to keep clean. Encourage your child to clean his teeth after every meal. Explain as much as possible the reasons for these measures so that they do not simply seem to be empty instructions. Sanitize a baby's diapers at each wash, and clean the baby's bottom at each diaper change.

Elderly people
Because of forgetfulness and decreased mobility, the hygiene routines of elderly people often suffer. Washing, tooth and gum care and careful food preparation may all be neglected. Those responsible for caring for elderly people should make sure that their food is fresh and that the surfaces and utensils used for preparing food are clean. Food should be bought in small quantities so that it will not be forgotten. Any hints of infestation by mice, cockroaches etc, which may not be noticed by someone with failing eyesight, should be dealt with professionally.

Illness
Hygiene during illness is a very important concern; good hygiene will help the invalid to recover more quickly, and also prevent (as far as possible) the spread of the illness to others. Keep the sick person isolated if he is very infectious; keep his dishes and cutlery separate from the rest of the family's, and launder his bed linen, washcloths and towels separately. Give him paper handkerchiefs instead of cloth, and discard them after one use. Place a large bag near the bed so that the patient can put tissues, soiled dressings etc in the bag; in that way, no one else needs to touch them.

Pets
Pets can harbor many diseases and parasites that they can transmit to humans, so good hygiene when there are pets in the house is essential. Don't allow pets to lick your face, or to lick family dishes clean after meals; give them separate dishes, and wash their food bowls separately. Keep your pets clean, and have them given any inoculations your veterinarian advises. Check them regularly for infestations. Don't allow pet cats or dogs to sleep on beds; they should have their own sleeping place elsewhere. Keep pets away from babies; if you have pets in the house, put a net over the crib.

Food preparation
Some of the hygiene concerns in food preparation are shown here.

a Wash your hands before doing any food preparation; the water should be hot and soapy to be effective.

b Cover any grazes or cuts on your hands with waterproof adhesive tape.

c Use clean utensils, and wash them or put them to soak in hot water as soon as possible after use.

d Thaw all frozen food slowly and thoroughly, unless the package specifically states it can be cooked when frozen. This inhibits harmful enzyme activity.

e Wash all raw food thoroughly under running water.

f Check cans for any unusual color or deposits inside; do not use any cans with domed ends as this often implies bacterial activity inside the can.

g Cook all pork, poultry and fish very thoroughly; do not eat these meats "rare."

h Do not keep food warm for long; if it must wait, keep it piping hot, and if it is not needed for an hour or more cool it as quickly as possible and refrigerate it.

i In general never refreeze food that has been frozen once. But food that has been frozen raw may be cooked and then refrozen in its cooked state.

j Don't leave food where flies or pets can get at it.

k Don't cough or sneeze over food.

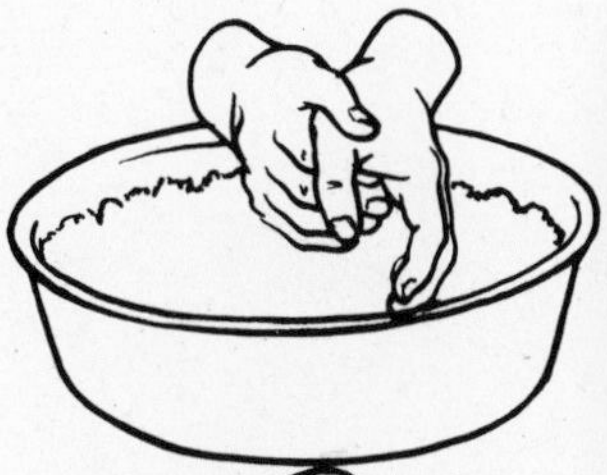

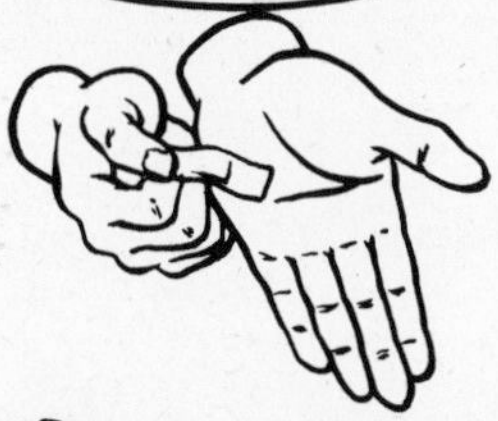

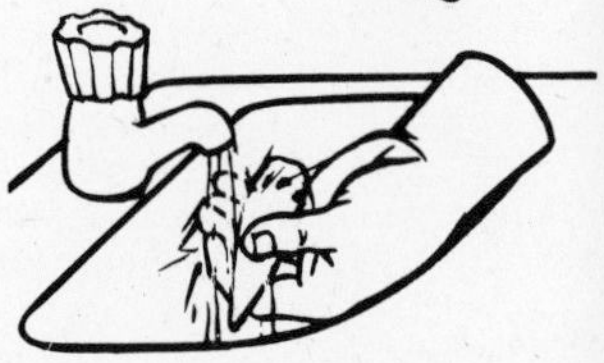

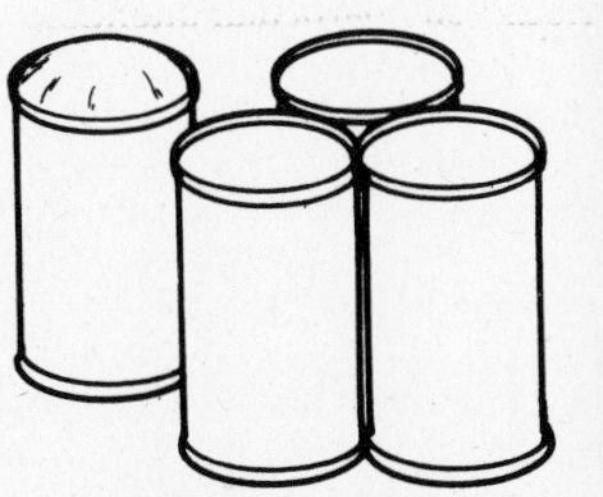

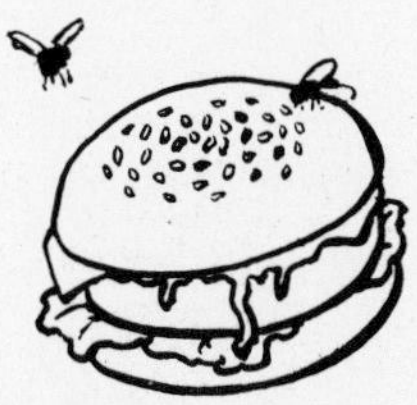

Travel
Travelers abroad are notorious for picking up any germs that happen to be in the area; if you are going abroad, follow these hygiene tips.

Do
- Have any necessary or advised vaccinations, inoculations etc.
- Carry a note in the relevant language(s) if you suffer from any condition that may affect hospital treatment, such as diabetes, hemophilia etc, or if you are pregnant.
- Have sufficient salt in your food; take salt tablets after a meal if you are in doubt.
- Equip yourself with protective items such as sunglasses, suntan filter oils etc, and use them when necessary.
- Wear shoes whenever possible to avoid transmission of disease from fecal matter or skin parasites.
- Wash yourself well and thoroughly, at least once a day, especially if you are using communal washrooms or swimming in dirty water.
- Sterilize or boil any water you use for cooking, washing food, or cleaning your teeth, and drink either sterilized water or bottled mineral water.
- Use mosquito nets in malarial areas.
- Wash any animal wound immediately, and try to trace the animal and its owner.

Don't
- Skimp on insurance against ill-health; it could ruin your holiday.
- Drink or cook with unboiled water.
- Drink unboiled milk.
- Buy ices, warmed-up meat or cold drinks from market or street vendors; go into a restaurant that looks clean and reputable.
- Eat unpeeled fruit or vegetables if you can possibly avoid it.
- Eat partially cooked or rare meat or fish.
- Eat shellfish, as this is a frequent harborer of food poisoning germs if improperly prepared.
- Walk barefoot, especially around streets, washrooms and potholes.
- Swim in water that is, or seems to be, polluted.
- Touch any local animals if you can avoid it.
- Neglect washing.
- Forget to take daily medication, such as anti-malarial tablets, if it has been prescribed.
- Suddenly change your eating, drinking or sleeping routine; plan your schedule so that there is as little disruption as possible.

Safety

Every day most of us successfully negotiate a world that is fraught with potential hazards, because we have been taught how to avoid danger areas, how to use equipment safely, how to use medicines, and how to use our bodies and their senses to alert us to danger. Unfortunately, it is also true that every day some people die as the result of accidents, and many others are injured or incapacitated. Most of these accidents could be prevented, especially those that involve young children, by following a safety code including the hints set out on these pages. Deal with any potential hazard as soon as you notice it: don't be tempted to leave it until later, or you may leave it until it is too late to prevent disaster.

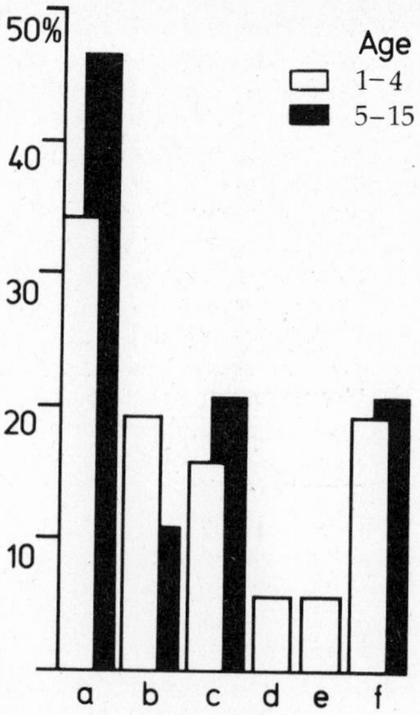

Accident statistics
Accidental death is one of the major causes of childhood mortality in the Western world. In the United States, 37% of all deaths in children aged 1–4 years are caused by accidents, and 46% of the deaths in the age group 5–15. The chart *left* shows the breakdown of these deaths into type of accident, and identifies the major areas for concern in each age group.

a Motor vehicle accidents
b Fire or burns
c Drowning
d Falls
e Poisoning
f Other

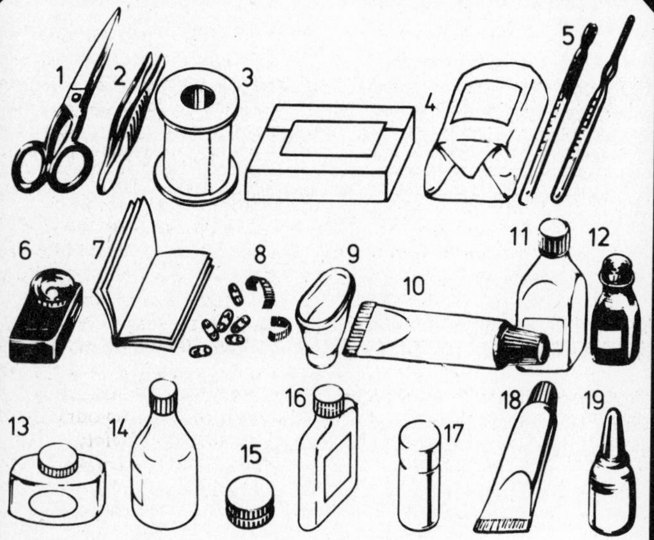

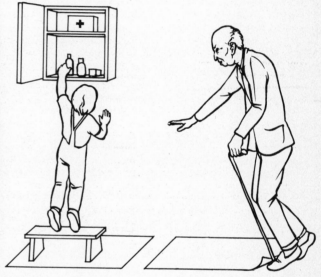

Medicine chest
Every home should be equipped with a medicine chest for dealing with minor emergencies and with common problems such as coughs, sore eyes, constipation, headaches etc. Here we list some of the items that could usefully be included in a family medicine chest. Remember, however, that the contents of a medicine chest could be fatal if they get into the hands of a curious young child; keep all your medicines and equipment in a lockable cabinet. Put the key in a place known by all adult members of the family and older children, but out of the reach of toddlers.

1 Scissors.
2 Tweezers.
3 Adhesive tape.
4 Gauze and bandages.
5 Thermometers.
6 Pocket flashlight.
7 First aid manual.
8 Safety pins or bandage clips.
9 Eyebath.
10 Antiseptic cream.
11 Rubbing alcohol.
12 Aspirin and junior aspirin.
13 Petroleum jelly.
14 Calamine lotion.
15 Sting reliever.
16 Mild laxative.
17 Indigestion remedy.
18 Antihistamine cream.
19 Nasal decongestant.

Children
Children, especially young children, are insatiably curious about the world around them, and are constantly exploring their surroundings. An infant or toddler is not old enough to understand why he should not open a particular closet or drink a particular liquid, so just telling him off when he tries to is not enough. You should make your house as childproof as is humanly possible; expect the worst, that is, imagine everything that your child could possibly harm himself with, and then make sure the danger is removed. Even very small children can move very quickly, so don't rely on watching their movements.

Elderly people
More accidents happen to the elderly than to any other age group. Since older people's bones become more brittle and their muscles less resilient, they may suffer fractures or other damage in falls that would scarcely affect a younger person. Failing eyesight and decreased coordination and balance make older people more prone to falls and slips; you can help to prevent such accidents by tacking down carpet edges, avoiding high polishes on floors, and keeping rooms tidy and uncluttered. Keep gas and electricity supplies well maintained so that danger from these is minimized.

Pets
As well as being potential carriers of disease (see p.19), pets can be a health hazard in other ways. Cats are notoriously fond of sleeping on beds, and this will include a crib or baby carriage if the opportunity arises; a cat is quite big and heavy enough to suffocate a baby, so put a net over the crib. While your children are small, don't have a dog big enough to knock down a toddler, and don't keep a dog with an uncertain temperament. Teach your children to respect animals and not to mistreat or frighten them; even placid dogs and cats may retaliate with a scratch or bite if suddenly disturbed.

Recreation
Sports and pastimes often have particular hazards associated with them. Of course it is unrealistic to try to take the danger out of all recreation; there will always be a risk in such activities as mountain climbing or hang-gliding, and even sports such as squash, hockey or track and field events carry the risk of accidents. However, you can minimize the risks by obeying all appropriate safety rules, such as leaving copies of walking, sailing or climbing itineraries, carrying safety signaling equipment etc. Also, make sure that you wear the clothing and footwear recommended for the specific activity.

Road safety
Children in particular frequently die in accidents on the road. Make sure that your child knows road safety rules, such as looking both ways when he crosses the street and not crossing from behind parked cars. Also, make sure that he uses this code every time he steps onto the street. Many children killed on the streets act carelessly or on impulse just that one time. If your child rides a bicycle, ensure that he keeps it in good repair and knows how to ride it properly. Never allow a baby or toddler to sit on your lap in the front seat of a car; always strap them into recommended safety seats.

Water safety
Water is a great danger to children, and to adults who are not strong swimmers. Teach your children to swim as young as possible, and learn basic lifesaving and resuscitation techniques. Put a fence round any pool, pond or river on your land, and drain pools when they are not in use. At the beach, find out about tides and currents and do not swim out of your depth. Always obey beach and pool safety rules, and never swim within an hour after a meal, as you are likely to develop stomach cramps. Check that any underwater equipment you use is in good repair.

Safety in the home
Most accidents happen in the home, with ordinary household equipment or objects that have been misused or are in bad condition. In this panel we look at some of the types of hazard encountered in the home, and give guidelines for making your home as safe as possible. In addition to these points, remember that most accidents happen when the person concerned is tired or ill, or, in the case of women, premenstrual or pregnant. Accidents happen to children most frequently when they are unsupervised or when supervision is inadequate, for instance when a babysitter is young or inexperienced.

Poisons
Keep all kitchen and bathroom cleaners, polishes, paints, perfumes, deodorants, medicines, contraceptive pills, matches, vermin poisons, weedkillers and chemicals out of the reach of children. Label all containers of such substances; never put chemicals in food or drink containers. Always put the light on to double-check the label of any medication given at night. Keep any gas supplies well-maintained, and do not allow children to play with the switches on gas stoves etc. Make sure all paints in the house and on toys and all water-pipes are lead-free.

Fires, burns and scalds
Use a fireguard in front of all fires, including gas and electric ones. Do not use the fireguard for drying laundry. Keep matches, cigarette lighters, firelighters and flammable liquids out of the reach of curious children. In the kitchen, turn pan handles toward the back of the stove and use the back burners when possible, so that children cannot easily reach the pans. Keep a heavy blanket in the kitchen for smothering fires, and always ensure that cigarette butts are properly extinguished.

Toys
Your child's toys should always be checked before he is allowed to play with them. Check animals and dolls for any small parts that can be detached and swallowed; see if there are any sharp projections or if truck wheels etc are attached by spikes. Make sure that your child's toys are suited to his age; do not give babies or toddlers toys small enough to be swallowed or ones that are too complicated for them to operate safely. If you buy a toy that is electrically operated, read the instructions with your child, along with any safety precautions, and make sure that he understands them fully.

Falls
Many falls can be prevented by anticipating and avoiding the circumstances in which they are likely to occur. Ensure that the stairway is well lit, and that it has a light switch at both top and bottom. Nail down any loose edge of carpet or linoleum (this applies to the rest of the house as well), and use safety gates at top and bottom to keep toddlers off the stairway. Do not carry large bundles in front of you when coming down the stairs, as they will block your view. Use a non-slip mat in the bathtub and shower, and do not place slippery rugs on highly polished floors.

Electricity
Make sure that all electricity supplies to your home are well-maintained. Check the leads and plugs of all electrical appliances regularly to make sure that they are in good order. Fit all electric outlets with childproof covers, and always unplug kettles, blenders, irons, electric blankets, televisions etc when not in use. Keep all electric appliances away from the bathtub, and never use an electric switch while your hands are wet. Before changing a light bulb or a fuse, switch off the current at the mains. Always switch off any electric appliance or tool before you make any alterations to it.

Tools and equipment
Store all adult hobby tools away from children, and make sure children do not have access to knives, parers, skewers, graters etc in the kitchen. Allow small children to use only scissors with rounded tips. Make sure that any tools you use are well sharpened; blunt tools require extra pressure for use, which often causes them to slip unpredictably. Dispose of any razor blades by wrapping them very thoroughly in thick paper before they are thrown away. If you own firearms, store guns and ammunition separately, with both under lock and key.

General safety for children
Always run cold water into the bathtub first and top up with hot to the required temperature rather than the other way around. Never leave a small child alone in the bathtub even for a second. Keep cribs away from drapes, blinds etc that the child may pull down on himself, and make sure the crib bars are sufficiently closely-spaced to prevent him from getting his head through the gaps. Always give small children unbreakable dishes and cups, and teach them never to walk, run or play with food or any other objects, especially sharp ones, in their mouths.

Nutrition 1

The human body needs food to maintain life processes and promote healthy cell growth. The substances required by the body in the form of food are proteins, carbohydrates, fats, vitamins and minerals. The body also requires about 2 quarts of water – some of which will be found in food – as roughly 75% of the body is water. The food is broken down and resynthesized in a form that the body can use. A wide variety of foods is more likely to provide all the essential nutrients than a limited diet. It is perfectly possible to be healthy on a balanced vegetarian diet, but some extreme diets can cause malnutrition because of deficiencies in essential nutrients.

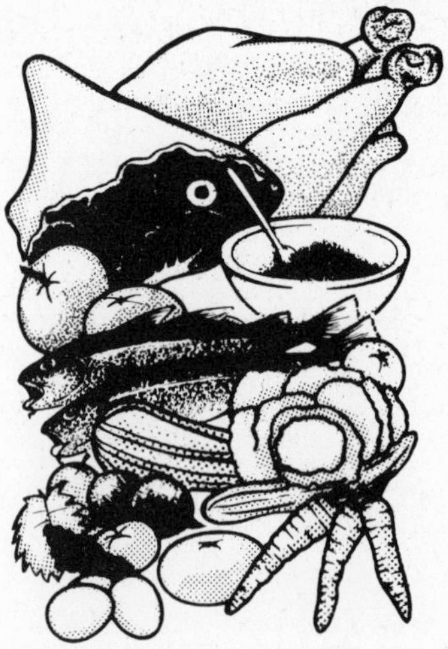

Omnivorous diets
Omnivores eat food from all the available sources, including meat, fish, poultry, eggs, vegetables, fruit and cereals. Most people in the Western world are omnivores, and in theory this should be the most nutritious diet possible as all the types of food source are available. In practice, however, many people do not think about planning out a healthy diet as food is so readily available, and fast foods and other convenience forms often replace fresh foods. This often means that some nutrients are not included in the diet at all, or not in sufficient quantities for optimal health.

Carbohydrates
Carbohydrates – chemical compounds of carbon, hydrogen and oxygen – are sources of energy and play a vital role in the functioning of internal organs, the central nervous system, and heart and muscle contraction. They should ideally make up 50–60% of the body's total daily calorie intake. After digestion and absorption as glucose into the bloodstream carbohydrates may be used directly, temporarily stored in the muscles and liver as glycogen (the only carbohydrate the body makes), or converted into fat and deposited in the adipose tissues of the body. The most important dietary carbohydrates are sugar, starch and fiber. Sugar comes in various forms, including sucrose (table sugar), fructose (in fruit), maltose (in malt), and lactose (in milk). In the Western world there has been a marked shift away from starch and toward sugar as the main source of carbohydrate in the diet. At the beginning of the century, 90% of the average cabohydrate intake was starch; now it is only 40%, with the other 60% being eaten in the form of sugar. Sugar contains no vitamins or minerals, whereas starchy foods such as potatoes and corn contain vitamins and protein, and so are more valuable sources of carbohydrate.

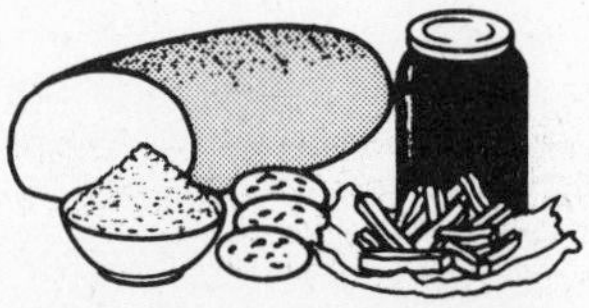

Foods high in carbohydrates
Listed *below* is a selection of common foods that are high in carbohydrates. Figures refer to the number of grams of carbohydrate per 100g of food, expressed for ready comparison as equivalents of simple sugars (monosaccharides).

g	
105	Sugar
87	Rice, uncooked
85	Cornflakes
84	Spaghetti, uncooked
80	Flour, white
76	Honey
73	Oatmeal
71	Ryvita
69	Jam
64	Dates, dried
62	Cookies, rich, sweet
59	Chocolate, semi-sweet
58	Plain cake, Madeira
55	Condensed milk, canned, sweetened
53	Figs, dried
50	Bread, white
49	Potato chips
45	Beans, haricot, dry
42	Bread, wholewheat

Fats
Fats in human nutrition are combinations of fatty acids and glycerol. They are energy sources, and they help to prevent heat loss from the body and to protect the body's structures. A small amount of "essential" fatty acids, not made in the body, is necessary for the maintenance of health; deficiencies may result in skin disorders and other problems. Fats contain twice as many calories per gram as either proteins or carbohydrates. They are major contributors to obesity, and have been implicated in heart disease. Many Americans eat too much fat; 30–35% of the total calorie intake should come from fat, but the average figure in America is about 40%. Fats are divided into two categories: saturated fats are found mainly in warm-blooded animals and include lard, suet and butter; unsaturated fats come mainly from plants and fish and include oils of maize and sunflower. A type of fat that does not contain fatty acid is cholesterol; this can be manufactured in the liver, and it builds brain tissue and hormones. A diet high in saturated fats is thought to increase cholesterol formation; high levels of cholesterol may in turn increase the plaques on the walls of arteries, possibly blocking the blood supply to the heart (see p. 80 and pp. 84–85).

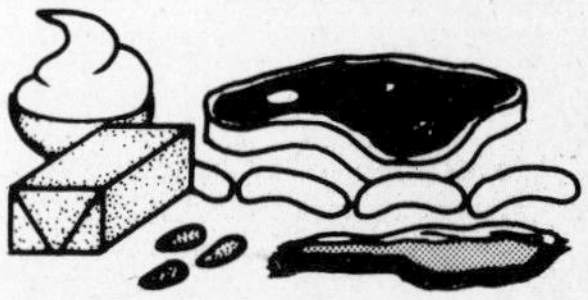

Foods high in fats
Included in the list *below* are selected common foods that are high in fats. Figures show the number of grams of fat for every 100g of food. (See also pp. 84–85.)

g	
100	Oils, cooking and salad
99	Cooking fat, dripping
82	Butter
81	Margarine, regular
79	Mayonnaise, home-made
62	Coconut, dried
54	Almonds
53	Bacon, rashers, fried
49	Peanuts, roasted
42	Sausage, pork, cooked
41	Low-fat spread
40	Potato chips
38	Cream, whipping
36	Chocolate, semi-sweet
32	Cheese, Cheddar
32	Sirloin steak, lean with fat, broiled
32	Pork chop, lean with fat
30	Cookies, chocolate-chip
29	Lamb chop, lean with fat
25	Luncheon meat, canned

Lacto-ovo-vegetarian diets
Lacto-ovo-vegetarians are those who eat all foods of plant origin and also dairy foods and eggs. This kind of diet is nutritionally sound as long as the ingredients are selected carefully. Eggs are an even better source of protein than meat, and also contain a complete protein rarely found in vegetables or fruit. People become vegetarians for various reasons. Some are philosophical, usually based on humanitarianism; some are religious, based on the sanctity of life; and some are economic – it is more economical to use land for growing crops than for feeding cattle. Other people find a diet that excludes animal protein more healthy.

Vegetarian diets
Strict vegetarians consume only plant products – fruit, vegetables and cereals. They do not eat any meat, poultry, fish, eggs, dairy produce or, in some cases, honey. Their main sources of nutrients are nuts, wholewheat flour, pulses, pasta, brown rice, unrefined sugars, fruit and vegetables (ideally eaten raw for maximum nutritional value) and unrefined vegetable oils. Soya-based milk can be substituted for cow's milk, and seaweed agar for gelatin. Strict vegetarians may need supplements of vitamin B_{12}, which can be taken in tablet form or added to the food.

Ch'ang Ming diet
The Ch'ang Ming diet, based on taoist long-life therapy, is a program of natural eating and herbal medication. Although its origins are ancient, the diet's emphasis on natural, whole foods free from chemical additives sounds extremely modern. Forbidden foods include white bread, refined and processed foods, coffee, alcohol, tobacco, chocolate, candy, fried foods, spices, rock salt, mustard, pepper, vinegar, pickles, pork and red meats, red and blue fish, sugar, tropical fruits, potatoes, dairy products, and any foods containing animal fat. With a little care over the balance of nutrients, this can be a healthy diet.

Macrobiotic diets
Foods in a macrobiotic diet are designated yin or yang, based on an acid-alkali contrast. For example, fruits and sugar are yin, meat and eggs are yang. The ratio in which these foods are eaten is supposed to be 5:1, yin to yang. Almost all foods may be eaten but there is a strong emphasis on the grains, particularly brown rice, which is thought to be an ideal food. Proponents of the diet suggest that it will cure every disease, including cancer. Critics, who include the American Medical Association, point out that in the 5:1 ratio the diet tends to be deficient in iron and most vitamins, and also distrust the medical claims for the diet.

Proteins
Proteins are complex organic compounds of numerous nitrogenous amino acids. Dietary protein is broken down by the body to liberate amino acids that pass into the blood and are rebuilt into whatever the body needs. There are 23 amino acids in nature that combine to make protein; 8 are essential in the diet of adults and 10 are essential for children because the body cannot synthesize them in sufficient quantity. Eggs and milk contain amino acids more suitable to human needs than others. Meat is the next best, then pulses, peas and nuts. Proteins in cereal, bread, vegetables and fruit are of a lower quality. Proteins regulate the internal water and acid base balance, and they provide energy and build enzymes, antibodies and some hormones. They are also needed for tissue repair, especially in cases of injury or blood loss. Extra protein is needed for growth in children, for pregnant women, and for nursing mothers. The recommended amount of protein needed by a man of 18–22 is 54 grams per day and 46 grams for a woman of the same age. The diet should contain about 15% protein. The body can tolerate 300 grams a day without harm if sufficient fluid is drunk to dispose of nitrogenous waste. Most Americans consume 2–3 times more protein than they need.

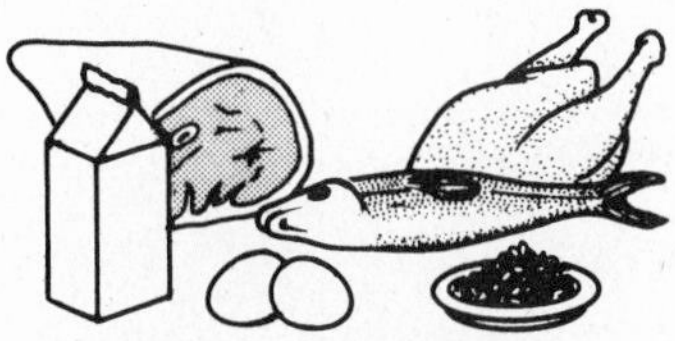

Foods high in proteins
The list *below* contains a selection of high-protein foods. Figures show grams of protein per 100g of food. Note that although eggs and milk are low in the list, they are both extremely good protein sources for humans.

g	
31	Beefsteak, stewed
28	Pork chop, broiled
26	Chicken, roast, white meat
26	Cheese, Cheddar
25	Liver, fried
25	Ham, cooked
24	Bacon, rashers, cooked
24	Peanuts, roasted
24	Lentils, dry
23	Lamb, roast
21	Beans, haricot, dry
20	Salmon, canned
17	Cod
17	Almonds
17	Herring
14	Spaghetti
12	Eggs
10	Flour, white
6	Rice
3	Milk, liquid, whole

Vitamins and minerals
Vitamins are coenzymes: they act in conjunction with enzymes to promote an increase in the rate of chemical reactions that occur in the body. Additional intakes of vitamins should not be necessary in a well-balanced diet, and in some cases an excess can cause harm, but deficiencies of certain vitamins cause serious diseases including beriberi, scurvy, night-blindness, rickets and pellagra. There are about 40 vitamins, of which 12 are essential in the diet. They can be divided into two classes: those that are soluble in fat (vitamins A,D,E and K), found for example in meat and oils; and those that are soluble in water (vitamin C and the B complex), mainly found in fruit and vegetables. Cooking vegetables in the minimum amount of water for only a short time will help to preserve the vitamins; the water can be used for a nutritious stock.
Minerals play a vital role in the regulation of body fluids and the balance of chemicals. Some are needed in comparatively large amounts; these are calcium, phosphorus, sodium, chlorine, potassium, sulfur and magnesium. Those that are needed in smaller quantities are iron, iodine and fluorine; deficiencies can cause serious illnesses such as anemia and goiter (enlargement of the thyroid gland). A varied diet is necessary to provide the essential vitamins and minerals.

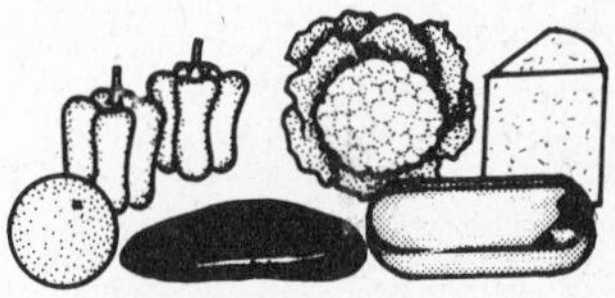

Calcium, iron, vitamin C
Listed *below* are good food sources for these three important nutrients. Most people in Western countries, however, will meet their daily requirements of these nutrients without special dietary planning. Note that figures given in each case are milligrams per 100g of food.

Calcium

800	Cheese, Cheddar
550	Sardines
280	Figs, dried
220	Chocolate, milk
180	Beans, haricot, dry
120	Milk, liquid, whole

Iron

9	Liver, fried
8	Lentils, dry
7	Beans, haricot, dry
4	Almonds
4	Figs, dried
3	Spinach

Vitamin C

200	Blackcurrants
100	Green peppers, raw
64	Cauliflower, raw
60	Spinach, raw
60	Strawberries
53	Cabbage, raw
50	Oranges

Nutrition 2

Malnutrition should not be a problem in the West, but ignorance of what nutrition the body needs may put some people at risk. Food habits are acquired early in life and it is difficult to change them. Age, sex, lifestyle, pregnancy and illness are factors that influence people's nutrition needs. Protein intake can be between 35 and 85 grams per day, fat between 55 and 130 grams per day and carbohydrates between 250 and 560 grams per day. The average person will be able to get all those nutrients, vitamins and minerals if his or her diet includes 2 servings of meat, fish, poultry, eggs, beans, peas or nuts per day; about ½ pint of milk or the equivalent in cheese or yoghurt; 4 servings of fruit or vegetables (to include both) per day, 4 servings of cereal, bread, pasta or rice per day and a little oil, lard, cream or sugar.

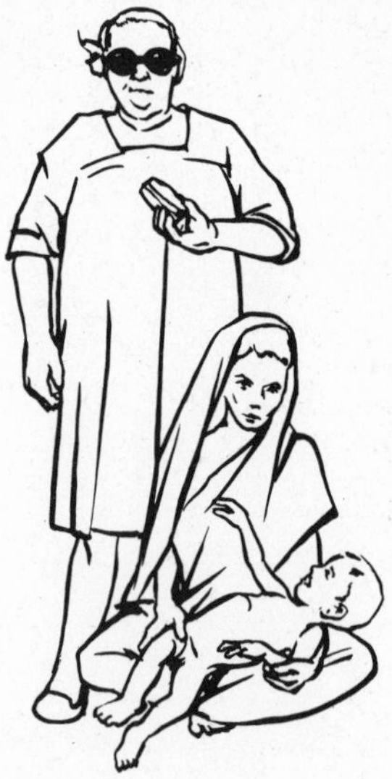

Western and Eastern diets
The West offers the most varied, cleanest and most readily available supply of food in the history of the world. Major nutrition problems include obesity, diabetes (associated in some cases with excessive carbohydrate intake) and digestive diseases associated with lack of fiber. Also, food additives may be overused in the West. 75% of the world's people live on a basic diet of one food, usually a cereal (rice). Deficiency diseases and lack of food because of crop failure are common in the East. But in times of plenty these diets often provide more nutrients than the average Westen diet.

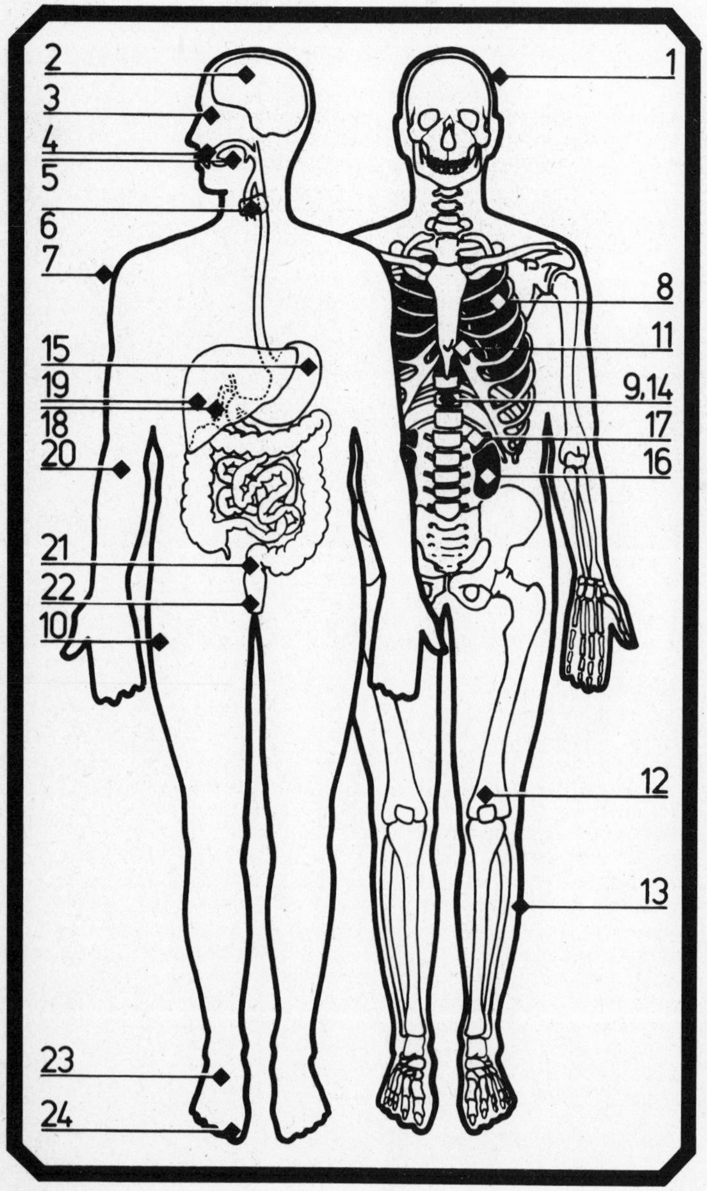

Effects of inadequate nutrition
There are many theories and much research into the link between diet and disease. We list some of the most commonly known effects of malnutrition.
1 The hair may become dull and brittle, or it may fall out or change color.
2 Headaches may be related to vitamin deficiency.
3 Nightblindness may arise from a lack of vitamin A.
4 The tongue may become inflamed as a result of a number of vitamin deficiencies.
5 Bleeding gums may be a sign of scurvy (vitamin C deficiency).
6 Enlargement of the thyroid gland (goiter) may be linked to iodine deficiency.
7 Rashes, itching, soreness, scaliness and cracking of the skin may be the sign of a number of vitamin deficiencies.
8 Obese people often experience breathing difficulties.
9 Backache may occur as a result of obesity.
10 Too much food, particularly fat and carbohydrate, will lead to obesity. Too little food will cause wasting of the tissues and ultimately starvation. Failure to thrive in children may be a sign of marasmus (too little energy intake) or kwashiorkor (too little protein and energy intake).
11 Heart disease can occur as a result of obesity, and heart failure may be a result of extreme anorexia nervosa (see p. 28) as the balance of electrolytes is disturbed.
12 Softening of the bones may be a sign of rickets (lack of vitamin D).
13 Loss of motor function in the legs may be sign of beriberi (lack of vitamin B_1, or thiamine).
14 Lesions in the spinal cord may be a sign of vitamin B_{12} deficiency.
15 There are a number of conditions affecting the stomach and digestive system as a result of diet. Symptoms may include diarrhea, nausea, vomiting, pain and cramps.
16 Stones may form in the kidneys as a result of insufficient fluid; obese people may be prone to kidney failure.
17 Adrenal glands may enlarge as a result of pantothenic salt deficiency (related to the B vitamins).
18 The formation of gallstones is associated with a fatty diet.
19 Too much alcohol may cause cirrhosis of the liver.
20 Insufficient iron will cause anemia.
21 Constipation can be caused by lack of fiber in the diet.
22 Piles (hemorrhoids) may also be a result of lack of fiber.
23 Swelling and painful feet may be a sign of vitamin B_{12} deficiency.
24 Numbness in the toes may be a sign of vitamin deficiency. Attacks of gout are connected with overindulgence in rich food and alcohol.

Children
Breast milk provides a baby with a complete diet. It also transmits immunological substances from mother to infant and is psychologically satisfying for both. The use of bottled cow's milk as a substitute depends on hygienic preparation to prevent gastroenteritis which can cause diarrhea, dehydration and death. Vitamin supplements may be given daily from 1 month. First solids of cereal and puréed or strained foods without sugar or salt are usually given at 4–6 months. From 1 year on the child can share in most of the dishes of the family but requires extra milk for growth.

Adolescents
The nutritional requirements of adolescents are conditioned primarily by the growth spurt at puberty. In boys this is responsible for a gain in height of about 8in and in weight of about 40lb. In girls the gains are usually less. The additional requirements are usually provided at mealtimes but if this is not done adolescents may have snacks between meals. These are usually sweet foods and may lead to an imbalance in the diet or obesity and dental decay – major problems in the USA and Europe. Young girls are particularly prone to anorexia nervosa, an aversion to food which may lead to self starvation (see p.28).

Adults
Eating habits begun in childhood tend to persist throughout adult life. With freedom to choose, an adult may tend to eat what he finds satisfying – sweet things, for example – rather than what is nutritionally sound. Lifestyle may dictate much of the daily food intake. People who are busy at work or in the home may feel too rushed or tired to prepare or eat a meal; some people may overindulge in rich, fatty foods and alcohol at business lunches or on other social occasions. Diet may also be influenced by social, psychological, religious, philosophical and economic factors.

Older people
Many elderly people remain active and so their diet is little different from the rest of the adult population. But as activity declines the need for food diminishes. If a man's intake is less than 2000 calories per day the diet may be deficient in minerals and vitamins, particularly calcium, folic acid, ascorbic acid and the B group of vitamins. Vitamin D may also be lacking without exposure to the sun. The diet should include fresh fruit, vegetables, milk, eggs and meat, with not too much bread and candy. Fiber is important to prevent constipation.

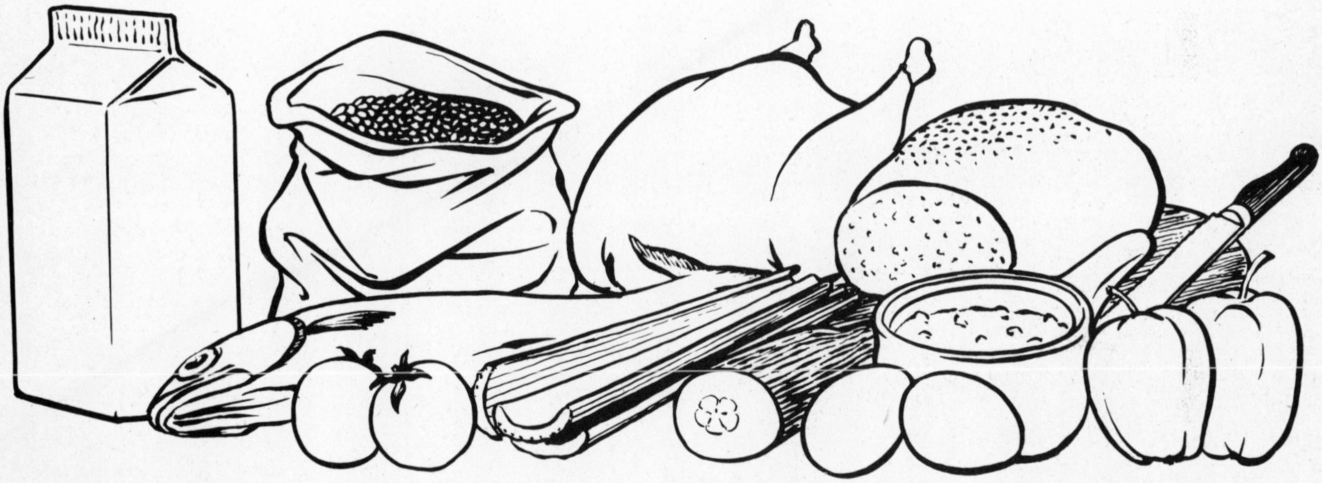

Pregnancy and nursing mothers
It is not necessary to eat for two during pregnancy but a woman needs about 15% more calories a day. A well-balanced diet is essential for the development of the fetus. Weight gain should be about 20 to 25 pounds. There may be a need for supplements of folic acid – the need in the body doubles in pregnancy – and iron. Extra calcium needs can be met in the diet. During lactation a women needs 500 more calories a day. At both times good sources of nutrients include milk, meat, fish, poultry, bread, potatoes, cereals, fruits and vegetables. Nursing mothers should have a high intake of fluid.

Illness and convalescence
People who are ill or convalescing may have little appetite and low food tolerance; the diet needs careful planning to be appealing and nutritious. Small helpings may tempt a wavering appetite. Ample protein and energy foods are needed to repair the drain on the body's reserves and to restore the person's strength. Immobilization in bed may have caused demineralization of the bones. Milk is a good source of calcium to correct this. Calcium from the bones is excreted in the urine and if the flow is sluggish calcium stones may develop. A high fluid intake – 2 or 3 liters daily – should prevent this.

Hypertension
Some degree of hypertension (abnormally high blood pressure in the arteries) is common in middle age. If untreated it may lead to cardiac failure. There are two dietary factors that may predispose a person to hypertension – obesity, and a high level of salt in the diet. Weight loss and a low sodium diet are usually recommended to reduce blood pressure. Sufferers are advised to eliminate table salt and reduce cooking salt and baking powder to a minimum and to select foods carefully. Among those that should be avoided are butter, bacon, sausages, canned meat and fish, and store-bought sauces.

Digestive problems
Dyspepsia or indigestion is one of the most common digestive problems. Symptoms are nausea, heartburn, epigastric pain, discomfort or distension. The cause may be psychological or intolerance to a particular type of food, or it may be a sign of an organic disease. It can be the result of overwork, overweight, bolting food and eating meals when excessively tired, or of smoking or drinking too much. If there is no organic disease sufferers are usually advised to have a bland diet, avoiding spices, fried foods, excess sugar, rich, heavy puddings and raw fruit and vegetables. Regular meals at short intervals are recommended.

Energy and calories

One of the main functions of food is to provide energy. This is necessary not only for strenuous activity, but also for the functioning of the internal organs. The amount of energy ingested in the form of food is measured in calories; if you take in more calories than you use you will put on weight, and if you take in fewer calories than you use you will lose weight. Carbohydrates and fats are the main sources of energy; protein can be used as an energy food, but is more useful to the body in other ways. Your daily calorie need will depend on your age, your sex, your lifestyle and activity level, the rate of your metabolism, and the climate in which you live. Here we look at calorie requirements and the calorie content of some foods.

Definition of a calorie
A calorie is the amount of energy needed to raise the temperature of 1cc of water by 1°C. The measure used for food is 1000 times that, a kilocalorie or kcal; here we follow common usage and refer to kcals as calories. One ounce of protein produces 113 calories, one ounce of carbohydrate the same and one ounce of fat produces 252 calories. The modern term for measuring energy is the joule. One calorie equals 4.2 joules.

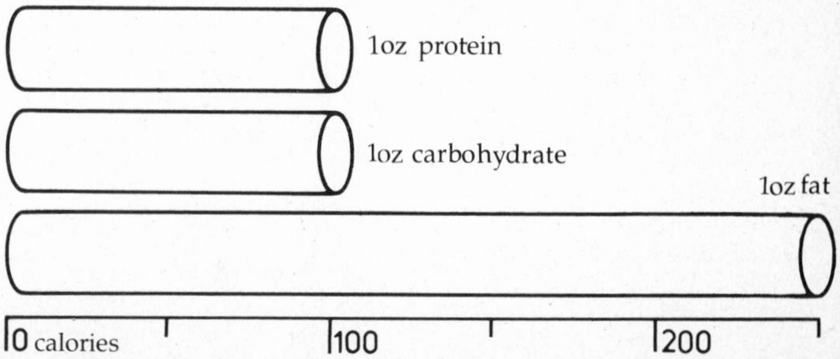

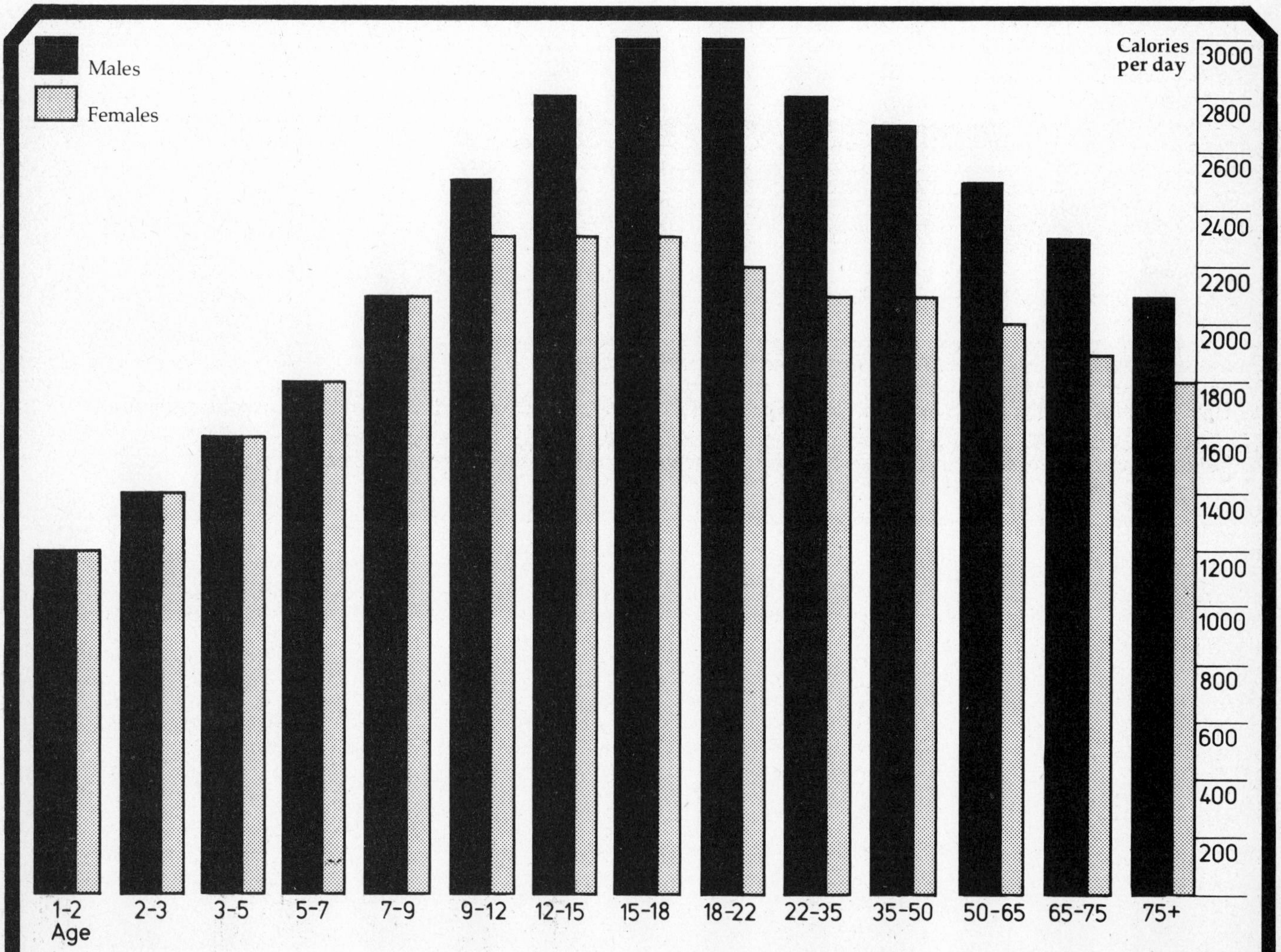

Calorie requirement chart
The chart *above* is based on the calorie requirements of a typical person living in a temperate climate. Children have a high calorie requirement for their size because energy is also needed for growth. Male and female needs are similar until puberty. Changes then bring differences in growth rate, body size and activity patterns; men need more energy from food than women. A man aged 75 requires the same number of calories per day as an 8 year old, but a woman aged 75 needs only as many calories as a 6 year old.

Energy needs of men
Most men use more energy than women doing the same activity because men's bodies are larger and need more energy to operate them. An average man uses up about 1650 calories a day just for basic life processes such as heartbeat, breathing, digestion and excretion. This is known as the basal metabolic rate. His work or other daily activities will use up at least 600 calories extra and about 2400 more if his job involves hard manual labor. When running a man consumes some 600 calories an hour, nearly twice as many as when he is walking. When driving he uses 170 calories per hour.

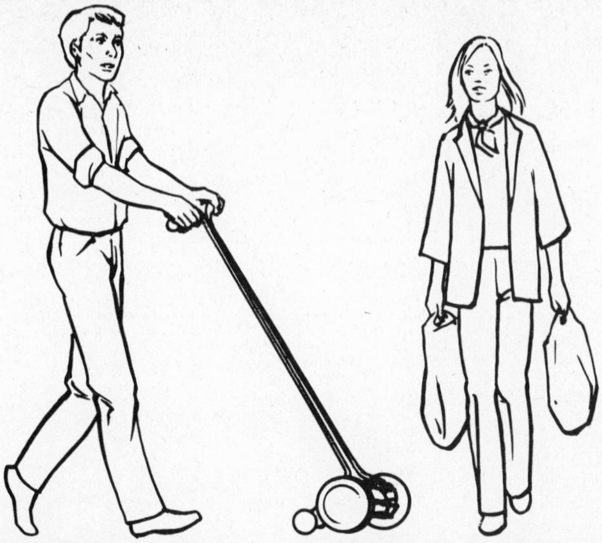

Energy needs of women
Women not only weigh less on average than men and so use less energy but their extra body fat traps heat and they need less energy to keep warm. An average woman uses up about 1400 calories a day to maintain basic life processes. A further 600 to 800 calories should provide the energy needed for all her other activities. During pregnancy calorie intake should be about 2250 and another 500 calories should be added during breastfeeding. A woman lying asleep uses up 55 calories an hour; doing sedentary work she uses about 70 calories an hour, and when climbing a slope about 360 calories an hour.

Calories in foods
The following tables show foods that contain specified numbers of calories based on single-portion quantities, in most cases after cooking. The method of cooking can change the calorie content. For example a large egg contains 90 calories if it is served boiled or poached, 108 calories if it is fried and 120 calories if it is scrambled. It is not necessary to count the exact number of calories that you need per day, unless you are on a strict reducing diet, but the rough guide provided here may be useful.

50–100 calories
3oz baked beans
2oz coleslaw
3oz olives
3½oz boiled potato
2oz potato salad
5oz cherries
8oz blackberries
8oz raspberries
1 apple
1 banana
2oz dates
1 pear
5oz fresh pineapple
1oz raisins
4oz cod
2oz smoked salmon
4oz clams
3oz crab meat
1 boiled or poached egg
2 plain crackers
2tsp honey

200–300 calories
3oz beef sausages
2oz chick peas
6oz tripe
4oz fish sticks
3½oz roast turkey*
3½oz canned tuna
¾pt milk
2tbsp cream
4oz processed cheese
1oz sunflower oil
1oz suet
1oz coconut oil
1oz peanut oil
1oz lard
1oz butter
1oz margarine
2tbsp mayonnaise
1pt sweet cider
6oz ham
4oz ice cream
6oz stewed lamb, lean only

400–500 calories
6oz ground beef
6oz fried liver
5oz fried brains
5oz roast duck*
5oz roast goose*
4oz pork sausages
5oz roast lamb
¼lb takeout hamburger
1 ice cream soda
4oz chocolate cake
4oz fruit cake
3oz salami
1 slice cheesecake
1 serving pumpkin pie
2oz chocolate
1 cup drinking chocolate
4oz pork paté

Under 50 calories
6oz cabbage
5oz carrot
5oz cauliflower
10oz cucumber
6oz lettuce
2½oz corn
3oz cottage cheese
1tsp sugar
5oz raw mushrooms
2oz boiled peas
4oz boiled spinach
8oz spring greens
7oz tomatoes
3oz apricots
4oz onion
8oz grapefruit
1 peach
6oz melon
3tsp caviar
2oz oysters
1tsp peanut butter

100–200 calories
2oz fried mushrooms
2oz fried onions
2oz dried peas
1oz potato chips
½ avocado pear
7oz canned raspberries
2oz prunes
2½oz corned beef
2½oz roast beef
4oz roast chicken*
2oz kidney
1oz fried bacon
½pt buttermilk
5oz boiled rice
3 chocolate cookies
5oz egg noodles
1pt beer
1 glass orange juice

300–400 calories
4oz fried potato
6oz roast venison
5oz lamb chops
4oz pork chops
6oz canned mackerel
6oz stewed rabbit
4oz veal steak
3oz condensed milk
4oz Cheddar cheese
4oz Camembert cheese
4oz Danish blue cheese
3oz cream cheese
3oz granola
4oz sago
2 doughnuts
1 serving apple pie
1 serving sponge cake

Over 500 calories
7oz beefsteak, lean and fat
1 serving beef curry
5oz roast pork
4oz fried whitebait
1 serving fish fried in batter
1 serving spaghetti bolognese
7oz frankfurters
1 serving chilli con carne
4oz hard candy
2oz olive oil
4oz fudge
1 fruit and nut chocolate bar
1 takeout hamburger and french fries
1 whole pizza

*Without skin

Eating problems

Occasionally the normal body cycle of hunger, eating and repletion becomes altered, perhaps by physical disturbances such as illness or at times by psychological disturbances, for example stress or depression. The hunger pangs that the body produces may be ignored, in an overenthusiastic attempt to lose weight or because of a psychological disturbance, and the condition known as anorexia nervosa may set in. Once anorexia is established, drastic and potentially fatal weight loss occurs. Other people may develop a psychological dependence on food even when their bodies do not need it, and ignore sensations of repletion; this situation can lead to chronic obesity. Here we look at some of the causes and effects of anorexia and overeating.

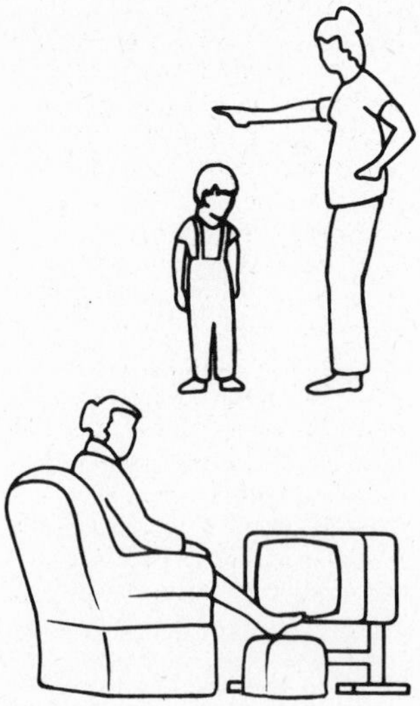

Types at risk
Children with dominating parents, particularly mothers, may be at risk from either overeating or anorexia nervosa; they may be forced to eat more than they want, or they may later use a refusal to eat as a means of rebellion. Mothers who are alone in the house all day may be tempted to nibble constantly; they may also find it hard to lose any weight gained during pregnancy. Lonely people of all ages run the risk of not bothering to eat much, or alternatively of eating too much through boredom; and those in occupations with irregular hours can easily fall into bad eating habits.

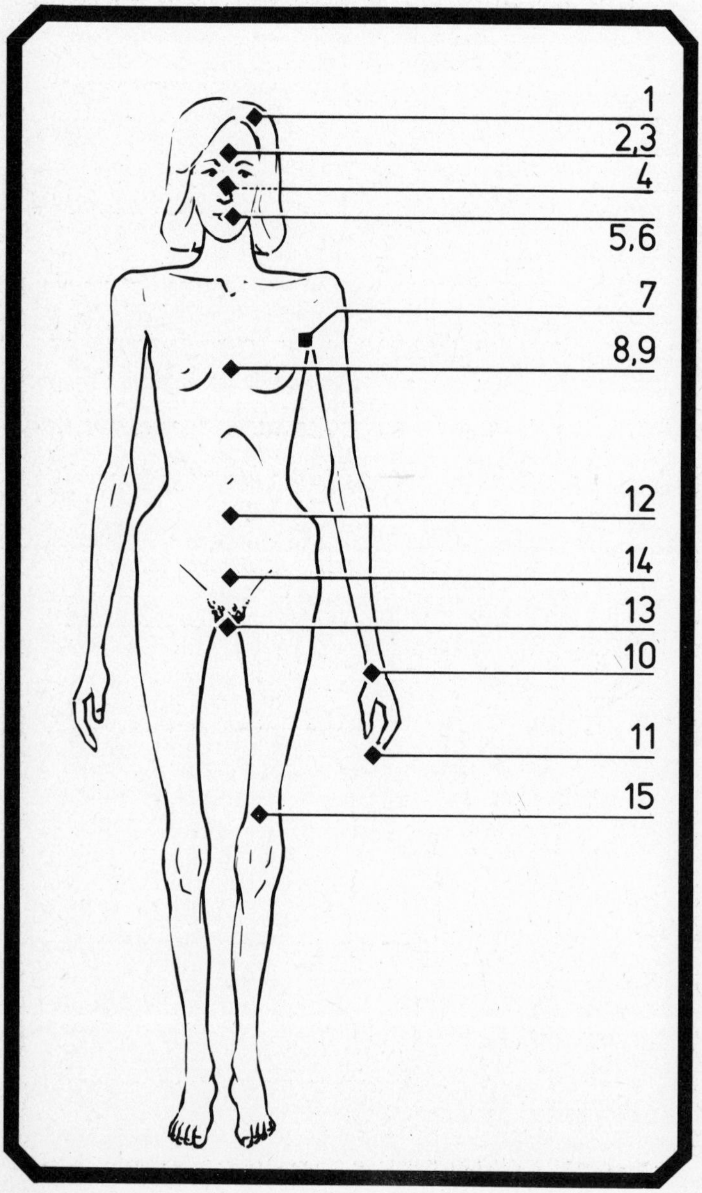

Effects of anorexia
The illustration shows some of the effects that prolonged anorexia nervosa can have on the body.

1 The hair changes texture and sometimes color because it lacks nourishment.
2 Dizziness and excessive fatigue may be felt as the muscles have no reserves of energy to call on.
3 Sleep disturbance often occurs; the person may be very active or excessively tired and lethargic.
4 Hormone imbalance arises because the body is not functioning healthily to produce and use hormones in the correct ratios.
5 Bad breath can be noticed because of the constantly empty stomach.
6 Decayed teeth occur in anorectics who persistently vomit; the tooth enamel is destroyed by stomach acid.
7 Hypothermia or low body temperature occurs as the body tries to conserve energy.
8 The electrolyte balance of the body is altered, and the blood becomes dangerously low in sodium and potassium. These conditions may have fatal effects.
9 The respiration slows.
10 The pulse slows, and the blood pressure drops.
11 The fingernails change in texture and become more brittle because they are not receiving nutrients.
12 Fine hair begins to grow in excess on the body as anorexia progresses.
13 Amenorrhea, or cessation of the menstrual periods, often occurs when a female has lost 25lb or more. Anorexia is often linked with a desire to reject adulthood and fertility, and so many anorectics are pleased when their periods stop.
14 Chronic constipation may occur as there is so little food in the system that the bowels cannot function properly.
15 Severe emaciation is one of the most obvious signs of the condition.

People who develop anorexia almost always insist that there is nothing wrong with them; they may explain away their weight loss, or even delude themselves into thinking that they are fat when in fact they are little more than skin and bones. Consequently it may be very hard to get treatment for an anorectic, as any successful treatment requires cooperation. If left untreated, however, the condition may well prove fatal.

Undereating in childhood
All children have phases when they either like or dislike certain foods intensely. If your child refuses certain foods point blank give others of similar nutritional value, such as cheese instead of milk, fish instead of eggs, soups instead of plain vegetables. Avoid confrontations over food, as once your child realizes that this is a way to gain your attention he will use the opportunity to the full. Don't give snacks between meals, even if he hasn't eaten at the previous meal; remember that a child will rarely go hungry from choice. If he begins to lose weight, consult a doctor.

Anorexia nervosa
This condition usually affects females between the ages of 14 and 18, although some may begin the condition in adulthood; it rarely begins before the onset of puberty. Boys and men are very rarely affected. A desire to lose weight is often the first stage, but soon gets out of hand, and the person either becomes physically incapable of eating or vomits the food after meals. Anorexia nearly always occurs in females who have been exemplary children, and may be a way of covertly rebelling against parents who have unrealistically high expectations of their daughters. Medical help should always be sought.

Overeating in childhood
Children who are deprived of affection, attention or a sense of worth often turn to food as a comforter, and this may lead to a dependence on food in all future times of stress. Parents should never feel that a child is rejecting them by rejecting their cooking, otherwise they can easily force the child into eating too much and suppress his body's signals of repletion. Don't encourage your child to eat between meals, and don't give him a diet rich in sugar and starch; if you teach him the value of a balanced diet he should grow up with healthy eating habits.

Overeating in adulthood
The danger situations likely to lead to overeating are rife in adulthood. After marriage people tend to take less care of their weight than when they were single; or their jobs may take them on an ever-increasing round of social functions and business lunches. Activity often declines during adulthood, but is not usually followed by a corresponding decrease in the amount of food eaten. Broken marriages, bereavement, family difficulties or work problems may all lead to the kind of stress that encourages overeating for comfort.

Effects of overweight
The illustration shows some of the effects of serious overweight.
1 Strokes are more likely in overweight people than in those of normal weight.
2 A double chin is one of the most immediately noticeable effects of overweight.
3 Hypertension, or high blood pressure, is more common.
4 Heart disease of many kinds, poor circulation, and palpitations of the heart are more common.
5 Breathlessness occurs on exertion, and respiratory disease is more likely than in a normal person.
6 Gallbladder diseases occur more often in overweight people.
7 Cirrhosis of the liver is more common.
8 Diabetes is more common.
9 Overweight may contribute to infertility in women.
10 Overweight may contribute to impotence in men.
11 Kidney disease of all types is more common.
12 Hernias are more frequent, especially in men.
13 Arthritis, especially of the hips and knee joints, is more common.
14 Varicose veins often occur.
15 Flat feet may develop as a consequence of carrying the excess weight.

Overweight people have a decreased life expectancy, and the more overweight you are the more your life expectancy decreases. If you began to be overweight before age 35, your life expectancy is even lower; and if you have been overweight since childhood the statistics are still more frightening. Overweight people are more accident-prone than those of normal weight, mainly because excess weight limits their mobility so that they cannot easily get out of the way of danger. Overweight may disguise symptoms of serious diseases and make it difficult for a doctor to make a diagnosis. Overweight also makes surgery more dangerous; some abdominal operations, such as appendectomy may be impossible in badly overweight people.

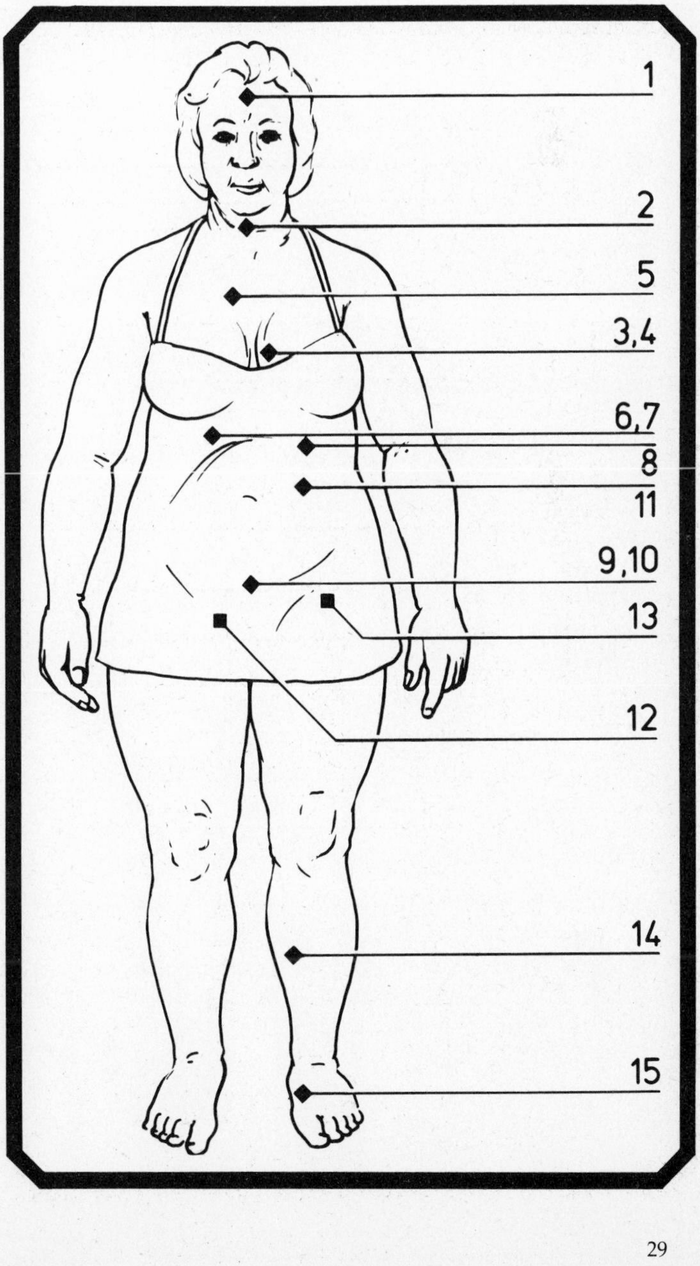

Reducing

Reducing weight and body size requires a good deal of commitment and planning in order to be effective. The only way to achieve a genuine weight loss – one resulting from the breakdown of body fat rather than the loss of fluid – is to use up more calories of energy than you take in by eating. A deficit of roughly 3500 calories is needed to lose one pound of body weight, so a person who would normally use 2000 calories per day should lose about 2lb per week on a 1000 calorie diet. This is the ideal rate of weight loss; if you lose weight more slowly you may become discouraged, and if you try to lose weight more quickly by eating less than 1000 calories per day you will damage the body tissues by breaking them down instead of your body fat.

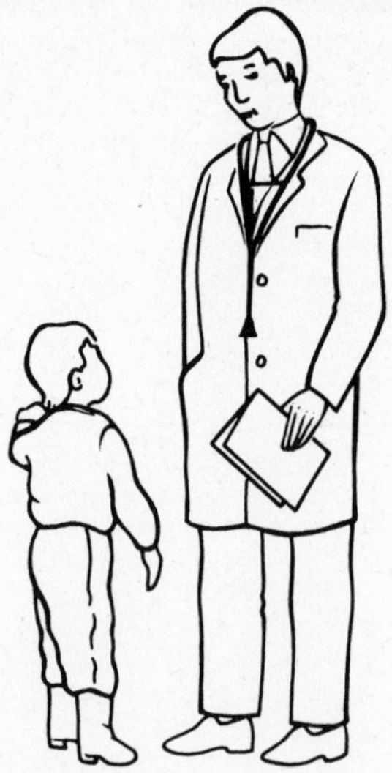

Age and reducing
People of all ages can go on reducing diets, provided that the diet is sensible and that the person's doctor agrees. In fact if you are overweight your doctor is likely to encourage you to reduce, and may give you a diet sheet and supervise it himself. Overweight children should reduce in order to avoid the possible miseries of a lifetime of obesity, and adults of every age will benefit from the advantages of being their correct weight, such as improved health and fitness and a more pleasing appearance.

Men		Women	
Height (ft:in)	Weight (lb)	Height (ft:in)	Weight (lb)
5:2	119–136	4:10	100–117
5:3	122–140	4:11	103–120
5:4	125–143	5:0	106–123
5:5	128–147	5:1	109–126
5:6	132–151	5:2	112–130
5:7	136–156	5:3	115–134
5:8	140–160	5:4	119–138
5:9	145–164	5:5	123–142
5:10	149–169	5:6	127–146
5:11	153–174	5:7	131–150
6:0	157–178	5:8	135–154
6:1	161–183	5:9	139–159
6:2	165–188	5:10	143–164

Weight table
The chart *above* shows desirable weights for men and women of various ages. During middle and old age people tend to put on about 10–20lb in weight, but there is no necessity for this; older people will find that they are healthier if they maintain roughly the same weight that they had in their 20s. Measure yourself without shoes, and weigh yourself without clothes. While reducing, always weigh yourself on the same scales, in the same room, at the same time of day, so that you have an accurate record of your loss.

Testing for obesity
Weight is not the only gauge of whether you need to reduce; body shape and condition will tell you a lot too. If you examine yourself honestly you may have to admit that you could do with losing some inches. If you stand relaxed, without pulling in your muscles, does your abdomen sag? Does your stomach bulge over a tight waistband? Can you pinch a roll of flesh on your midriff, upper arm or thigh? Do you deliberately wear loose clothes so that your real shape is hidden? Are your body measurements larger than they used to be? If so, think seriously about reducing for the sake of your health and appearance.

Food groups
The no-counting method of dieting is basically a calorie-controlled diet, but one in which you do not need to weigh all your portions of food. The foods are divided into three groups, by high, medium and low calorific value, and the aim is to eat as much as you please of the lower group and avoid the foods in the high group. Foods in the middle group should be eaten only in moderation.
A This is the group of forbidden foods, and contains such things as cakes, cookies, candy, pastries, chocolate, nuts, cream, sugar, fried foods, sausages, salami and bologna, avocado pears, puddings, sauces, jellies, honey, mayonnaise and oily salad dressings.
B This is the group of medium calorific value, and contains such foods as lean meat, mackerel, herring, anchovies, bananas, crackers, bread, rice, pasta, whole milk, eggs, cheese, duck, goose, and ryvita.
C This is the group of very low-calorie foods, and contains such things as onions, peppers, tomatoes, mushrooms, lettuce and other salad greens, beet, apples, oranges, lemons, grapefruit, tangerines, melon, strawberries, raspberries, blackberries, peaches, nectarines, loganberries, sugar substitutes, diet soda, skim milk, black tea and coffee, unsweetened fruit juice and water.

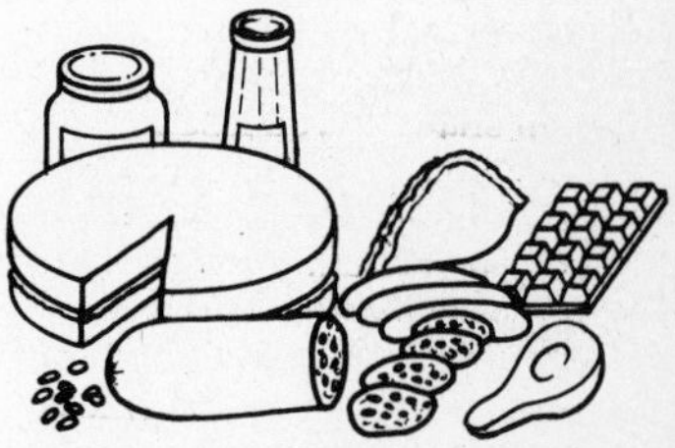

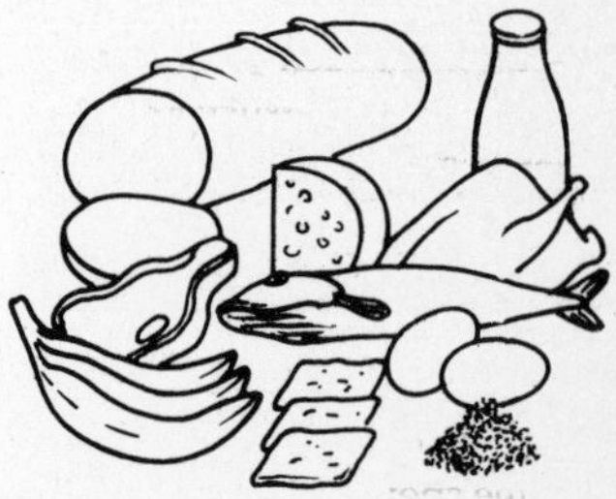

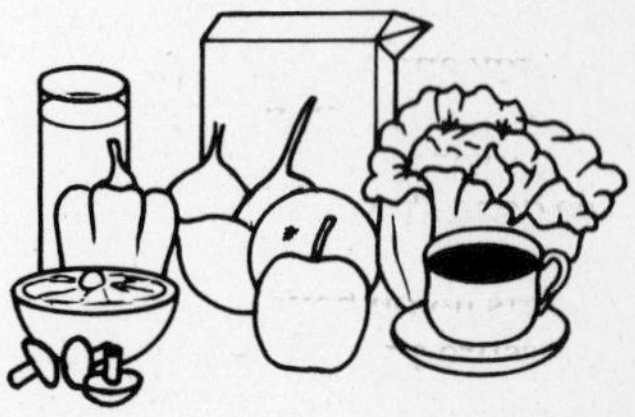

Attitude to eating
If you are trying to lose weight and then to maintain that weight loss afterward, it will probably be necessary to alter the role that food plays in your life. Studies of overweight people show that they generally do not eat to satisfy hunger, but rather they eat because they have uncontrolled urges for a particular food or because food is too readily available. An overeater will not stop when his or her body has had enough, but will continue until the food is finished. Your body will need gradual re-education until you eat only when hungry, and stop when your hunger has been satisfied.

Eating patterns
Overweight people often tend to eat whenever food is available; they are open to temptation from snacks, candy stores, takeout foods, leftovers on plates, and food in the kitchen when they are working there. One of the keys to successful reducing – and maintaining your recommended weight – is to remove sources of temptation or to learn to overcome them. Help yourself to stop snacking by removing all tempting food from the kitchen; keep only low-calorie foods readily available. Never buy food when you are hungry; go shopping after a meal so that your appetite will not be stimulated.

Family attitudes
Your family may be your biggest help or your biggest hindrance in your reducing plan. If other members of the family are overweight they are likely to feel threatened by your hopes of being slim; or your family may resent missing out on their favorite fattening foods if you stop preparing or buying them. Try to enlist your family's support, and also try preparing tempting low-calorie dishes so that they still feel that they are having appetizing food; don't become obsessive about your diet or about calorie counting.

Clubs
Mutual support clubs exist in many areas to help their members to reduce in company. The clubs provide diet sheets that recommend good, balanced diets, and may also provide cooking tips, discussion groups so that individual problems can be aired, regular weighing sessions at which progress can be charted, and sometimes even prizes for achieving your target weight. Many people who lack the willpower to reduce on their own have benefited tremendously from such clubs; meeting with people who share the same problems and temptations helps them to carry on under difficulties rather than giving up.

Exercise
Exercise is an aid to reducing, and can help you to tone up flabby muscles and improve your shape as you lose weight, but it is not a substitute for dieting. Very strenuous exercise is needed to burn up even 1lb of body weight, but exercises such as these can help to make certain areas of your body look trimmer. Don't waste your money on steam treatments, so-called "reducing garments" or vibrating belts, as these will not make you lose weight, but equipment such as that shown *right* – exercise wheels and exercise machines – may help to trim your figure.

Sport and reducing
Some sports are particularly good for helping you to trim your figure. Sports such as sprinting, rowing, cycling, racket sports, and competitive canoeing, swimming or skiing use up quite a few calories of energy and so may help you to lose weight, but they need to be a regular part of your life and to be done strenuously for this effect; do not engage in these sports if you have high blood pressure or any problems with your heart. Other sports, such as ice and roller skating, fencing, walking, volleyball, basketball and jogging, provide overall muscle exercise and so will improve your figure and, in conjunction with a diet, help you to lose inches.

Reducing exercises
These exercises may help you to trim inches from various parts of your body. Repeat each exercise several times.
1 Stand with your hands under your chin and your elbows horizontal; draw your elbows back as far as possible.
2 Stand with your fingertips on your shoulders and your elbows to the sides, and rotate your elbows forward and back.
3 Stand with your feet apart and one arm raised; bend to the opposite side, then change arms and repeat.
4 Stand with your feet apart and your arms stretched out to the front; swing your arms and trunk to each side.
5 With your back straight, move your head around in large circles as shown.
6 Lie on your back with your knees bent and your arms out to the sides, holding a book in each hand. Slowly raise your arms to bring the books together.
7 Lie on one side with your head resting on one hand; raise your upper leg slowly as high as you can, then lower. Repeat on the other side.
8 Lie on your back with your arms at your sides. Keeping your legs straight, slowly raise them a few inches off the ground and hold the position for several seconds.

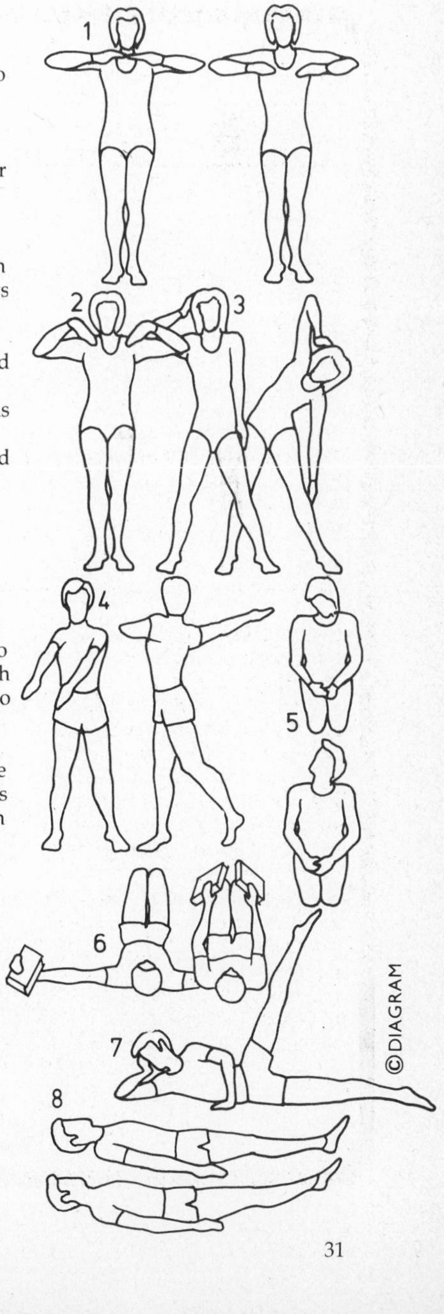

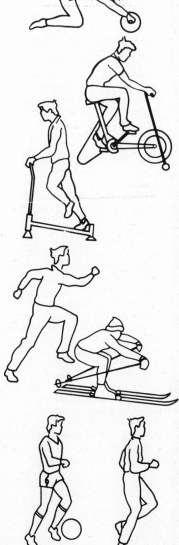

Exercise

Exercise is a vital ingredient for keeping the human body in good health. Muscles, lungs and heart are built to work; an inactive lifestyle makes them ineffective and out of condition, but exercise can help to remedy these ill effects and promote a sense of health and wellbeing. As your physical fitness increases you will find that your work and leisure activities become less tiring, and also that your capacity for activity of all kinds increases. Exercise also helps to make your internal organs work more efficiently, and so makes you less likely to succumb to poor health and disease. Exercise improves muscle tone, skin tone and general appearance, and helps to delay the physical effects of aging.

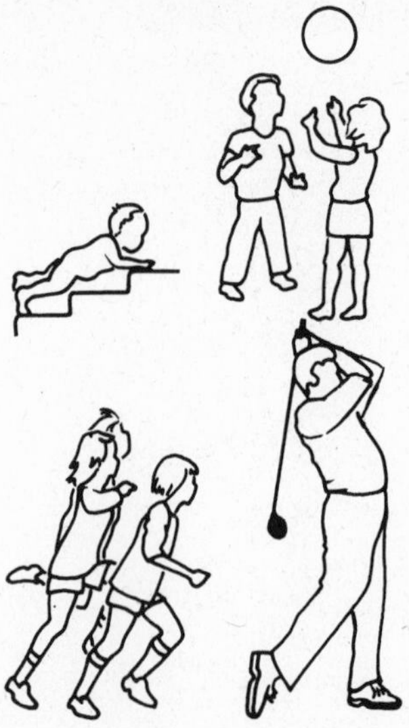

Exercise and age
Exercise of some sort is possible whatever your age, and in fact suitable exercises are desirable at every age. Babies should receive exercise through play and through movements that increase the range of activities they are capable of; older children usually get plenty of exercise through play and sport. In middle and old age, a conscious effort may be needed to ensure that exercise is a regular part of life. Always check with your doctor before you embark on any exercise program or take up a new sport, especially if you are 35 or over.

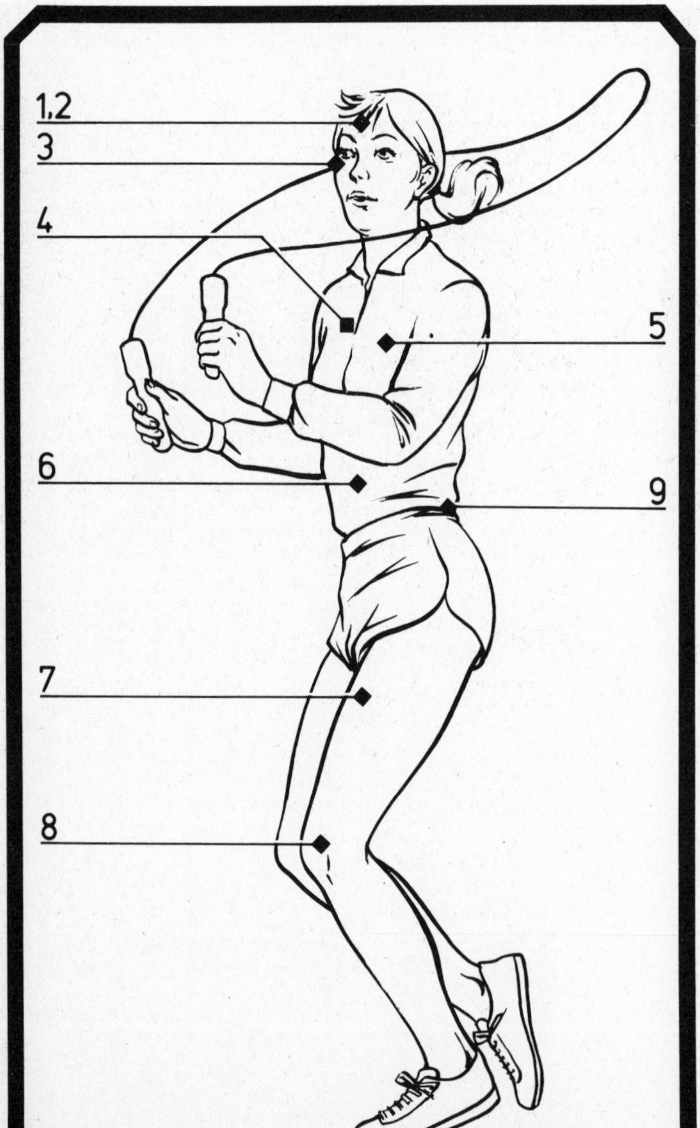

Benefits of exercise
The illustration shows some of the parts of the body benefited by regular exercise.
1 Mental wellbeing is improved as stress decreases and the physical benefits of exercise become noticeable. Increased capacity for activity can help to decrease fatigue and depression.
2 The coordination and responses of the nervous system improve as the body gets more accustomed to obeying mental signals promptly.
3 The skin tone is improved as the increased circulation to the skin disperses waste products and impurities more quickly.
4 The efficiency of the heart increases a great deal. The volume of blood pumped per beat increases, so that the heart does not have to work so hard to pump the blood around the body, and the heart rate decreases as a result. This new efficient circulation causes more capillaries to form in the body tissue and therefore improves the blood supply to internal organs.
5 The efficiency of the lungs also increases. The improved blood supply enables them to exchange carbon dioxide for oxygen at a faster rate, and their capacity is enlarged.
6 The metabolism alters as physical activity increases. The body may use up food more quickly, which combined with increased energy output makes overweight less likely; also, the fats and sugars in the blood are reduced.
7 The contours of the body alter as the muscles and ligaments strengthen. Body tissue is prevented from sagging when the muscles are in good condition, and weight may be lost as body fat is burned up in strenuous exercise.
8 The bones and joints of the body strengthen so that they are less liable to injury and debilitation.
9 The posture improves as the overall condition of the muscles and joints is improved; as a result, problems such as back trouble and flat feet may be avoided.

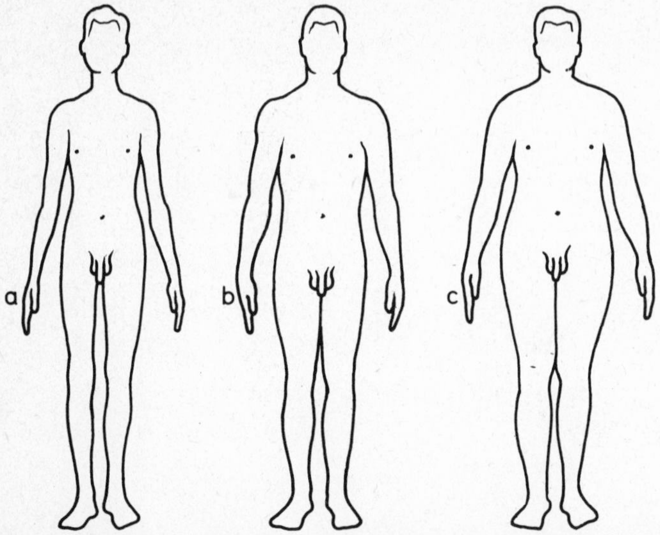

Body type and exercise
Body shapes and physiques are classified into three main types: ectomorphs (**a**) who are lean and rangy, with no excess body fat or weight; mesomorphs (**b**) who have a good balance of muscle and weight; and endomorphs (**c**) who tend to be bulky and rounded in shape. The type of exercise that will be best for you depends to some extent on your body type. If you are an ectomorph you have very little excess weight or bulk to carry around, and so will probably do very well at exercises and sports that require endurance and stamina; you may also find that you can sprint and cycle rapidly. If you are endomorphic your natural range of activities may be somewhat limited and exercises of most kinds may be awkward; endomorphs with a great deal of muscle may be well equipped for weightlifting and sports such as football, wrestling and boxing. Mesomorphs are generally suited to most kinds of exercise and sport, especially those where both muscle power and endurance are required. Whatever your body type, try to include several types of exercise – mobility, strength, endurance, isometric etc – in your health program.

Exercise chart
This chart shows the parts of the body that are benefited by various kinds of exercise. The type of benefit the body receives is keyed as follows:
△ Muscle strength
■ Muscle endurance
▲ Mobility and flexibility
□ Heart/lung endurance

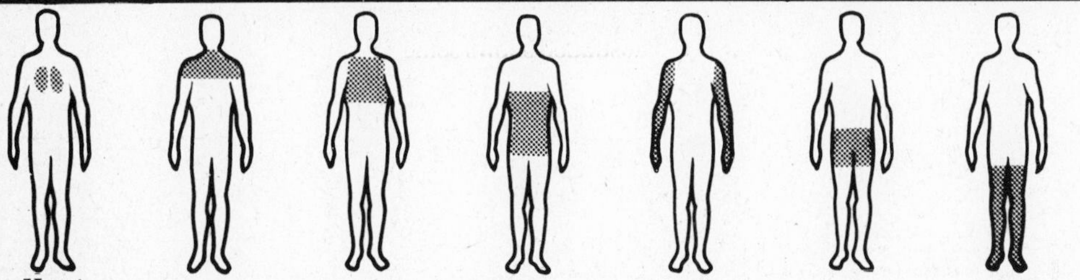

	Heart and lungs	Shoulders	Back	Trunk	Arms	Hips	Legs
Baseball		▲			▲		▲
Basketball	□						△ ■ ▲
Beam (gymnastics)			△	△	▲	▲	△ ▲
Boxing	□		△ ■	△ ■	△ ■ ▲		△ ■ ▲
Cross-country running	□		■	■			△ ■ ▲
Fencing	□				▲	▲	△ ▲
Field hockey	□		■		▲	▲	△ ■ ▲
Floor exercises (gymnastics)		▲	△	△	△ ■ ▲	▲	△ ▲
Football	□		△ ■	△	△	▲	△ ■
Handball	□	▲			△ ▲		△ ■ ▲
High jump			△	△		▲	△
Horizontal bar (gymnastics)		△ ■ ▲	△	△	△ ■ ▲		
Horse (gymnastics)		△ ■	△	△	△ ■ ▲	▲	
Ice hockey	□		△	△	△	▲	△ ■
Judo	□		△ ■	△ ■	△ ■ ▲	▲	△ ■ ▲
Karate	□		△ ■	△ ■	△ ■ ▲	▲	△ ■ ▲
Long jump			△	△		▲	△ ▲
Parallel bars (gymnastics)		△ ■ ▲	△	△	△ ■ ▲	▲	▲
Pole vault		△ ▲	△ ▲	△ ▲	△ ▲	▲	△ ■ ▲
Racketball	□	△ ▲			△ ▲		△ ■ ▲
Rings (gymnastics)		△ ■ ▲	△	△	△ ■ ▲	▲	
Rowing	□	△ ■	△ ■	△ ■ ▲	△ ■		■
Skiing (cross-country)	□	△ ▲	▲	▲	△ ▲	▲	△ ■ ▲
Sprinting						▲	△ ▲
Soccer	□						△ ■ ▲
Squash	□	△ ▲			△ ▲		△ ■ ▲
Swimming	□	△ ■ ▲	△ ■	△ ■	△ ■ ▲	▲	△ ■ ▲
Tennis	□	△ ▲			△ ▲		△ ■ ▲
Throwing events		△ ■ ▲	△		△ ▲	▲	△ ▲
Volleyball	□	▲			△ ■ ▲		△ ■
Water polo	□	▲	■		△ ■		■
Water skiing	□	△ ■	■	■	△ ■		△ ■
Weightlifting		△ ■	△ ■	△ ■	△ ■		△ ■
Wrestling	□	△ ■ ▲	△ ■ ▲	△ ■ ▲	△ ■ ▲	▲	△ ■ ▲

Mobility exercises

Mobility exercises help to improve the flexibility and range of movements of the muscles and joints. People who lead a sedentary life often have very little mobility in their joints, and as a result their bodies are limited in efficiency and movement and prone to various joint and muscle problems. General "aches and pains" can often be removed by a course of mobility exercises, and this kind of exercise is used in physiotherapy for rehabilitating weakened muscles. Always be very careful when beginning mobility exercises; muscles that are unused to strenuous movement can easily be damaged or torn. Begin any course of exercises very gently, to avoid stiff and painful muscles the following day, and never stretch your muscles to the point of discomfort.

Arm and shoulder flexibility
These tests will enable you to see how well you are progressing as you use the mobility exercises to increase your flexibility. Try the tests before you begin your exercise program, and then do them at weekly or two-weekly intervals and note your improvement.
a Stand with your arms at your sides; keeping them straight from the shoulders, move them forward and up and then down and back as far as possible.
b Stand with your arms straight out to the sides; move them first up, and then down and across your body, as far as possible.
c Start as for **b** and reach behind you as far as you can.

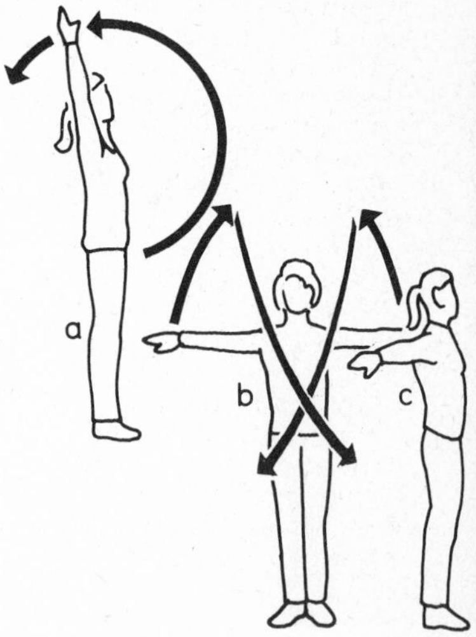

Mobility activities
Yoga (see p. 150) is very good for improving mobility and flexibility, as it stretches and loosens muscles and joints. T'ai Chi and K'ai Men sequences of exercises are also good for making the muscles more mobile, as they involve a series of stretching poses that exercise the whole body. Jumping rope improves the flexibility of the arms and shoulders, and will also tone up the muscles of the hips, thighs and calves. Sports such as swimming, golf, gymnastics, racket sports and track and field events all promote mobility as they tend to require the use of many of the muscles in the body for coordinated movements. Exercising with Indian clubs or ribbons, and gymnastic floor exercises and movement sequences, will also tone up and flex the muscles.

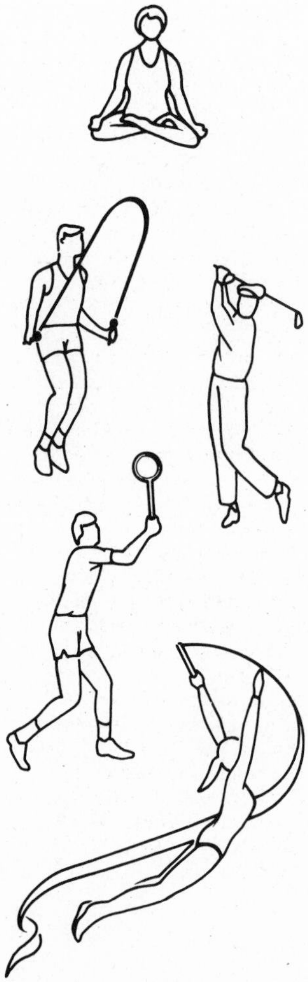

Arm and shoulder exercises
For exercises **1** to **22**, begin with one or two repetitions each day and work up slowly to a maximum of 30 repetitions.
1 Stand upright, with your arms loosely at your sides. Bend your trunk first forward and then backward.
2 Move your head first forward and back, and then from side to side, to loosen your neck and shoulder muscles.
3 Stand upright with your arms stretched above your head. Cross your arms in front of your face, and then behind your head.
4 Stand with your arms at your sides. Cross your arms first in front of your body then behind your back.
5 Stand with your arms at your sides and make giant circles first forward and then backward.
6 Stand with your feet together and your arms against a wall; bend your arms so that your chest is lowered to the wall, and then straighten your arms again. This is a modified push-up; when you are more flexible you will be able to do full push-ups.
7 Stand with your feet apart and your elbows raised to shoulder level; clench your fists in front of your chest. Push your elbows back as far as possible, keeping your back straight.

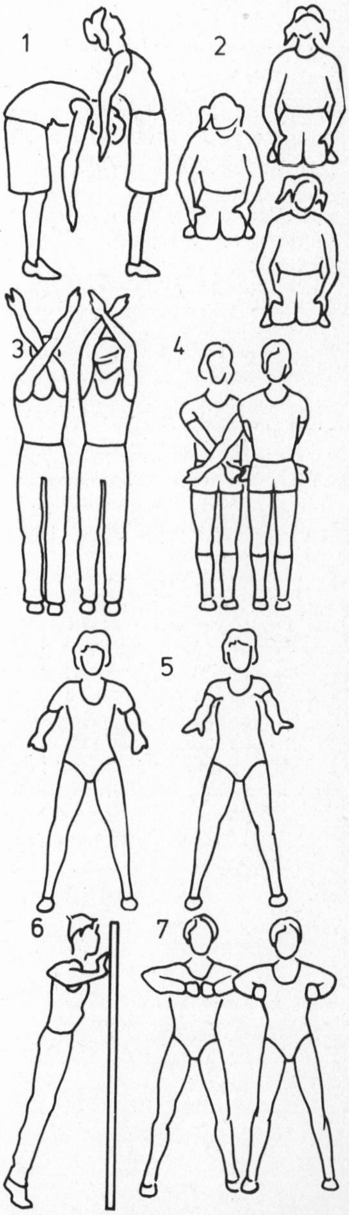

Waist and trunk flexibility
These tests will show you the improvements in mobility of your waist and trunk if you do them at regular intervals.
d Sit with your legs apart; put your hands over your head as shown, and then lean your trunk forward to try and touch each foot in turn.
e Sit with your legs stretched out in front of you, then lean forward and try to put your head on your knees. This will be impossible at first, but you will gradually get nearer over the weeks.
f Stand with your legs apart and your arms over your head; bend as far as possible to each side.

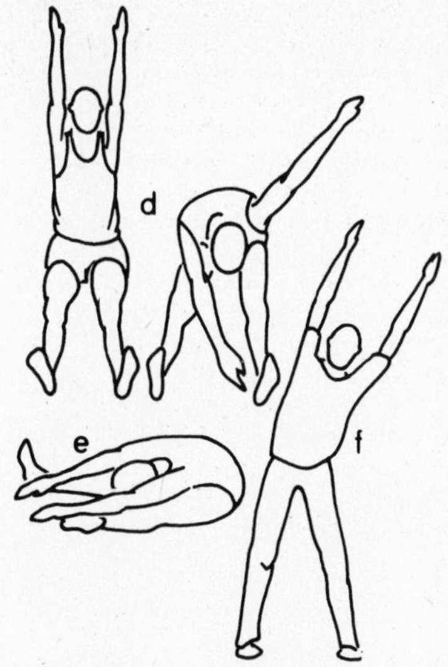

Waist and trunk exercises
8 Stand facing forward with your arms loosely crossed, and then twist your trunk to first one side then the other as far as possible, keeping your feet flat on the floor.
9 Stand with your arms stretched out in front and your feet apart, then swing your arms around as far as possible to the left, then to the right.
10 Stand with your legs apart and your arms loosely at your sides; bend as far as possible to each side, keeping your trunk facing the front.
11 Lie on your front with your knees bent up as shown; try to clasp your ankles and raise your thighs. This will become easier as you progress.
12 Stand upright with your arms at your sides, then flop forward to touch your toes.
13 Sit with your legs apart, then lean forward and reach your arms out as far as you can.
14 Stand with your legs apart and your arms by your sides; bend forward to touch one foot with the opposite hand, swinging the other arm back. Straighten up and repeat to the other side.

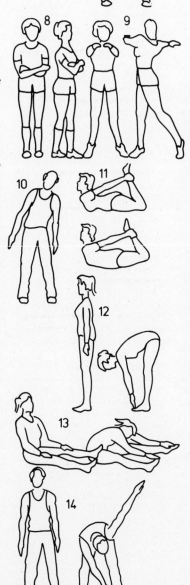

Leg and hip flexibility
Use these flexibility tests in the same way as the others, to test the progress of your body mobility.
g Stand upright against a wall; raise one leg out to the side and then across your body as far as it will go, keeping it straight at the knee.
h With your arms out to the sides for balance, take a small step forward and then kick the other leg into the air as high as you comfortably can, keeping it straight.
i Sit with your knees apart and your feet together; hold your ankles and see how near you can press your knees to the floor.

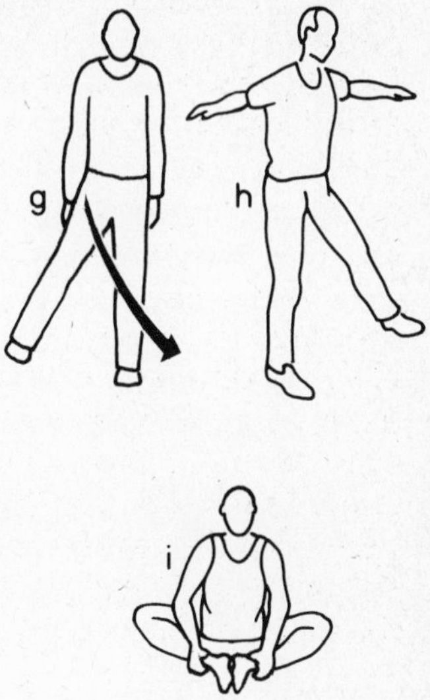

Leg and hip exercises
15 Stand on one leg, supported by leaning your hand on a wall or table, then lift your free leg as high as possible to the side.
16 Stand as in **15**, and swing your free leg forward and back as far as possible.
17 Lie on your back with your buttocks touching a wall and your legs raised, then open your legs as wide as you can.
18 Stand with your arms behind your head as shown, then lunge forward onto each leg in turn.
19 Stand with your feet together; keeping your feet flat on the ground, bend your knees while at the same time twisting them to the left. Straighten up, then repeat twisting them to the right.
20 Stand with your feet together, then jump as high as you can to one side as though jumping a fence, keeping your feet together. Repeat to the other side.
21 Lie on one side with your arms positioned as shown. Lift your upper leg as far as possible in the air, then lower it.
22 Lie face down with your arms at your sides, then lift each leg in turn as high as possible off the floor.

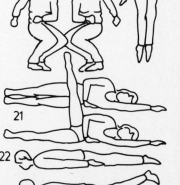

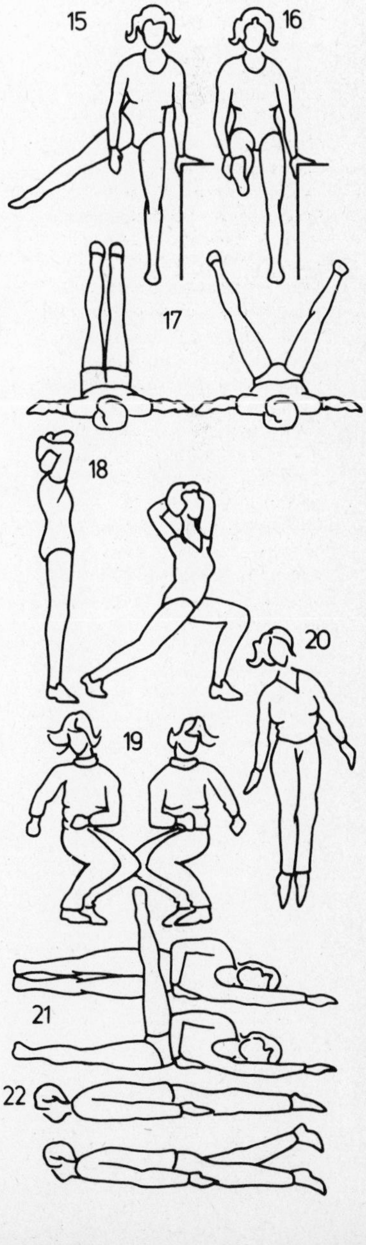

Strength exercises

Strength exercises are not just for wrestlers and bodybuilders; they are beneficial exercises that will improve the health of most people's bodies. They impart shape and tone to the body muscles, and enable the body to cope with situations that call for more than usual physical effort, such as carrying or pushing heavy objects and taking part in certain strenuous sports. Strengthening exercises also make the muscles more capable of protecting the joints and the internal organs; as a result these parts of the body are less liable to injury. Strengthening exercises usually build up the weight and power of the muscles by repeating various strenuous actions; using weights while exercising is one very common way of increasing the effects of strengthening exercises (see p.74).

Sports and activities
Various sports increase strength by repeatedly exercising one or more sets of muscles. Boxing, shot put and hammer throwing pay particular attention to the arm muscles, but the legs and trunk will gain some benefit at the same time. Competitive swimming (especially the butterfly stroke), rowing and wrestling have greater all-round effects on the body's strength, as most of the body's muscles are exercised.

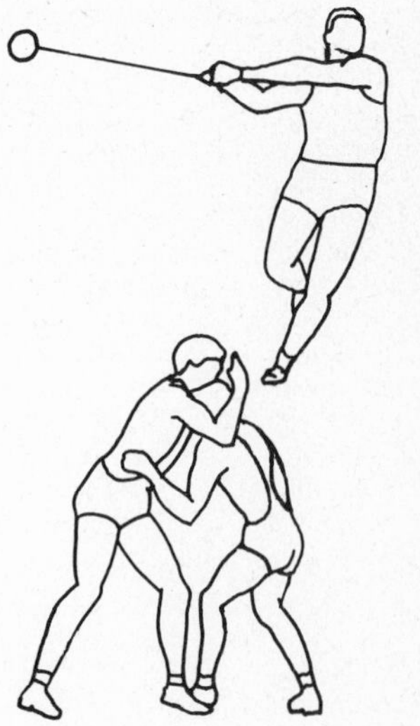

Arm and shoulder exercises
For exercises **1** to **22**, begin with one or two repetitions and build up slowly each day to a maximum of 20 repetitions.
1 Balance your body weight on your hands and toes as shown; keeping your back straight, lower your body by bending your elbows. Straighten your arms to return to the original position.
2 Lie on your back with your knees bent up, clasping a heavy book in each hand as shown. Keeping your arms straight, slowly raise them to bring the books together, then lower them again.
3 Stand facing a partner with your feet touching. Hold hands, then both lean back, keeping your backs straight, until your arms are fully extended.
4 Holding Indian clubs (or you can use heavy books or rolled magazines), stand with your arms raised; lower your arms, keeping them straight, out to the sides and down, then return to the starting position.
5 Throw and catch a large, heavy ball, such as a medicine ball, until your arms are tired (this can also be done from one partner to another).
6 Stand back to back with a partner, linking your arms. Lean forward to raise your partner off the ground, then repeat with the roles reversed.

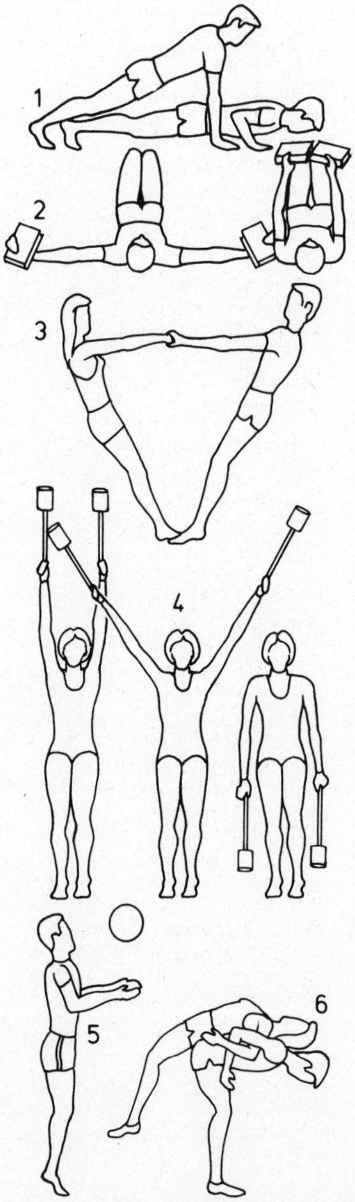

Abdominal exercises
7 Lie face down with your hands under your chin; lift first one leg and then the other as high as possible.
8 Lie face down with your hands clasped behind your head; raise your head and chest as high as possible.
9 Lie on your back with your feet hooked under a piece of furniture or held by a partner; lift your head and shoulders off the ground.
10 Sit at the front of a chair, gripping the sides with your hands; lift your feet and bend your knees up to touch your chest, then lower them slowly.
11 Start as for **10**, then lift your legs while keeping them straight; hold them in this position as long as you can.
12 Lie on your stomach over a chair, as shown, and raise your arms and legs so that your entire body is in a straight line. Hold for as long as you can.
13 Lie face down with your arms outstretched and your hands holding a towel as shown. Raise your legs and arms simultaneously.
14 Sit with your weight balanced over your bottom, then raise your legs and try to hold your ankles as shown. Eventually you will be able to hold this position for several seconds.

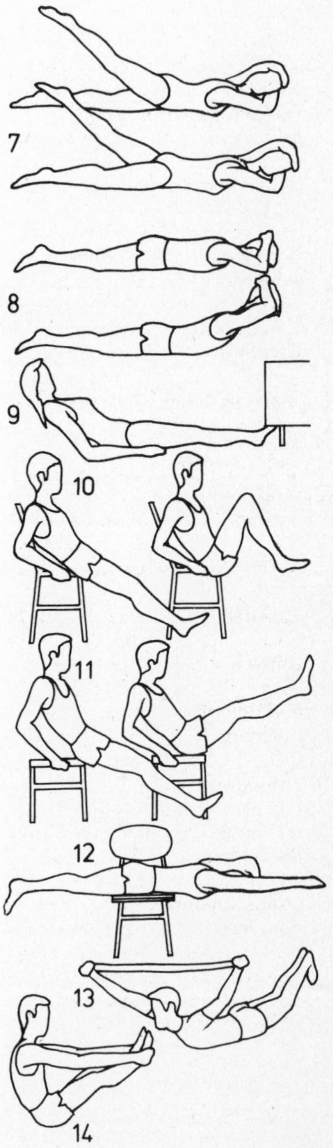

Throwing tests
Test the improvement in your muscle strength every few weeks by these tests; the more you exercise your muscles, the better you will be able to perform.
a Stand at a fixed point and throw a medicine ball, holding it first against your chest and then throwing it by levering your arms away from you. Measure the distance thrown.
b Hold a small ball in your right hand (or your left, if you are left-handed), and throw it overarm as far as possible. Measure the distance achieved.

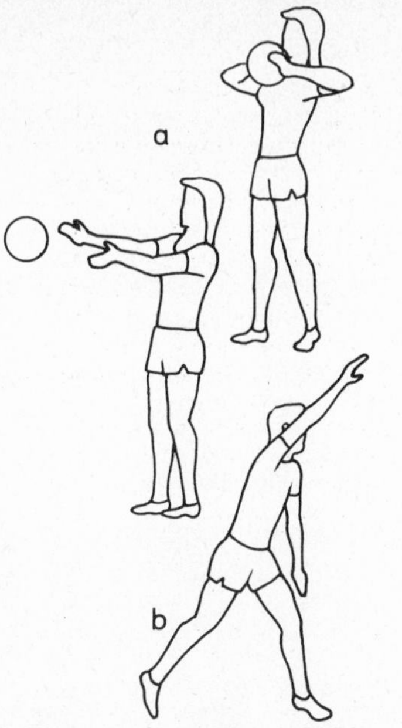

Jumping tests
Measure the improvement in the strength of your leg muscles by doing these tests every few weeks.
c Without a run-up, jump as high as you can with your arm stretched up to touch a mark on the wall. Measure the height jumped.
d Repeat **c**, but with a run-up this time; you should be able to jump considerably higher with the extra impetus.
e Stand at a fixed point, with your feet together. Bend your knees, and jump as far forward as you can; measure the distance jumped.

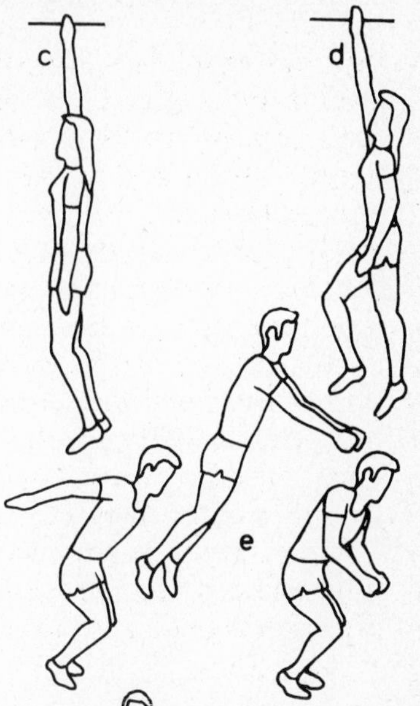

Leg exercises
15 Stand facing a firm chair with your hands on your hips, then swiftly step up onto it; step down with the other leg.
16 Run up and down a staircase quickly, as often as you can before you feel out of breath.
17 With a partner, sit on the floor and raise your legs so that your feet meet as shown. Push your legs away from you as your partner resists the pressure, then repeat with the roles reversed.
18 Start from the same position as for **17**, but this time move your right and left leg alternately.
19 Sit on one step of a staircase with your feet on the step below and your arms outstretched. Raise your legs until they are horizontal, and balance in this position.
20 Attach light ankle weights to your feet (or use a heavy book or rolled magazines) and sit as shown; lift your feet and legs and hold them in the raised position.
21 Lie face down with your arms at your sides. Lift both legs together as high as possible, and hold them in this position for as long as you can.
22 Lie on your back with your hands at your sides. Keeping your legs straight and your toes slightly pointed, raise your legs slowly until they are vertical. Hold in that position, then lower them slowly.

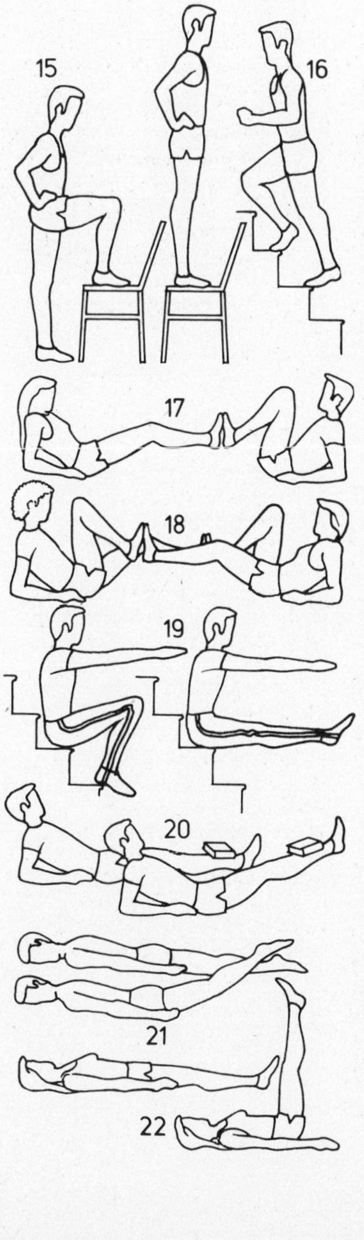

Isometric exercises
Isometric exercises are exercises without body movement; one group of muscles exerts pressure against an immovable object or an opposing group of muscles. Isometric exercises exert a great deal of force on the muscles, and the positions should be held for a maximum of only six seconds; do each exercise only once a day.
23 Sit with your legs apart and your hands on your knees, and try to push your knees together; resist the pressure with your legs.
24 Sit with your legs apart and your hands crossed as shown; try to push your knees apart as you resist the pressure with your legs.
25 Place the palms of your hands together and push them against each other.
26 Clasp your hands behind your head, and resist the pressure as you try to push your head forward.
27 Sit well back in a chair with your legs raised and your hands on your shins as shown; press downward with your hands and upward with your legs.
28 Stand in a doorway with your hands resting on the inside of the door frame; push against the frame as hard as you can.
29 Lie on your back with your hands under your head, and press your stomach downward as hard as possible.

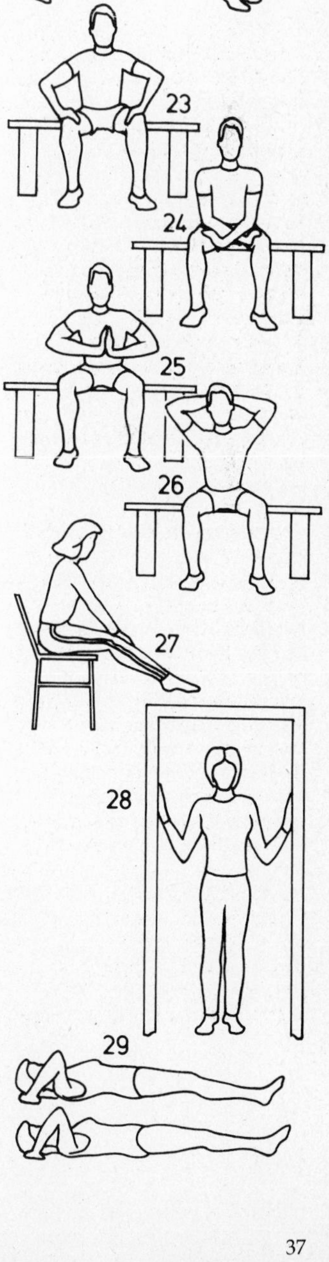

Aerobic exercises

Aerobic exercises are those that improve the performance and endurance of the heart and lungs, or cardiovascular system. Mobility and strength exercises alone will have little effect on your overall bodily fitness unless you include some aerobic exercise in your fitness program. Whether your lifestyle is completely sedentary or whether you engage in a lot of active sports and pastimes, your system will benefit from an improvement in the cardiovascular system; your heart and lungs will work more efficiently and become more resistant to disease and disorders, and your circulation in general will be improved. Regular aerobic exercise will also help you in the fight against heart disease; your heart will be stronger and have a more efficient blood supply.

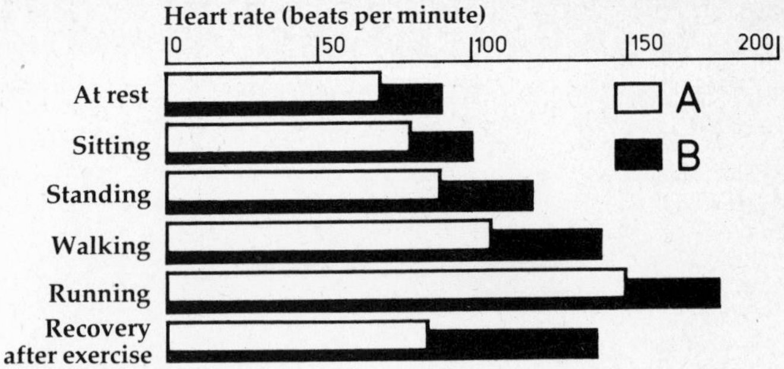

The fit and unfit heart
The diagram shows the comparative amounts of work done by a fit heart (**A**) and an unfit heart (**B**) during various activities. The higher the heart rate, the harder the heart is having to work; when the heart rate is low, the heart is being used efficiently. The unfit heart has to work much harder all the time, and so may be under a constant strain. A healthy heart works under a self-imposed maximum pulse rate of about 190 beats per minute, which means that even under severe, unplanned stress it is unlikely to increase its work to a dangerously fast rate.

Ways of improving fitness
Even before your exercise program begins, there are ways in which you can improve your fitness in other areas of your life. Smoking and drinking in excess reduce drastically your body's efficiency, and the direct effect of tobacco smoke on the lungs makes them less capable of exchanging carbon dioxide for oxygen. Because the blood carries less oxygen, the muscles tire more easily. Giving up smoking will add enormously to the benefits of aerobic exercise. Overweight will hamper you in efforts to become fit; lose the excess weight gradually and safely (see p.31). Even if you are not overweight, eating large meals will make you less inclined to exercise; try to eat several smaller meals a day rather than one or two large ones. Make sure you get enough sleep; if your body is run down it will not be able to function efficiently. Stress also has an effect on your physical wellbeing; learn to relax so your body is not overtaxed in the wrong ways (see pp. 150–151). A sedentary life will increase any tendency to eat, drink or smoke too much; develop hobbies that are as active as possible.

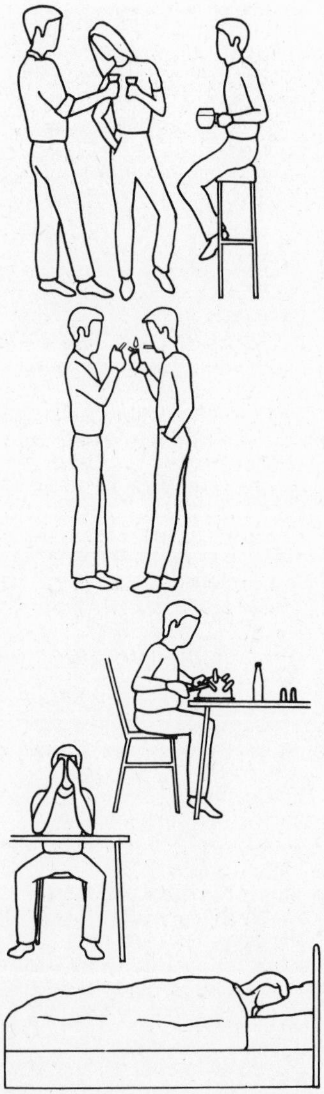

Gentle aerobic activities
If you are very unfit, and cannot perform even the simple aerobic tests well, then your body will need to be eased very gradually into exercise. Never go above your maximum recommended pulse rate (see p. 81), and have a thorough physical examination before you embark on any kind of exercise. Once your doctor has given the go-ahead, try some of these activities.

1 Walking is perhaps the best way to ease your system into aerobic exercise. On your first day, walk as far as you can without excessive tiredness, and then increase the distance gradually each day. Once you can walk several miles, increase the speed of your walking so that your lungs are exercised.

2 Swimming is another activity that can be increased gradually as your fitness improves.

3 Cycling will probably make you out of breath very quickly, but is good exercise. Start with a gentle ride on level ground, and increase the distance each day; try uphill terrain when you are ready.

4 Jogging can be started as part of your walk; jog for a few yards every 5 or 10 minutes, and make the jogging stretches gradually longer as your fitness improves.

1
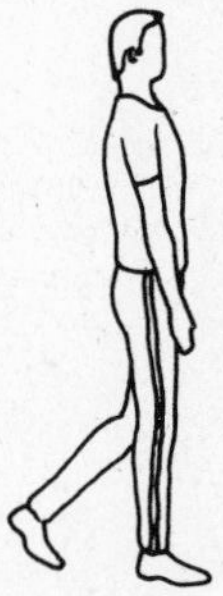

2
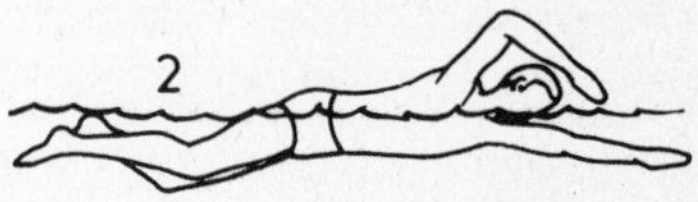

3
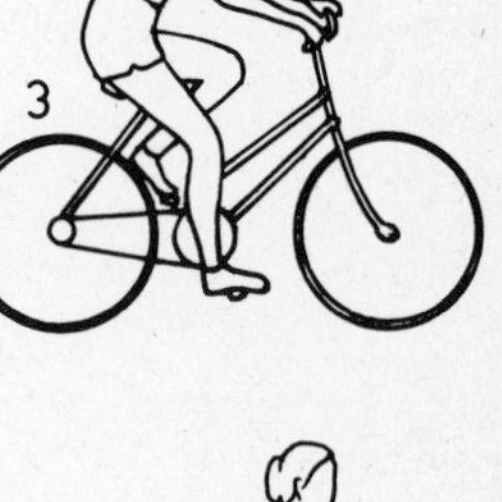

4
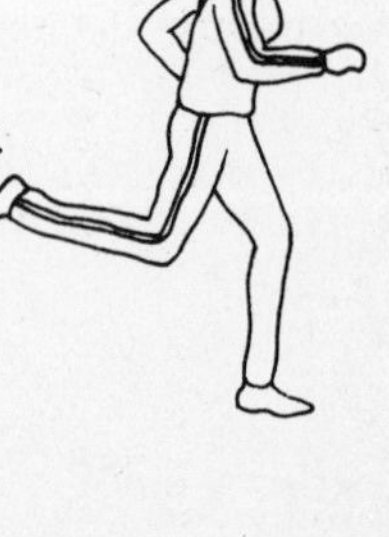

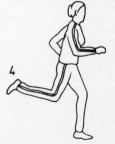

Signs of unfitness
If you suffer from any of the following problems, your body will not be working at maximum efficiency – in other words you are unfit and your body would benefit greatly from an aerobic exercise program.
a Breathlessness and a pounding heart after even very short bursts of exercise such as running for a bus or lifting a trash can.
b Bad posture caused by weak muscles or laziness.
c General aches and pains, especially in the back and legs, caused by weak muscles.
d Aching muscles after mild exercise.
e Excess weight caused by lack of exercise or overeating.

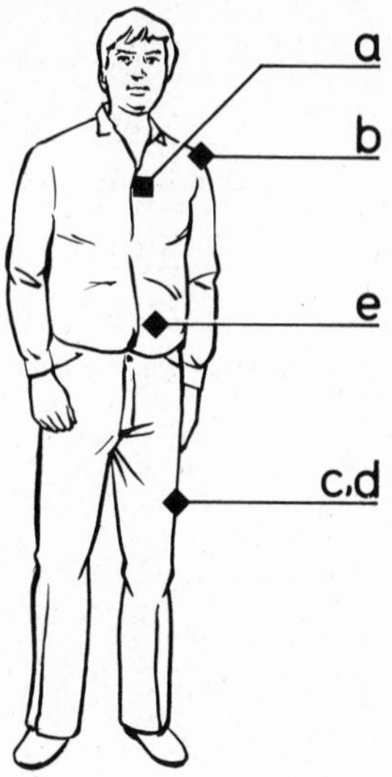

Aerobic tests
You can judge the condition of your circulatory-respiratory system by your performance in simple tests such as these. If you are very unfit you will find even these tests strenuous; stop as soon as you feel out of breath or if your heart begins to race uncomfortably.
f Walk up and down an average staircase at normal speed three times. Can you do this without feeling out of breath, and can you hold a normal conversation immediately without gasping?
g Can you easily walk for one mile at your normal speed?
h Can you run for 50 yards?

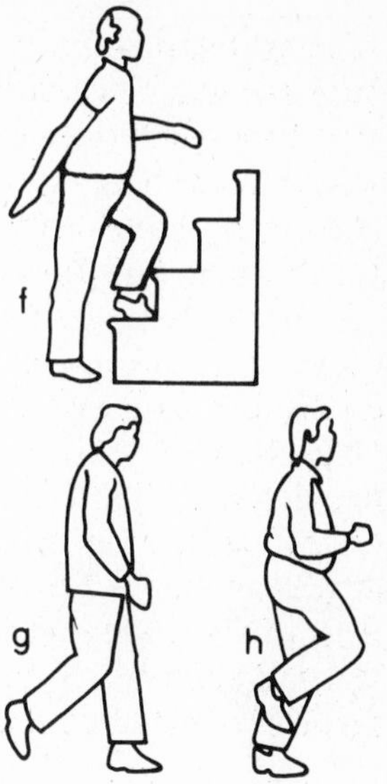

Strenuous aerobic activities
When you have gradually built up your fitness and capabilities through walking, jogging or cycling, you will find that the following activities provide more strenuous aerobic exercise.
5 Racket sports provide good exercise because of the amount of running that they entail.
6 The same is true of most ball games such as football, soccer, hockey, basketball and volleyball.
7 Competitive sports such as canoeing, rowing, skiing, swimming, hurdling, skating and cycling tend to provide aerobic exercise because of the speed at which they are executed in competition, but they are not recommended for people with heart trouble or for those past middle age. If you do the same activities non-competitively you will not gain so much benefit aerobically.
8 Hill-walking, or walking over any rough terrain, will provide good aerobic exercise if you keep up a brisk walking pace and cover several miles or more.
9 Vigorous repetition of many exercise movements, as in a step test (see p. 81), will provide aerobic exercise if the movement is repeated many times in a row.

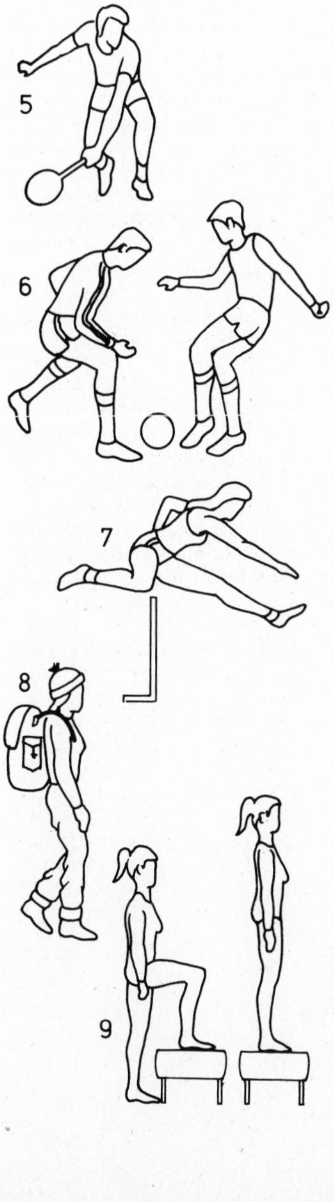

Running and jumping
Running and jumping rope (skipping) provide very good aerobic exercise for people who are fit.
10 Jogging over long distances will improve your circulatory-respiratory system considerably as both your heart and your lungs are working hard.
11 Sprinting requires short bursts of immense energy, and will tax your lungs and your heart with the extra oxygen required and the speed at which your heart needs to pump the blood around your body.
12 Long-distance running is excellent exercise for the lungs and heart as it requires a continuous, sustained effort.
13 Orienteering and cross-country running are pleasant ways of getting aerobic exercise; hard running will alternate with easier terrain.
14 Running in place is an indoor alternative to ordinary running in bad weather; or you could use a running machine that measures the number of steps you have taken and converts them into mileage equivalents.
15 Jumping rope (skipping) provides very vigorous aerobic exercise if it is done strenuously. Try turning the rope backward for variety, or turn the rope extra fast so that it passes under your feet twice before you land back on the ground.

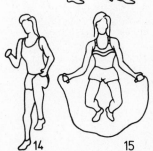

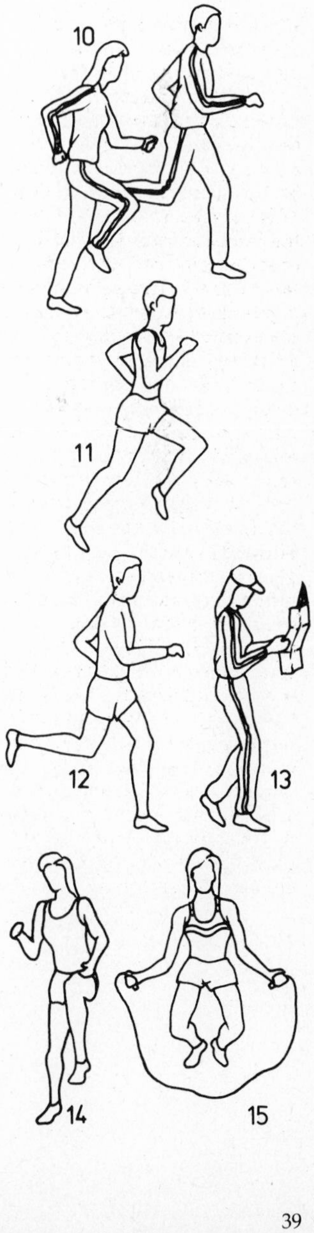

Advanced exercises

Here are some advanced exercises that can be undertaken when you have increased your mobility, strength and aerobic endurance. If you already have a high level of fitness, you could go straight on to these exercises, but never try to do them before your body is ready. You cannot take short cuts to fitness, and if you try to do too much too quickly you will strain your body and possibly cause it permanent damage; your muscles and joints need to be conditioned slowly. If you feel you are ready, try one of these activities slowly and gently, and stop if you feel that you are taxing your body too much. The tests of strength and endurance given will help to tell you if your body is in good condition.

Strength tests
Although these tests may appear to test only the strength of the arms, they actually test the muscles of the whole body, as all are required for the completion of the tasks.
a With the backs of your hands facing you, hang from a high bar with your arms straight. Pull yourself up until your chin is level with the bar.
b Stand between standard parallel bars, holding one with each hand; straighten your arms until your feet are off the ground. Lower yourself until your elbows form a right angle, then straighten your arms.
For men, 10 repetitions of each is good, 20 very good; most women do less well.

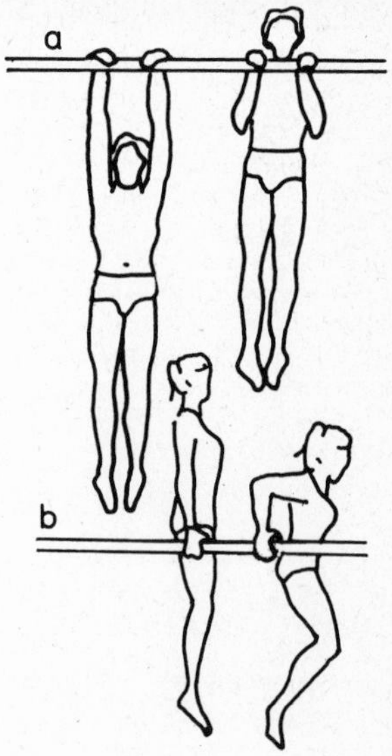

Strenuous abdominal exercises
1 Lie on your back with your knees bent, your feet flat and your arms and hands placed as shown. Slowly lever yourself into an arch by raising your body, keeping your feet flat on the floor. Hold for 10 seconds.
2 Lie on your back with your knees bent, your feet flat on the floor and your hands behind your head as shown. Without using your arms to help you, roll up into a sitting position.
3 Lie face down with your hands clasped behind your head and a pillow cushioning your hips and abdomen. With your feet held down by a partner, raise your head and chest off the ground and hold the position for 10 seconds.
4 Lie on your back with your legs extended and your hands behind your head. Lift your feet 10in off the ground, keeping your legs straight, and hold this position for 10 seconds.
5 Lie face down with your hands under your shoulders and push your chest off the floor as shown; raise your head to look upward, and hold for as long as comfortable.
6 Start as for **3** but with your head resting on your arms as shown. With a partner holding your waist and chest down, lift your legs and feet off the ground and hold that position for 10 seconds.

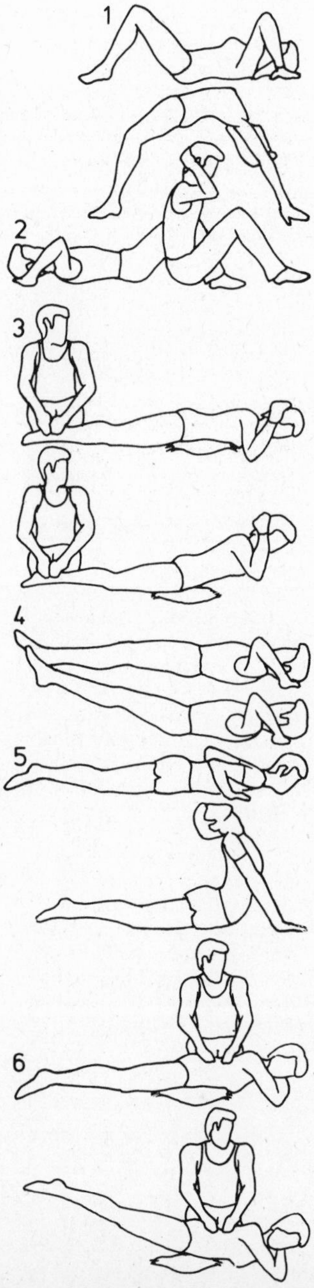

Strenuous flexibility exercises
7 Lie face down with your knees bent up and your hands clasping your ankles. Keeping your knees together, pull on your feet to raise your trunk and knees from the floor; hold this position for as long as possible.
8 Lie on your side with one hand supporting your head and the other in front of you as shown. Keeping your legs straight and your feet together, raise both as high as possible off the ground and hold in this position.
9 Sit with your legs stretched out in front and your feet together. Lean forward to grasp your ankles and pull your head down onto your knees; hold for as long as possible.
10 Lie on your back with your legs straight and gradually raise your legs and trunk until they are vertical. Resting on your shoulders, take your legs over your head to touch the floor if possible.
11 Stand upright and clasp your hands straight out behind your back. Lean forward until your body is horizontal and your arms vertical.
12 Lie face down with your arms outstretched to the sides, palms down. Raise your arms, chest and head while simultaneously raising your legs; hold for as long as possible.

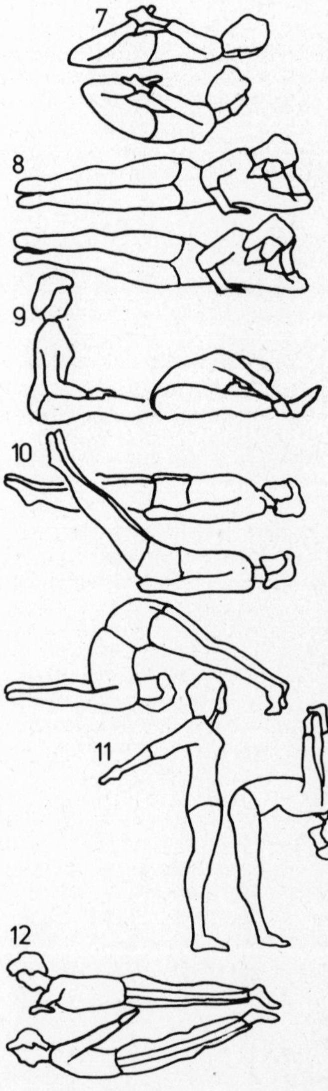

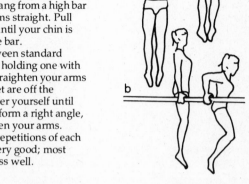

Endurance tests
Muscle endurance is tested by the following tasks.
c Stand upright, then bend your knees and lean forward so that your hands are flat on the ground. Kick your legs back as shown, then return to the squatting position and stand upright again. You should be able to do this 10 times without stopping.
d Lie face down with your legs straight, your toes tucked under, and your hands flat under your shoulders. Raise your body into the push-up position by straightening your arms, then lower again. For men, 20 is good and 30 very good; for women, 10 is good, 15 very good.

c
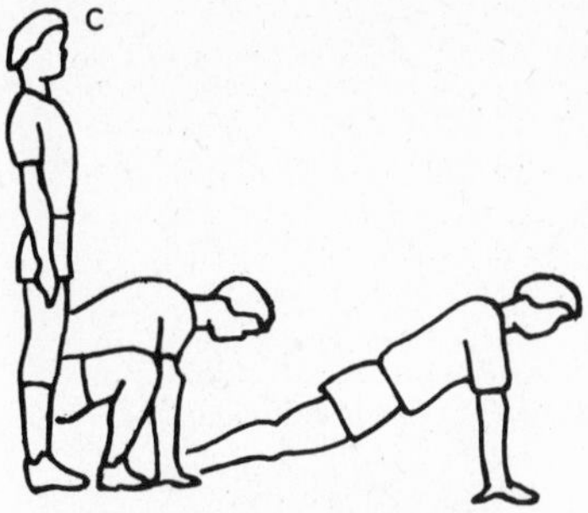

d
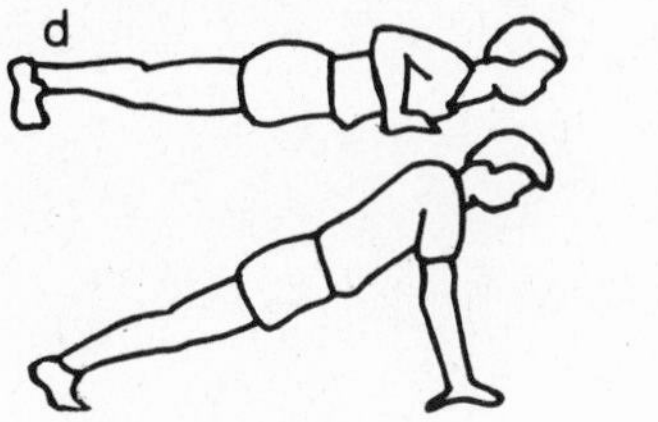

Aerobic fitness test
The table *right* shows "good" fitness ratings for men and women of different ages taking part in a test run/walk. Do not do this test unless you have been taking part in an aerobic fitness program for at least three months. To do the test, cover 1½ miles of level ground in your own mixture of running, jogging and walking; time yourself, or have somebody else time you, and compare your time with the time for your age and sex on the table.

	Age	Time (mins:secs)
Men	13–19	9:41 – 10:48
	20–29	10:46 – 12:00
	30–39	11:01 – 12:30
	40–49	11:31 – 13:00
	50–59	12:31 – 14:30
	60+	14:00 – 16:15
Women	13–19	12:30 – 14:30
	20–29	13:31 – 15:54
	30–39	14:31 – 16:30
	40–49	15:56 – 17:30
	50–59	16:31 – 19:00
	60+	17:31 – 19:30

Further strenuous exercises
13 Stand on your toes on the edge of a stair or a thick book; stretch your arms out, then raise and lower your heels. This will stretch the backs of your calves.
14 Lean with your body supported on one hand as shown. Raise your upper leg as high as possible, and hold this position.
15 Lie on your back with your arms stretched out above your head. Raise your legs, arms and trunk simultaneously to balance on your hips, touching your hands as far down your legs as possible. Hold this position, then slowly relax.
16 Stand with your feet wide apart, holding a barbell with your knuckles facing forward. Bend your elbows to bring the weight up to your chest.
17 Stand with a barbell behind your neck as shown. Slowly bend your knees and sink down until your thighs are horizontal, then rise up onto your toes.
18 Stand with your feet apart; hold one end of a small towel in your right hand and put your right heel on the other end. Place your left hand on your hip and pull up with your right hand as hard as possible. Repeat to the other side.

13
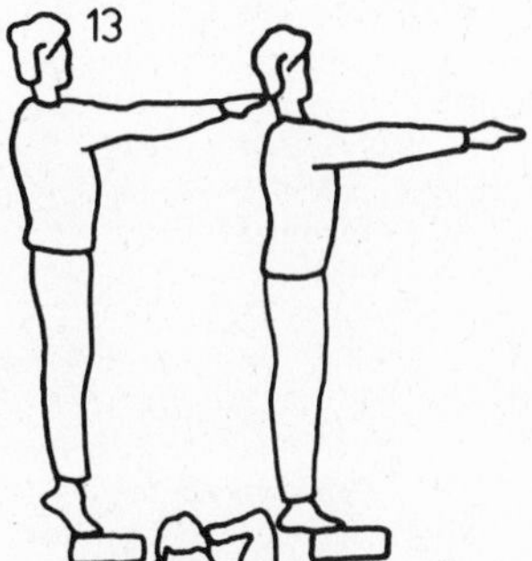

14
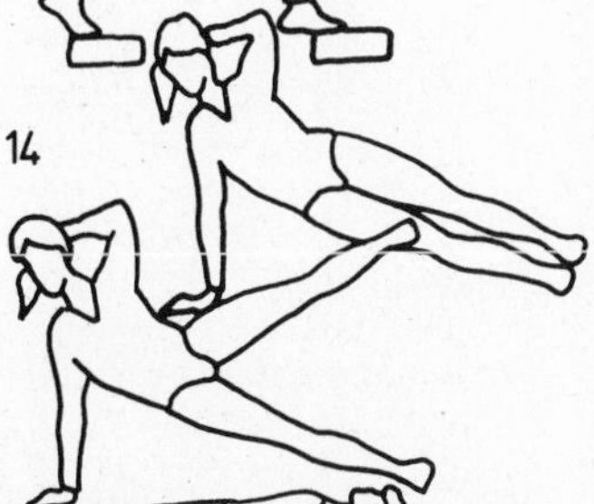

15
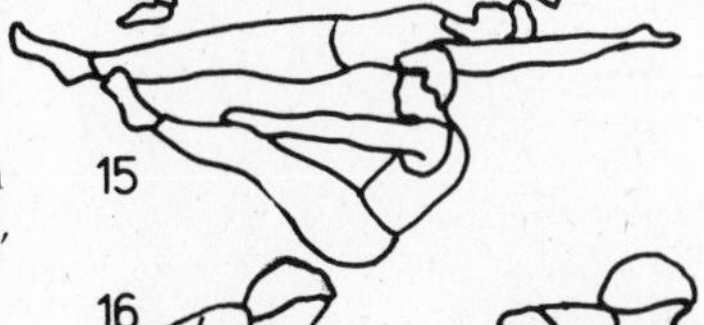

16
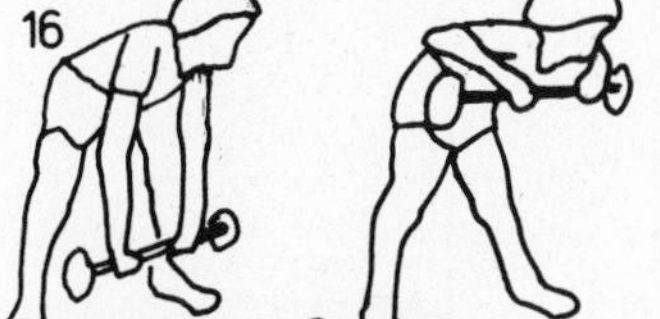

17
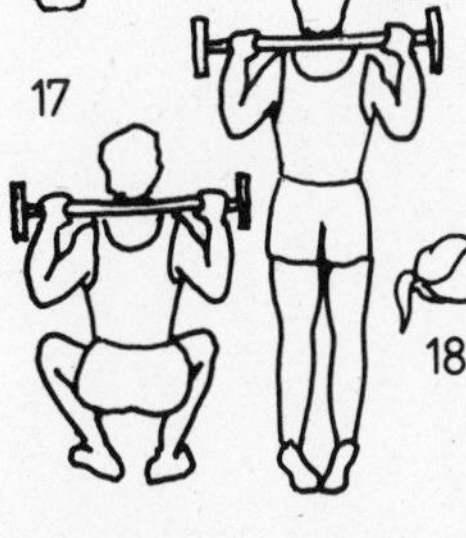

18
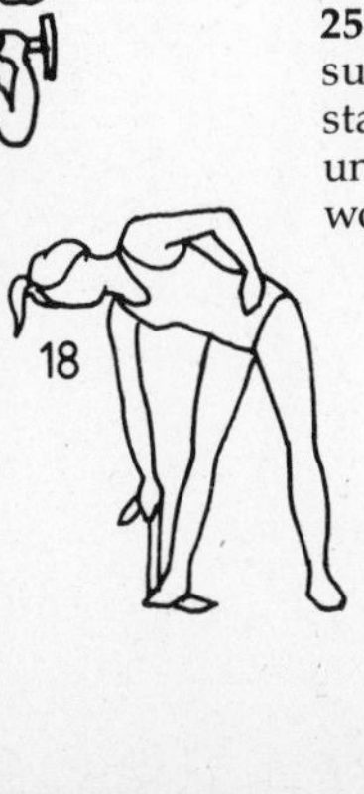

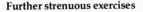

Gymnasium activities
The equipment available in gymnasiums often requires a high level of fitness, strength and flexibility in order to make proper use of it. Always use equipment under supervision, and obey all safety rules.
19 Sloping benches may be used in many strengthening exercise programs; weights on the legs and arms are often used in conjunction with these benches.
20 Gymnastics using equipment such as rings, the horse, the parallel bars and the asymmetric bars can be very strenuous.
21 Rowing and cycling machines simulate these activities and are ideal for use in confined spaces.
22 The wall bars of a gymnasium provide ideal equipment for improving muscle strength in various areas of the body.
23 Field events such as pole vault and triple jump require great strength and flexibility.
24 Treadmills or joggers are a series of rollers used to simulate outdoor running; the rollers can be inclined to make the task more difficult.
25 Sophisticated equipment such as leg presses, chinning stations and combined exercise units can be used for strenuous workouts.

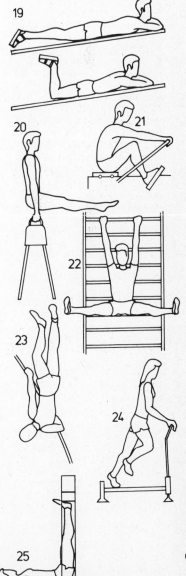

19
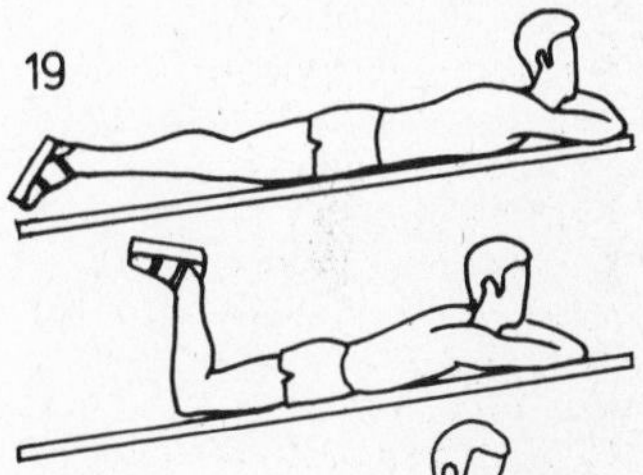

21

20
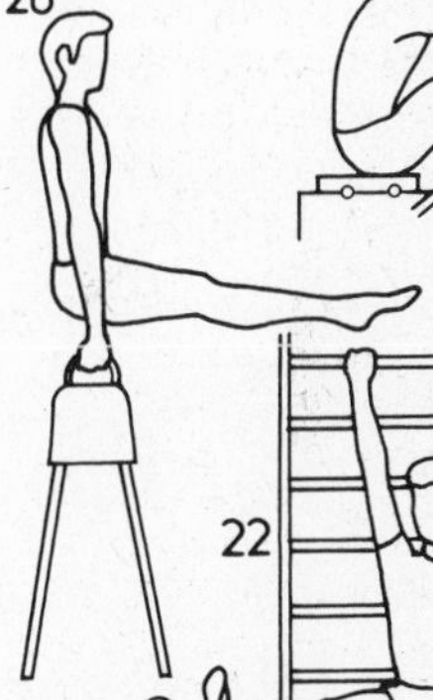

22
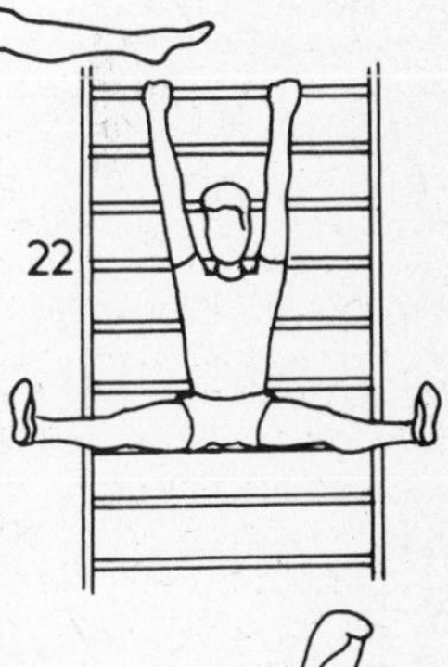

23

24

25
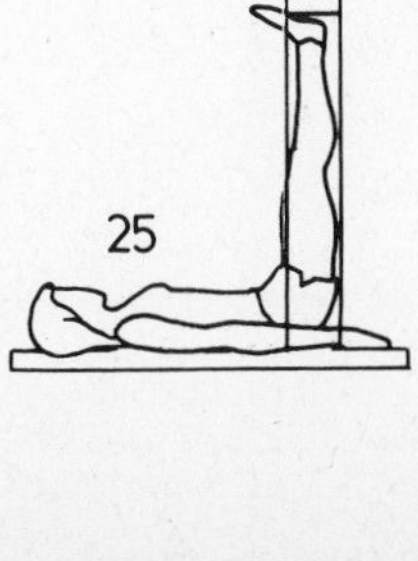

Sleep

The mechanism of sleep is by no means fully understood by scientists or doctors, but certain facts about sleep have been ascertained. First, sleep is necessary to support human life; lack of sleep kills faster than lack of food. Everyone dreams during a normal night's sleep, although the dreams are very often not remembered in the morning, but there are periods of dreamless sleep as well. If deprived of normal sleep the body undergoes dangerous changes that will eventually prove fatal if they are allowed to continue, and most people are familiar with the personality disturbances and coordination and concentration problems caused by sleeping poorly for one or two nights in a row. On these pages we look at normal sleep and various sleeping problems.

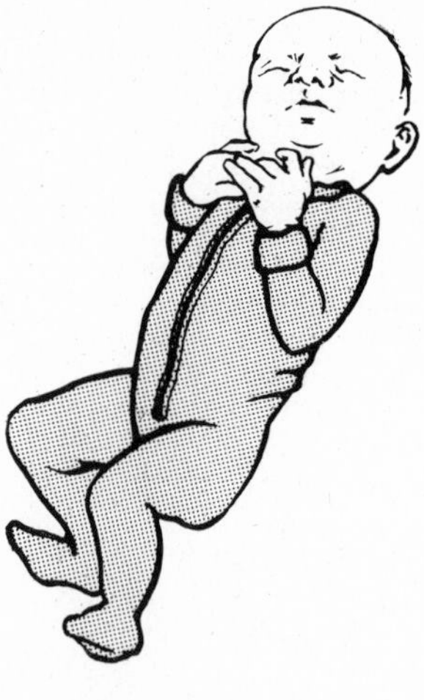

Sleep and age
Sleep requirements vary a great deal with age. Babies require far more sleep than adults, although not as much as is often supposed; some leaflets for new mothers tell them to expect their babies to sleep for nearly 24 hours, but the reality is an average of 16 hours a day. A 6-year-old child should sleep an average of about 10 hours a night, a 12-year-old about 9 hours, and an adult about 7½ hours, but needs depend on individuals; some people can survive on 2 or 3 hours of sleep a day, whereas others need to average 9 or 10 hours. Older people's sleep needs may be broken into several shorter periods.

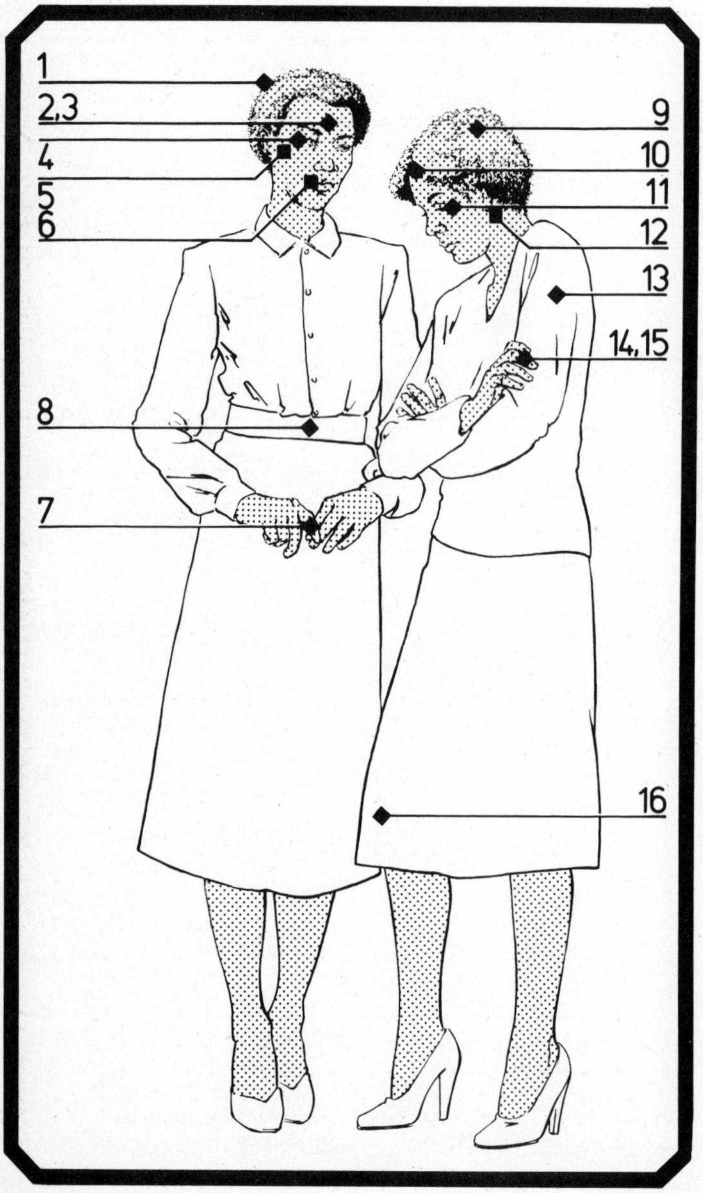

Benefits of sleep
The whole of the body is benefited by regular periods of satisfying sleep. Some parts of the body where the benefits are particularly noticeable include the following.

1 The hair is shiny and healthy looking rather than dull and brittle.
2 The mind is better prepared for any mental task, and is as free as possible from confusion and lethargy.
3 A feeling of wellbeing pervades the senses after a solid night's sleep; this is caused in part by the release of a growth hormone into the blood. The growth hormone is necessary for the maintenance of a healthy body.
4 The eyes are bright and lively.
5 The skin is clear and smooth rather than dull and mottled.
6 The appetite is healthy.
7 The muscles are relaxed and rejuvenated by a night's rest, and no tension is present.
8 The digestion functions healthily, having continued to work while the remainder of the body was at rest.

Effects of lack of sleep
The effects of lack of sleep on the body can range from inconvenience to crippling, depending whether the lack of sleep is temporary or whether it is long-term sleep deprivation.

9 Mental disturbances occur. These range from fatigue, depression, irritability and lack of concentration in mild cases through to hallucinations and neuroses in severe cases.
10 Headaches occur when the body is crying out for sleep, and become more severe the longer sleep is withheld.
11 Focusing becomes difficult when the body needs sleep, and eventually visual perception becomes completely distorted.
12 Hearing is also distorted when the body is severely deprived of sleep.
13 Muscle tension is both a cause and a result of lack of sleep, and helps to perpetuate a vicious circle of sleeplessness.
14 The performance of tasks requiring manual precision becomes increasingly erratic the more sleep is needed.
15 Coordination deteriorates first mildly, then severely if the body is still denied sleep.
16 Restlessness is a common feature of the body that is in need of sleep.

Requirements for sleep
In order to obtain a good night's sleep, various conditions have to be met. Most people sleep better in the dark; if you work shifts and have to sleep during the day, it may be advisable to wear eye pads. Make sure that your bed is comfortable and provides firm but even support, with no lumps or hollows. Wear comfortable nightclothes and try different kinds of bedcovers until you find the best type. Although people living near railroads or airports learn to sleep through the noise, quiet is more conducive to sleep. Your room and bed should be neither too hot nor too cold, and you should have some ventilation.

Snoring
Snoring can occur in phases or be a part of every night's sleep. Snoring in children often occurs as a result of a mouth, nose or throat infection that blocks the nasal passages and causes mouth breathing; the snoring will stop once the infection clears up. Snoring in adults occurs most often in those who sleep on their back and breathe through the mouth; avoiding both these circumstances may cure the problem. If you are kept awake by your partner's snores, a gentle shake may cause him or her to rise to a lighter level of sleep and solve the problem.

Sleepwalking
Sleepwalking (somnambulism) usually occurs during the dreaming portions of sleep and is often associated with the actions being dreamed of. Sleepwalking phases may also be associated with problems that are worrying the person concerned. Sleepwalking can be dangerous, as the person's perception of the surroundings is impaired, and accidents such as falling downstairs or stumbling over furniture may occur. If you come across a member of your household sleepwalking, try to lead him or her back to bed by persuasion.

Insomnia
Insomnia (lack of sleep) takes various forms. First it is important to realize that the body will eventually take over and force you to sleep if you are seriously deprived of sleep, so insomnia generally takes the form of unsatisfactory sleep, or a difficulty in getting to sleep or staying asleep. Occasional insomnia is common, but chronic insomnia often has a psychological root such as worries about money, family relationships, sex etc. In these cases it is important to sort out the problem before the insomnia can be cured. Constantly waking early may be a symptom of depression.

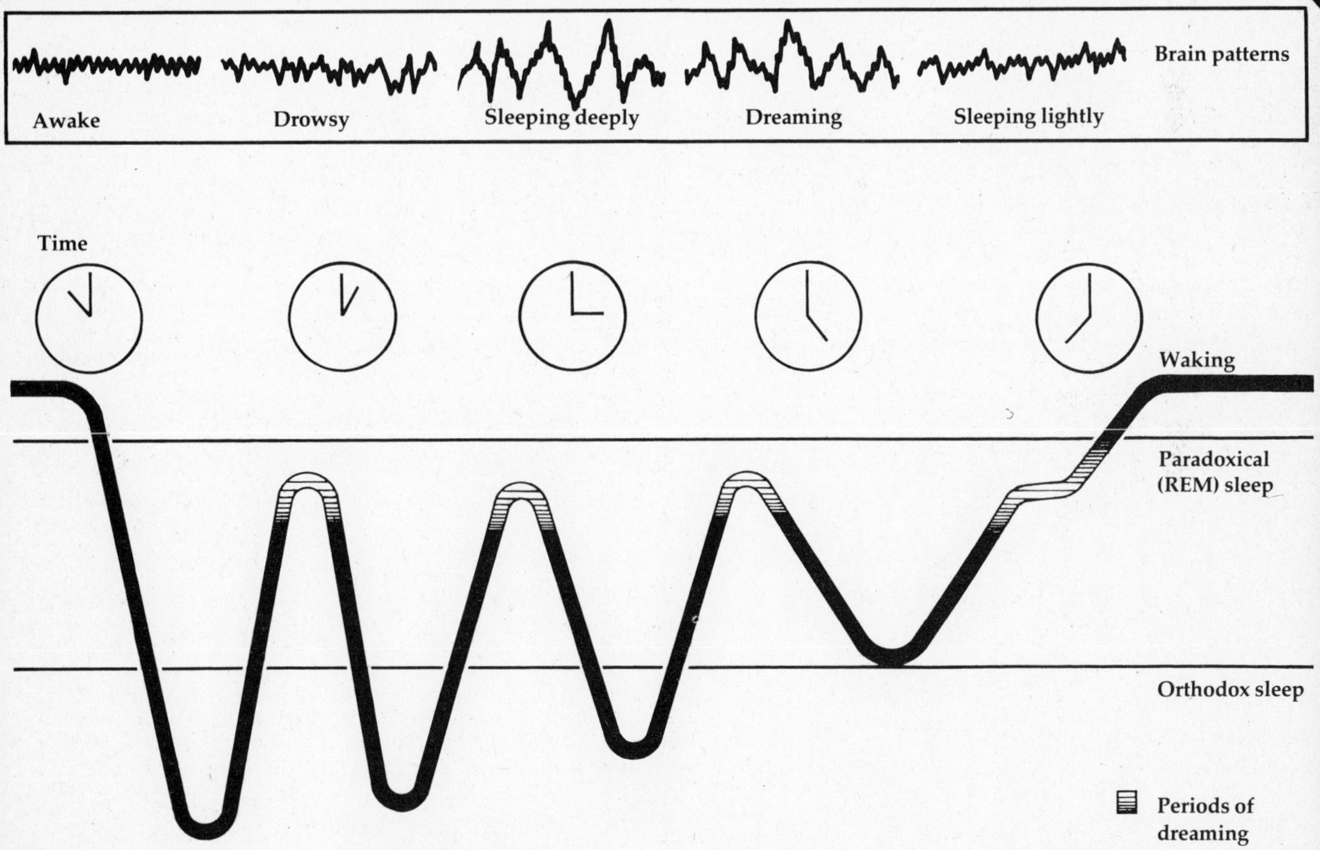

Sleep chart
The chart *above* shows the normal pattern of a healthy night's sleep. Sleep is divided into two kinds, orthodox sleep and paradoxical sleep. Orthodox sleep forms roughly three quarters of our total sleeping time; it is a deep sleep, during which the body is relaxed and works hardest to produce protein and growth hormone and to replace damaged body tissue. The other quarter of our sleeping time is taken up by paradoxical (REM) sleep. It is in this stage of sleep that dreams occur, and there is also rapid eye movement (REM) behind the closed eyelids. The heartbeat and breathing rate become irregular, and more blood is diverted to the brain than it generally receives during the daytime. Electrical activity is equal to that observed during waking hours. Paradoxical sleep, although it is not the major part of the night's sleep, is essential for our wellbeing; people deprived of paradoxical sleep and its dreams become emotionally disturbed. Sleeping pills do not induce periods of paradoxical sleep, and therefore can often leave a person still feeling tired and washed out in the morning rather than refreshed and rejuvenated.

Relaxation

Relaxation should be a concern of everyone who wants to maintain a healthy body. Relaxation enables the body to rest from the stresses and pressures of everyday life; the muscles are given an opportunity to relax, and you should use your period of relaxation as a time to remove all worrying thoughts from your mind, since physical relaxation cannot be effectively achieved in the absence of mental relaxation. On these pages we talk about some of the problems caused by lack of relaxation, and also look at some of the ways in which you can help your body and your mind to relax. Try to spend at least 30 minutes relaxing every day, ideally alone so that you can be as free as possible from interruptions.

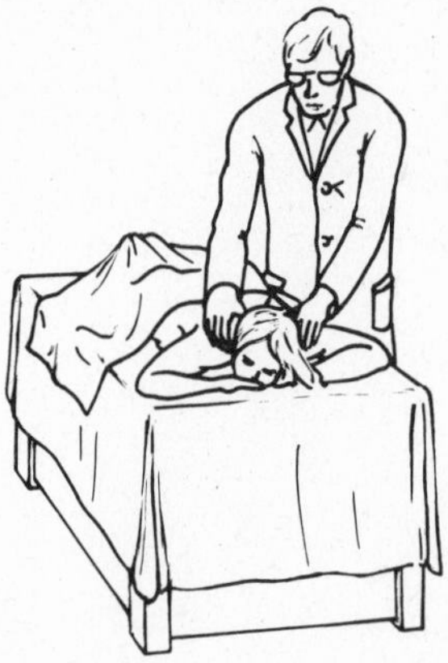

Massage
Massage is one of the most effective ways of relieving tension in tired, knotted muscles. Techniques of massage vary greatly (see p.73) but the most straightforward ones used for physical relaxation are mainly concerned with manipulating the muscle tissues in order to increase the blood supply to that area and restore suppleness to the muscle. The increased blood flow speeds the removal of impurities from aching muscles, which helps to relieve the pain. The masseur usually rubs the affected muscles with slow, even pressure without losing contact with the skin until the massage is complete.

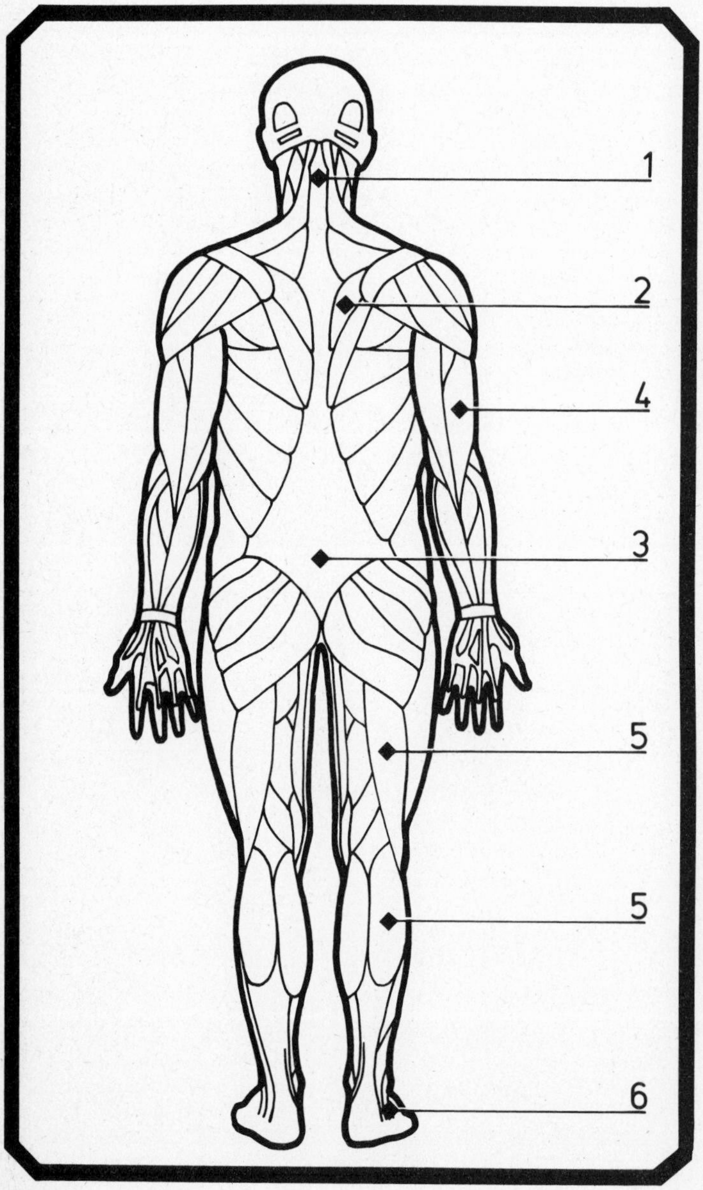

Areas of tension
The illustration shows some of the main areas of muscle tension that frequently affect the body.
1 Tension in the back of the neck is frequently a result of psychological conditions such as anxiety or stress; tension in the muscles here often leads to the so-called tense, nervous headache. Massaging the back of the neck with your fingertips may relieve the tension.
2 Tension in the shoulders may often occur after overwork, or if your desk or workbench is at the wrong height. Stretching and easing the muscles with exercise will often prove effective.
3 Pain and muscle tension in the small of the back may be a result of poor posture – for instance, wearing high-heeled shoes too frequently – or may be caused by sagging muscles in the back and abdomen that fail to give proper support to the spine. Menstrual problems, pregnancy or hormonal disorders can cause low backache in women.
4 Muscle tension and aches in the arms are usually caused by overworking the muscles concerned – carrying heavy objects, digging, shoveling, pushing, or pulling. Massaging and resting the affected muscles should ease the problem.
5 Tension and stiffness of the thigh and calf muscles is usually caused by strain. Over-enthusiastic exercising such as running or cycling will often produce stiffness the following day, which can be eased by using the muscles gently, for instance in walking or gentle jogging. Pregnancy and its related circulatory problems in the legs will often cause muscle aching; resting with the legs raised will ease the discomfort.
6 Aching muscles in the feet result from overwork. Walking, running or even standing for long periods may interfere with the efficient circulation in the feet and lead to tenderness and fatigue in the muscles. Warm footbaths are often soothing.

Tension in all parts of the body can very often be relieved by taking a long, warm bath. If the water is too hot it will be tiring, and if it is too cool it will not have the desired relaxing effect. Bath salts and other preparations for use in the water will not help your muscles to relax; the relief of tension is gained from the warm water. For muscles that are very painful and stiff, preparations can be bought for massaging into the affected muscles and producing localized heat; these can be very effective.

Sitting positions
Relaxation is possible in many positions. One of the best ways to learn to relax is to discover some of the positions that enable your body to rest itself without strain. If you are sitting in a chair, make sure that it gives adequate support; sit well back on the seat with your back straight and your head supported (**a**). In this position you can watch television, listen to music, meditate, or just recover from a busy day. The classic lotus position of yoga (**b**) is a good sitting position to use when relaxing.

a
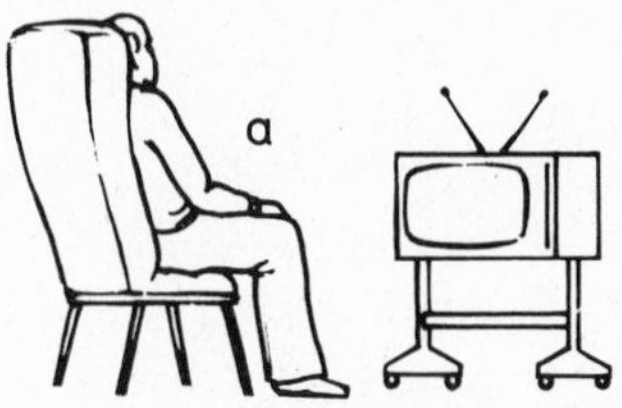

b
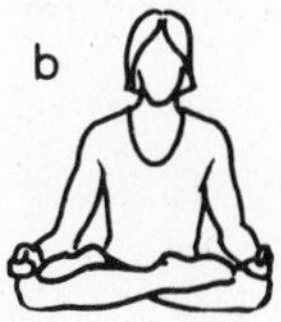

Lying positions
Lying down is one of the most effective ways to relax the entire body completely, and need not be reserved only for sleep. Lying on your right side ensures that your heart is not constricted and enables you to relax better than lying on your left; bend your left knee up and cushion your head on a pillow (**c**). Alternatively you could try the yoga corpse position. Lie flat on your back with your arms by your sides, palms up; allow your arms and legs to go limp so that your feet fall gently apart (**d**). Raise your chin and breathe deeply. Good relaxing positions for pregnant women are shown on p.135.

c
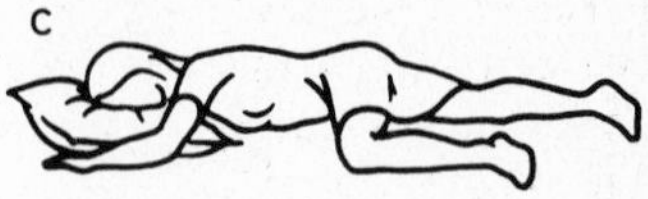

d
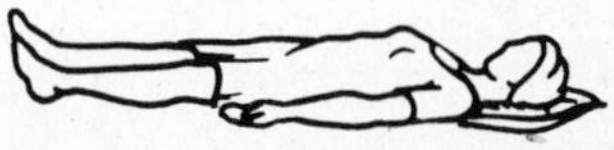

Relaxation exercises
1 Stand upright, as relaxed as possible, and shake each arm in turn; shake first from your wrist, then from your elbow, then from your shoulder. Then repeat with each leg in turn, shaking from the ankle, the knee, and then the hip.
2 Stand with your feet apart and your arms by your sides. Take a deep breath as you slowly raise your arms out to shoulder level, then hold your breath as you maintain this position for a few seconds. Breathe out as you lower your arms slowly.
3 Loosen your neck muscles by tilting your head down, to the right, to the back, to the left, then down again.
4 Loosen your shoulder muscles by standing with your arms by your sides and then shrugging your shoulders as high as you can. Hold this position briefly, then relax; repeat several times.
5 Stand with your arms at your sides. With the backs of the hands leading, move your arms forward, up, back, then down again so that they trace large circles; this will help to relieve tension in the shoulder muscles.
6 This is a good exercise for relieving stiff back muscles. Kneel on all fours as shown, then alternately hollow and hump your back.

1 2
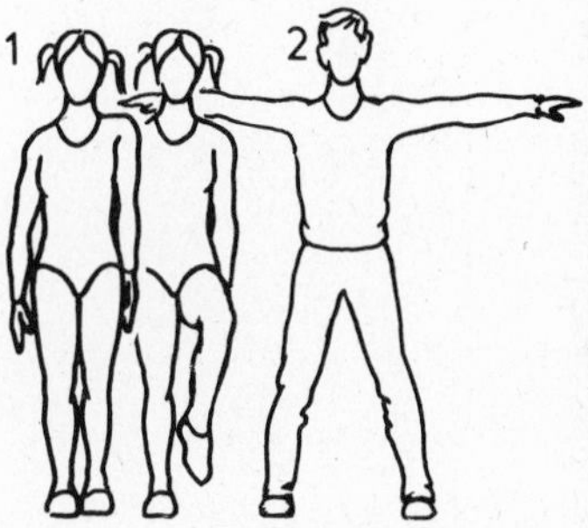 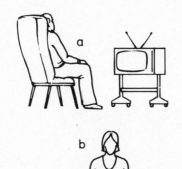 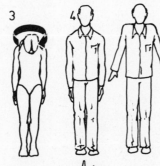

3

4
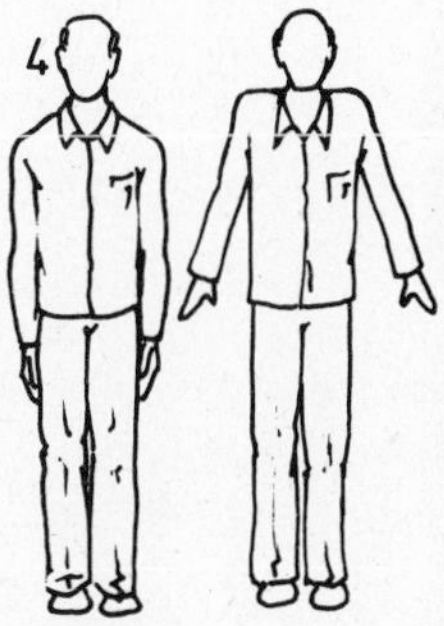

5
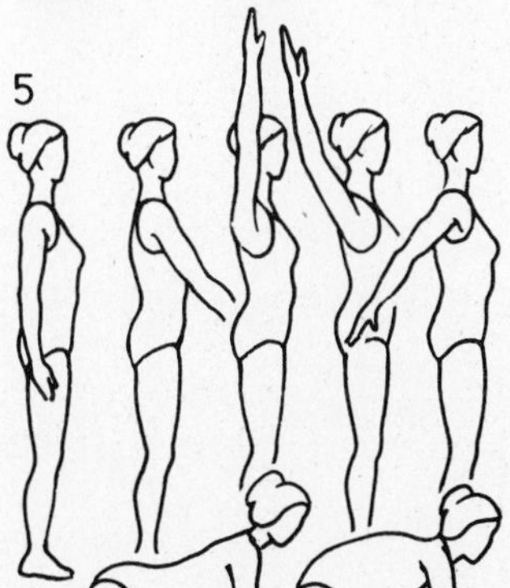

6
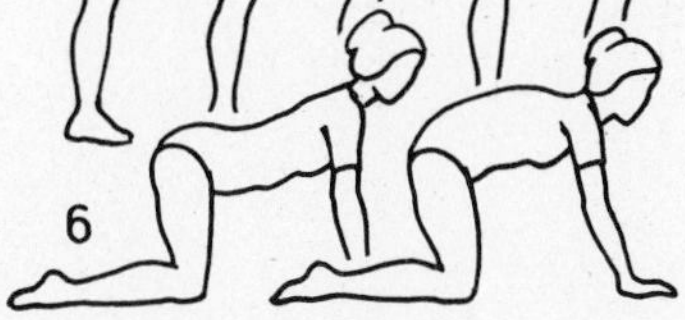

Relaxation exercises
7 Sit back to back with a partner and hold hands above your heads. Alternately pull and push forward and back; this will help to stretch and relax your back muscles.
8 Kneel on the floor and bring your head down until it touches your knees as shown; this will begin to loosen up your back muscles. Then swing your head and trunk backward slowly until your head and outstretched arms are resting on the floor. Relax in this position.
9 First massage your thigh muscles to loosen them slightly, then sit on a chair with your feet slightly apart. Keeping the toes on the ground, move the thigh and knee of one leg from side to side several times until the muscles feel looser; repeat with the other leg.
10 To relieve tension in your calf muscles, stand upright with your feet flat on the floor. Keeping your heels on the floor, slowly bend your knees and sink down as far as you can; you will feel the muscles of your thighs and calves being stretched.
11 To relieve shoulder tension, do modified push-ups against a wall as shown.

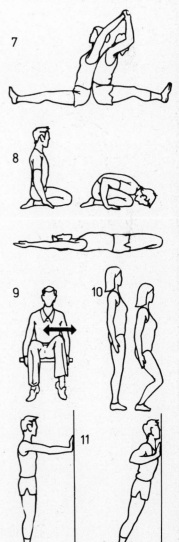

7

8

9
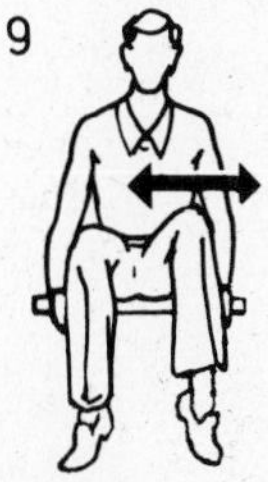

10
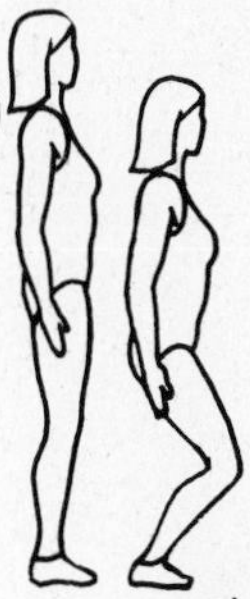

11

CHAPTER 2

HEAD TO TOE

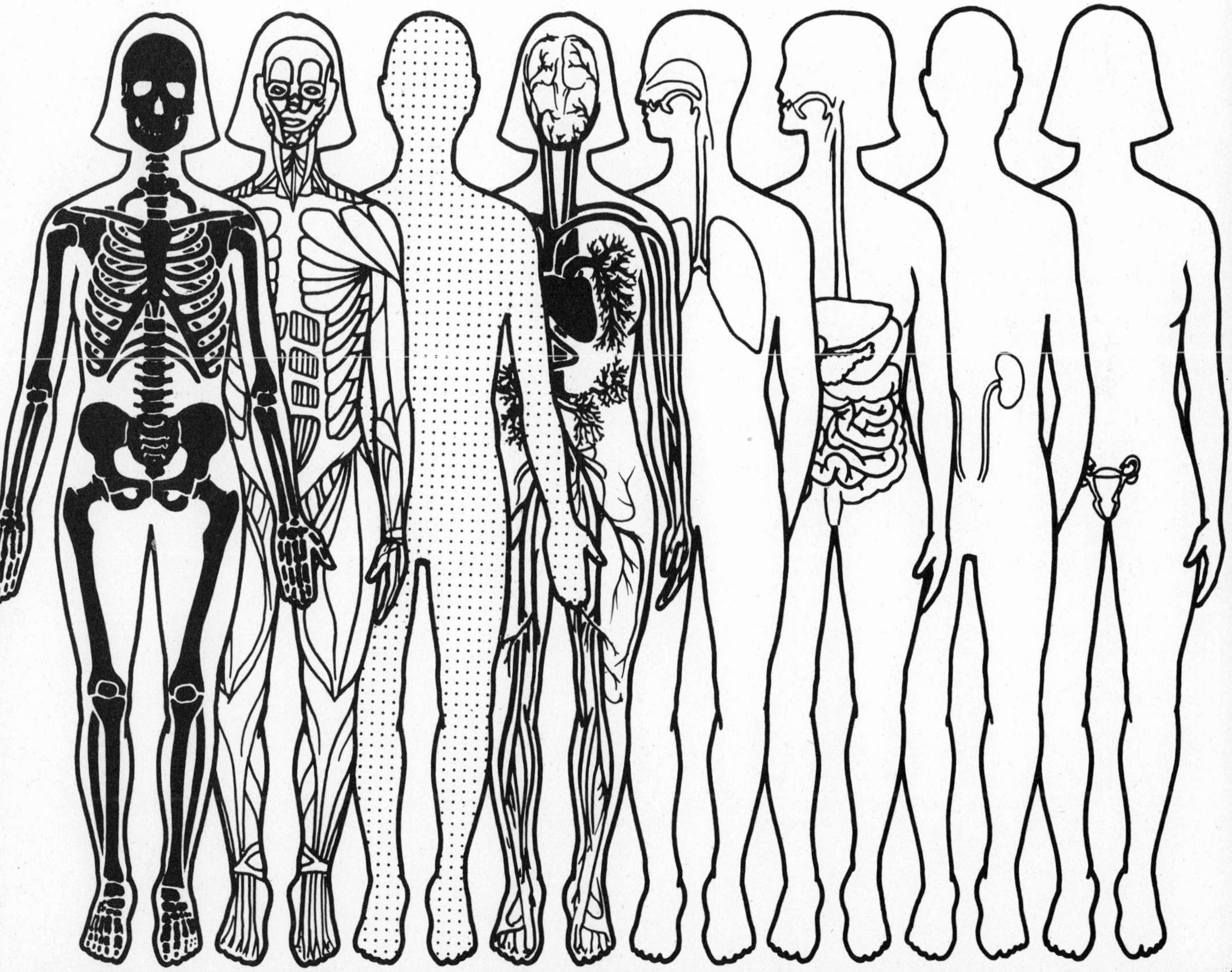

Introduction

In this chapter we look at each section of the body in turn, considering health problems and ways of avoiding or alleviating those problems.
The conditions we talk about are those that you can do something about at home: either taking preventive measures, or relieving the symptoms of medical problems, perhaps in conjunction with medical treatment. Severe medical problems are outside the scope of this book, as the individual can rarely prevent them or treat them himself. The sections in this chapter, however, will help you to learn more about the way each part of your body works, and show you many ways in which you can keep your body healthy.

Head
This section covers the hair and scalp, the face, the ears, the eyes, the nose and mouth and the teeth and gums. Each of these areas has its own problems and concerns that need to be borne in mind when aiming to keep the body healthy. Ears can be very badly infected; hair may develop infestations, or baldness may be a concern; eyes are very delicate organs that need scrupulous care; the skin of the face reflects the welfare of the rest of the body; and the nose, mouth, teeth, and gums are prone to a variety of annoying or damaging conditions.

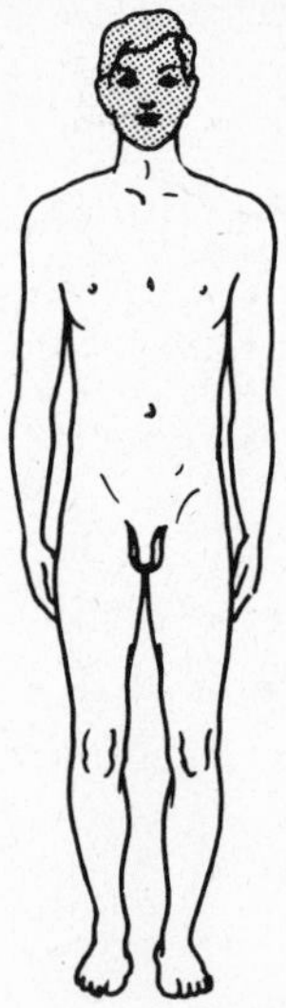

Bones and joints
The skeleton acts as a supporting frame for all the muscles and tissues of the body. It protects the vital organs and enables us to move with precision and control. Because of its importance, the body's efficiency is greatly reduced when any part of the skeleton fails to function properly. In this section we look at the components of the skeleton, the various types of joint in the body, and the problems that can affect bones and joints. We also look at posture and the effect that it has on the skeleton and the rest of the body.

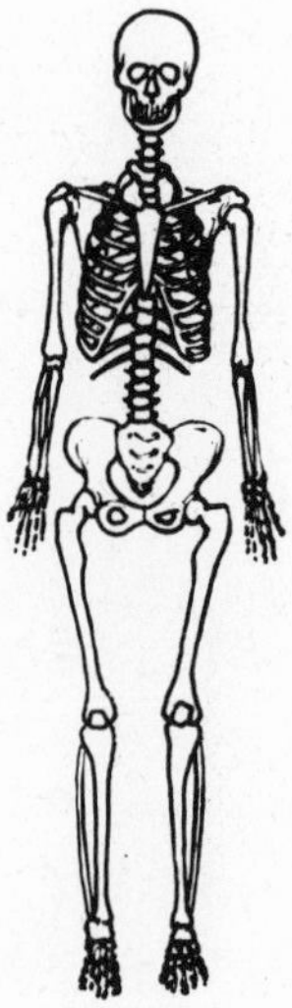

Muscles
The body's system of muscles enables it to perform a wide range of movements, from assembling a complicated piece of machinery to lifting a heavy weight. The muscles provide the body's power to perform tasks, and work in conjunction with the skeleton and the joints to carry out movements. In this section we look at the body's muscles and their functions, and some of the problems that can affect them.

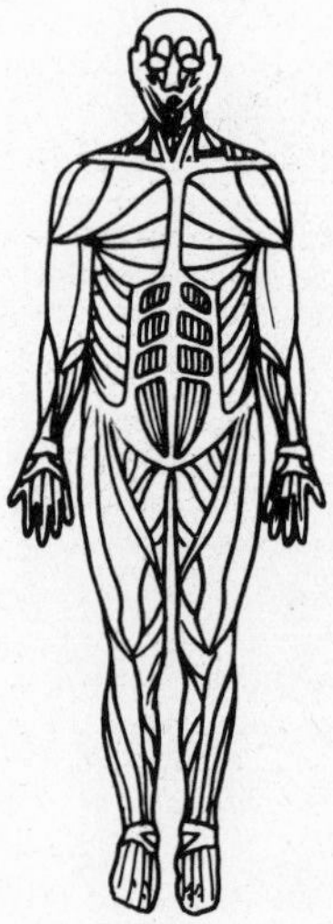

Skin
The skin covering the body is prone to many different ills. Infestations such as fleas, ringworm, ticks etc manifest themselves in or on the skin and cause various kinds of misery or embarrassment. The skin may be dry or greasy; it may be prone to nervous or allergic reactions such as dermatitis, eczema, heat rash or food allergies. It can become burned, blistered, inflamed, chafed or infected in numerous ways, and it can also show signs of infectious diseases such as measles or chicken pox, or conditions such as anemia or poor circulation. In this section we look at common skin problems.

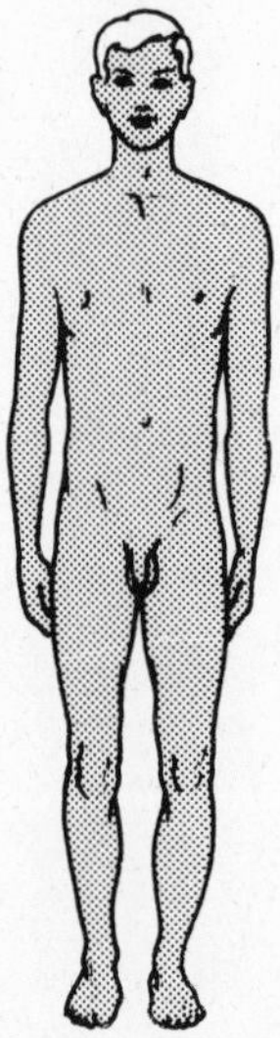

Heart and circulation
The circulatory system is made up of countless blood vessels – the veins and arteries and their branches – through which blood is pumped by the heart. All parts of the body system require blood for their healthy functioning, so if any adverse condition affects the heart or the circulation the entire body is affected. The heart can become diseased or inefficient for many reasons, and the blood can be deficient in its components or in its performance of the task of keeping the body supplied with nutrients and removing waste products.

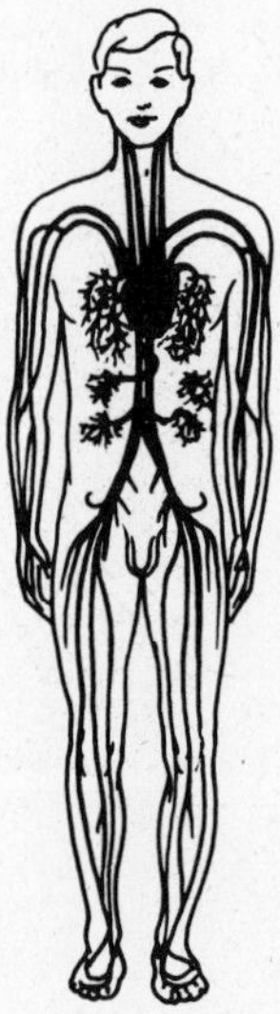

Respiratory system
The respiratory system is the part of the body concerned with taking in air and exchanging oxygen from it for carbon dioxide produced as the body carries out its work. The system comprises the nose, mouth, windpipe and lungs; each of these sections is prone to particular ills or problems. Many malfunctions of the respiratory system are hard to detect because they occur in the lungs and have no sudden or startling effect on the body. In this section we look at some of the things that can go wrong with the respiratory system and how many of them can be prevented.

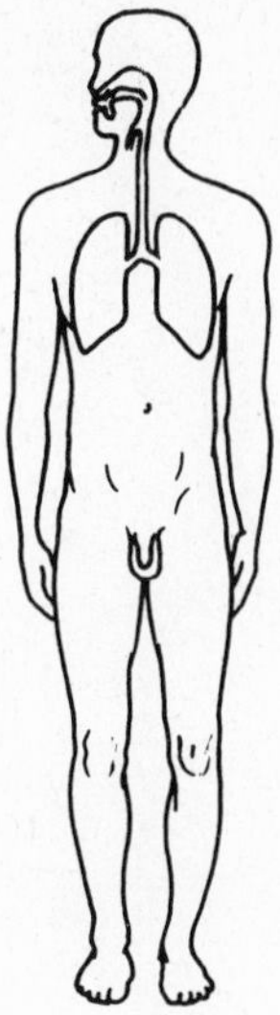

Digestive system
The digestive system is concerned with breaking down the food taken into the body and using it to supply the fuel the body needs for its work. The system also helps in the elimination of toxins and waste from the body. The main parts of the digestive system are the mouth, the gullet, the stomach, the intestines, the colon and the anus; the food is processed as it passes through these parts of the body. In this section we look at some of the many common ailments that affect the digestive system.

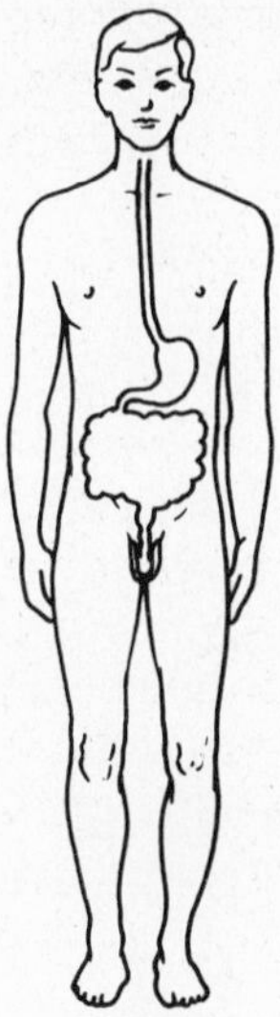

Urinary system
The urinary system is involved in ridding the body of waste products. The system comprises the kidneys, the tubes leading from them to the bladder, the bladder itself and the tube by which urine leaves the body. The kidneys process the blood through filters; if a health problem affects the functioning of the kidneys, then effects are likely in the rest of the body also. Infections of the urinary system are relatively common, and tend to be very painful, so we emphasize particularly ways of avoiding urinary tract infections.

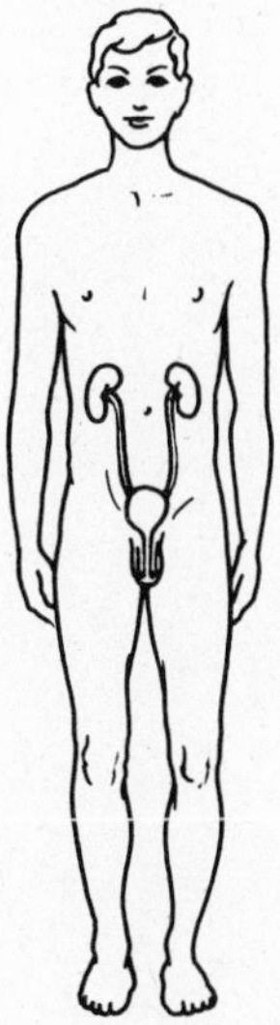

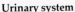

Glands
Many glandular malfunctions can only be treated medically, and few of them can be foreseen or prevented; as a result, many glandular disorders are outside the scope of this book. The glands covered in detail here are the liver, the pancreas, the gallbladder and the breasts. All of these are liable to particular disorders, many of which can be prevented or at least caught in their early stages by good health care. We look at some of the ways in which you can keep these glands functioning well.

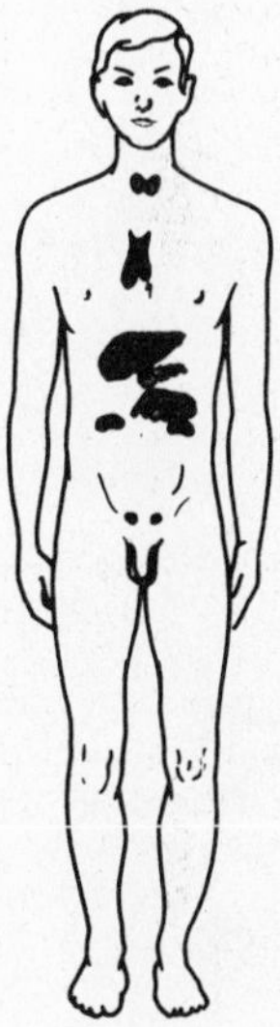

Arms and hands
The arms and hands perform an astonishing range of functions in most people's lives. They clothe us, feed us, wash us, lift, push, pull, carry, hold and move objects, and perform numerous tasks in our day's work. Strains, sprains and dislocations are fairly common in the arm and hand because of the variety of situations that they meet; in this section we talk about some of the most frequently occurring hand and arm problems and the ways in which they can be avoided. We also cover the topic of fingernails, and show you how to make them an attractive part of your hands.

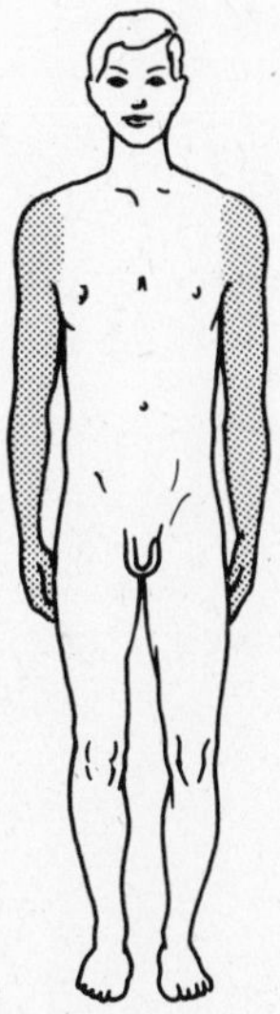

Legs and feet
The legs and feet take a good deal of punishment during our everyday lives. They support our weight, move us around, and perform tasks such as climbing, cycling and kicking. Problems in the legs and feet have a marked effect on the rest of the body; pain makes you limp or walk slowly, or perhaps stand awkwardly, which in turn puts strain on other parts of your body. In this section we look at some common leg and foot problems, their effects on general health, and ways in which you can avoid them.

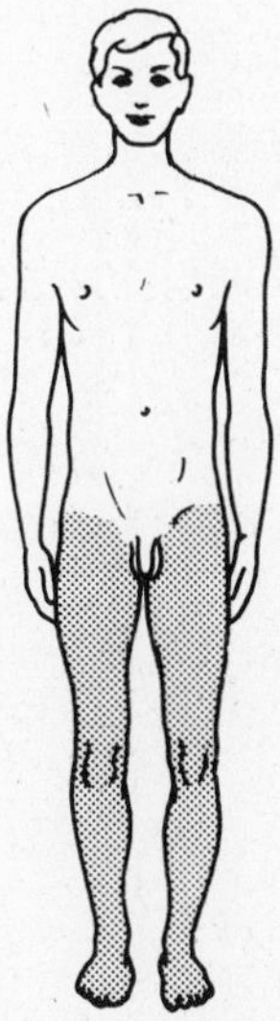

Hair and scalp 1

Humans have hair follicles all over their bodies except on the lips, the palms of the hands and the soles of the feet, with the densest growth from the scalp; men and women have between 100,000 and 200,000 hairs on their heads. Although the part of the hair that is visible is dead, it can nevertheless be in good or in poor condition, and so can the scalp from which it grows. Cleanliness is an obvious part of hair and scalp health, but on these pages we also cover some of the common problems that may arise with your hair and scalp but can easily be dealt with in your hair care routine. Care is both internal, affecting the growth of the hair in the follicle, and external, affecting the condition and appearance of the visible part of the hair.

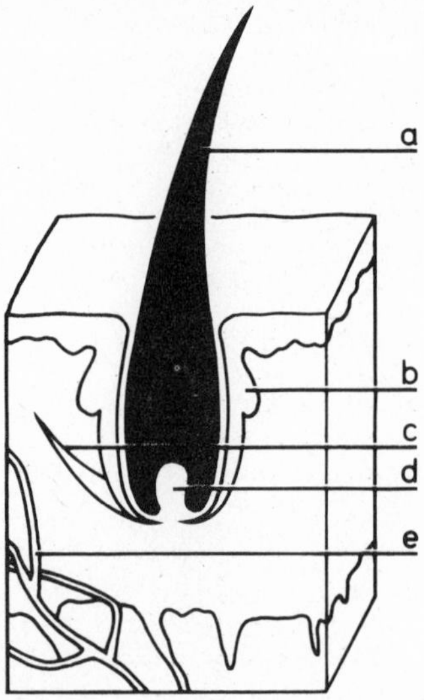

Hair follicle
This diagram shows a cross-section of a hair follicle – the part of the skin from which the hair grows.
a Hair shaft.
b Sebaceous gland; this produces a greasy substance which mildly "waterproofs" the hair.
c Muscle, controlling the erector or "goose-pimple" reaction to cold or fear.
d The root of the hair.
e Blood capillary, supplying nutrients to the growing part of the hair.

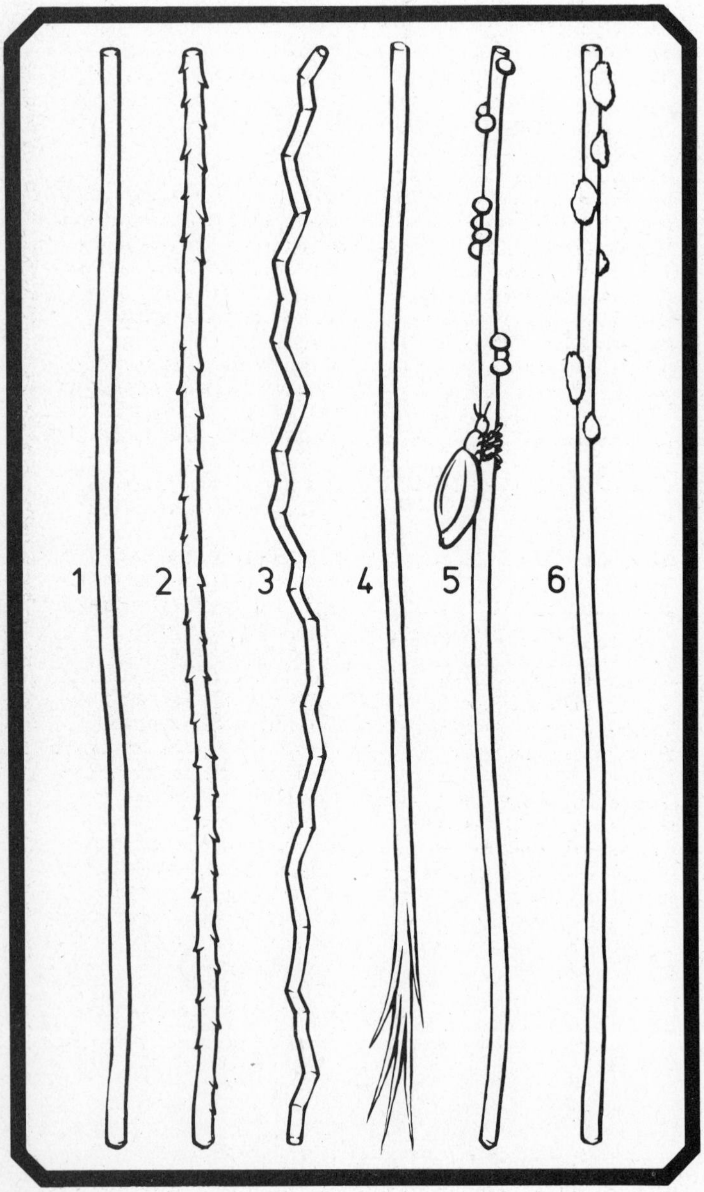

Common hair problems
The illustration *left* compares a healthy hair with others showing some of the common problems that may affect your hair.
1 Healthy hair; the coating of the hair is smooth, giving it a shiny appearance, and there are no kinks or broken portions in the hair. Healthy hair is either slightly pointed at the end, or blunt if it has recently been cut or trimmed.
2 Dry, brittle hair, with a ruffled appearance caused by the disturbance of the tiny scales that coat the shaft of the hair. This kind of damage may be caused by overheating with dryers or heated rollers, or by frequent bleaching or lightening of the hair which dries out natural oils.
3 Damaged and frizzy hair. The hair can be damaged in this way by too-frequent use of permanent waves or by careless combing. Back-combing ruffles the scales of the hair; vigorous brushing while the hair is wet damages and stretches it. Hair should always be combed gently, beginning at the tips and slowly working further up the hair as the tangles are removed.
4 Split ends, caused by the use of rubber bands or by careless combing. The only cure is a trim; lotions which purport to "re-seal" split ends are ineffective, and so are attempts to burn them off.
5 Hair with nits and lice. Once these are contracted they can be very difficult to remove, so if there is an epidemic, for instance at a child's school, keep all the family's hair short and inspect it regularly.
6 Hair with flakes of dandruff attached.

Lack of growth
An apparent lack of growth of the hair may be caused by one of several factors. If little blood is reaching the follicles, then growth may be slowed; ensure that you have plenty of sleep, since blood is diverted to the skin during sleep and will help to supply nutrients to the follicles. Massage of the scalp has the same effect, and so may speed up hair growth. Apparent halting of growth may simply be the result of brittle hair; if the hair is blunt and broken at the ends, it could be a sign that the hairs are snapping near the scalp before they have completed their full growth cycle.

Coloring and bleaching
Hair colorants can be natural or chemical, temporary, semipermanent or permanent. Of course, even permanent color has to be supplemented by painting over the regrowth at the roots every few weeks, but the main body color is not washed out with shampoo as it is with other types of colorant. Chemical colors and bleaches often contain harsh ingredients such as peroxides, shellac and alcohol solvents, and frequent use damages and dries out the hair; a conditioner should be used at every shampoo to counteract this effect. Natural or vegetable colors generally have no ill effects, but their color is impermanent.

Drying
The method of drying is very important to the health of the hair in general. Ideally, the hair should be combed into shape when wet and then left to dry naturally, but this is often not practical. Dryers that blow cold or cool air, although slower than hot-air dryers, are better for your hair as prolonged heat makes the hair weak and brittle. Always put your dryer on its coolest setting, and hold it at least six inches from your hair. If you blow-dry your hair after every shampoo, make sure that you give it a thorough conditioning treatment regularly so that the natural oils are not dried out.

Dandruff
Dandruff, or scurf, is the flaking of dead skin from the scalp, which causes an unsightly white dust on the scalp and hair. Dandruff is a very common complaint; most people are likely to experience this problem at some time in their lives. Most cases of dandruff can be controlled by washing the hair frequently, perhaps every three or four days, and by using a medicated dandruff shampoo. Severe dandruff is probably associated with a medical condition, and should be brought to the attention of your doctor. Excess use of hairspray, and inefficient rinsing after shampooing, can cause residues on the scalp.

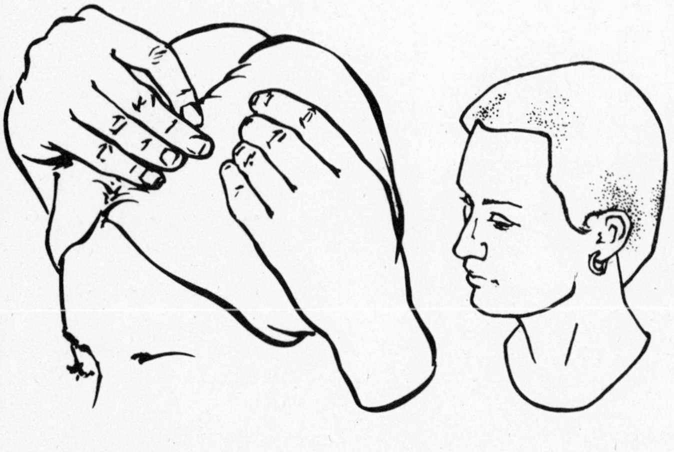

Scalp massage
There is considerable controversy over the efficacy of scalp massage for the treatment and prevention of baldness, but it certainly appears to be true that scalp massage can help to stimulate blood flow to the scalp and improve the general condition of the hair. The scalp should be gently massaged with the fingertips, as shown in the illustration *above*, until the skin feels loose and elastic, and glows with the fresh blood being diverted to feed it.

Lice
Lice are small, six-legged parasites that feed off the blood in the scalp. It is not true that only dirty people catch lice; on the contrary, lice prefer clean hair as the scalp is more readily accessible. The lice are spread by head-to-head contact, and no one is immune. The females lay pinhead-sized eggs which stick to the roots and shafts of the hair; these are the nits. Lice and nits can be removed by applying a prescribed insecticide and combing out the eggs with a fine metal comb. The most likely sites for nits are shown *above*.

Do
- Wash your hair regularly; for greasy hair, every 1–3 days is advisable, but if your hair is dry every 4–6 days is preferable.
- Use a mild shampoo that does not contain a lot of detergent, so that the natural oils of the hair will be retained.
- Use a conditioner after shampooing if your hair tends to be dry and frizzy, or if you regularly color or bleach it.
- Pat your hair dry with a soft towel rather than rubbing it.
- Eat a balanced diet, with plenty of vitamins, to keep your hair in good health.
- Keep your brush and comb scrupulously clean, ideally washing them each day.
- Keep your hair trimmed regularly, whether it is long or short, so that it retains a good shape and has the minimum of split ends.
- Change your hairstyle occasionally so that your hair is brushed in a different direction; this has quite a rejuvenating effect.
- Examine your hair regularly if you think you may have been exposed to lice and nits.
- Rinse all shampoo out of your hair thoroughly.
- Massage your scalp occasionally to stimulate the blood supply.

Don't
- Pull or stretch the hair or brush it vigorously while it is wet, as wet hair is more easily damaged.
- Use hairstyles that tug the hair back from the face, as this can lead to temporary hair loss.
- Swim in chlorinated or salt water unless there is provision for you to rinse your hair in fresh water immediately afterward.
- Use too much heat on your hair; heated rollers should only be used occasionally, and your hairdryer should be switched to its coolest setting.
- Use rubber bands on your hair, as these can cause split ends.
- Tug or twist your hair.
- Neglect shampooing in the hope that this will alleviate baldness or dandruff.
- Singe split ends.
- Sunbathe without adequate protection for your hair; the sun dries hair out very rapidly.
- Use color, bleach, permanent waves or hair straightener too frequently, as over-use damages the hair.
- Lend your brush or comb to anyone else, or borrow theirs.
- Waste money on "miracle" hair restorers or colorants; there is no cure for natural baldness or natural graying.
- Permanently cover up your hair with a wig, headscarf or hat; air is vital to the wellbeing of your hair and scalp.

Hair and scalp 2

Hair loss in general is a natural and inevitable process. Some 100 hairs are lost from the head each day as a result of the natural growth cycle of the hair and scalp; usually these hairs are pushed out and replaced by new growth from the follicle, but if this fails to happen a minute area of skin is left without a hair. If several or many follicles stop producing hair in one area of the scalp, then a bald area results. As a rule this process increases with age, although some men and most women will keep a fairly thick mop of hair into old age whereas some men can be bald from natural causes by the age of 30.

The individual's attitude to hair loss, and the nature and extent of the loss, will determine the way in which the problem is tackled. Hair loss should not become an over-important consideration in your life; the middle-aged man who combs his few remaining strands strategically over the bald spot and then avoids exercise or walking in the wind for fear of having the bald spot exposed is an unhappy man. If hair loss is that important to you, then have something done about it by an expert; if not, then comb your hair naturally. In any case, never neglect washing and conditioning the hair; this will only draw attention to the area where you least want it.

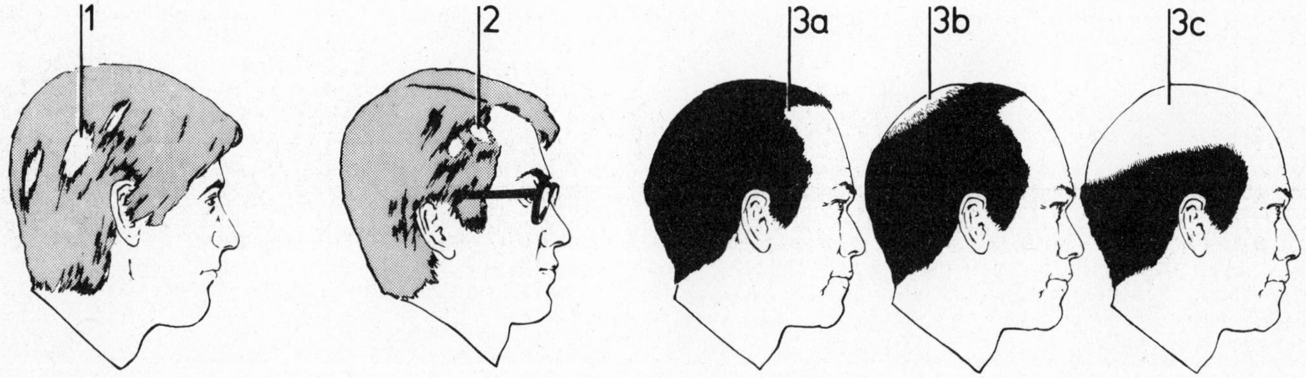

Unnatural baldness
Unnatural hair loss can be caused by illness or by bad living habits or poor hair care. A bald patch on the back of a baby's head may simply be a result of rubbing on a crib mattress. A disease that often first presents itself in older children is alopecia areata; this disease can also occur, or recur, later in life. It leads to partial or total baldness, with the hair first dropping out in isolated patches on any part of the head; this random appearance (**1**) distinguishes alopecia from natural balding in men. The causes of alopecia areata are unknown, but the condition usually disappears of its own accord in time.

Ringworm, a parasitic eruption, can cause localized baldness as the hair breaks off short in affected areas (**2**). Baldness may also be a result of chemotherapy or radiation treatment. Stress can contribute indirectly to hair loss; the person under stress does not pay sufficient attention to good eating, sleeping and relaxing habits, and so his hair quickly becomes brittle and dull from lack of nutrients. Hairstyles that pull the hair tightly off the face have been known to cause temporary hair loss (traction alopecia) in affected areas, and nervous habits of tugging and twisting the hair can pull the hairs out eventually.

Male pattern baldness
Male pattern baldness is the result of a hereditary balding "program" dictated by the man's genes, and is virtually impossible to halt. The balding pattern may begin as young as the early 20s, or may not appear until old age, but most men have experienced some degree of this kind of balding by middle age. The balding usually begins around the hairline at the temples, as shown *above* (**3a**), and is then followed by balding around the crown of the scalp (**3b**). In the final stages, all the hair from the front and crown of the head is lost (**3c**). Male pattern baldness may stop entirely of its own accord at any of these stages, so the loss of hair from the temples need not mean that a man will end up completely bald. Many preparations are sold that purport to stop baldness and make the hair grow naturally again; if they do appear to be working, you can almost take it for granted that the balding would have stopped in any case without the preparation. There is some evidence that wearing a hat very frequently or neglecting to wash the hair may aggravate balding once the condition is established, but as yet there is no proven method of preventing it.

Wigs
A wig is a cap of false hair designed to cover the entire scalp (*right*). Wigs can be made for men or women, and can be used either in cases of baldness or as cosmetics to change a person's appearance temporarily. A wig to be worn over a bald head should be well-fitting and should match your natural coloring as closely as possible. Before you buy a wig, make sure that you know how to look after it; buy a wig stand such as the one shown here, in order to keep the wig in shape while it is not being worn. Do not wear a wig too often if you have some natural hair left, as your hair and scalp need to breathe to keep healthy.

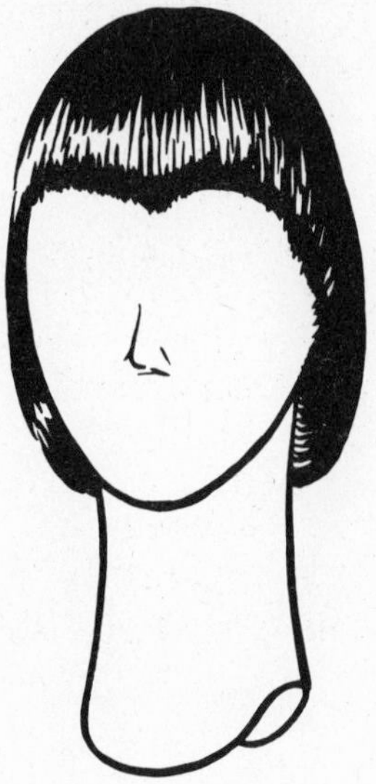

Hairpieces
Hairpieces are sections of false hair designed to cover only a part of the head (*right*), and are usually used to supplement natural hair or to change the hairstyle temporarily. A hairpiece may be used to give more fullness to fine hair or to bulk out a bouffant hairstyle; in this case the false hair is arranged so that it can be styled with the natural hair. Some hairpieces are made so that they are permanently set in a particular style, such as a group of curls or a traditional plain bob. Smaller hairpieces, such as pre-worked braids, may be used for decorating an elaborate hairstyle.

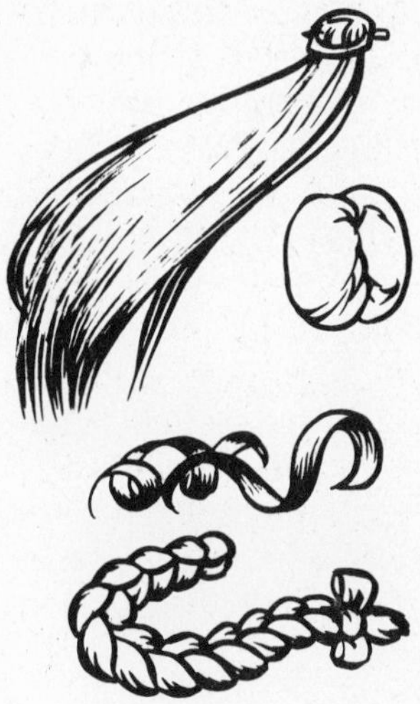

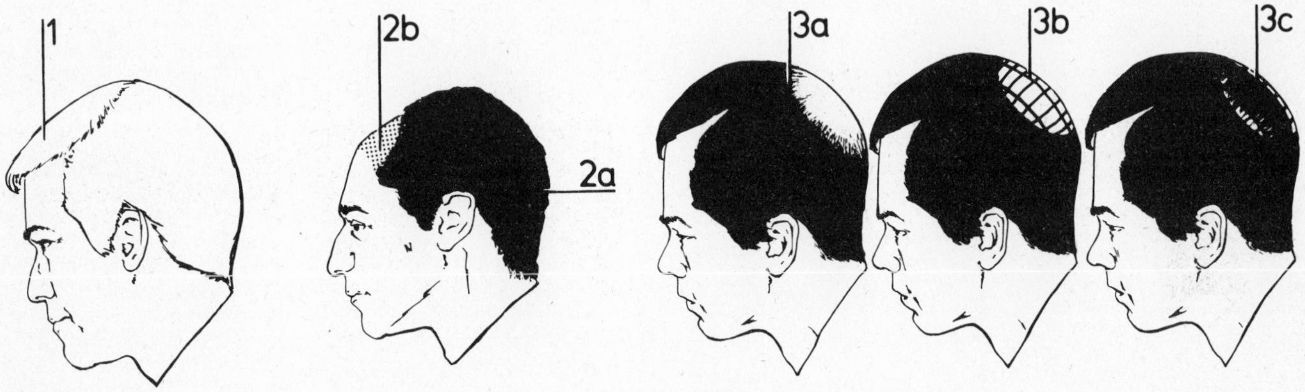

Toupées
These are small hairpieces, often made to cover the front and top of the scalp (**1**), since this is where hair loss first shows itself. A good toupée should be made to measure, or at least tinted and cut to match your own hair color and style. Toupées may be attached to the surrounding hairs, or they may be stitched to anchor points made in your scalp by a doctor. Stitching can produce many problems, such as difficulty in keeping the scalp underneath clean, and strain on the sutures which may cause soreness and irritation.

Hair transplants
Hair transplants have received a good deal of publicity recently, as many men see them as an ideal solution to baldness. Small areas of scalp are taken from parts where the hair is thick (**2a**), and tufts are transplanted into balder areas (**2b**), where they continue growing. Drawbacks are that the process is time-consuming and expensive, and requires extreme care of the sites until they are healed. Some patients have developed serious complications after hair transplantation, and the process is currently under review in the medical profession.

Hair weaving
The process of hair weaving is shown in the sequence of diagrams *above*. Hair weaving is a mixture of your own hair and some from the specialist's stock, either natural or synthetic. First, strands of hair are chosen around the bald site (**3a**), and stretched across the bald area to form a web of hair that is, of course, securely anchored to the scalp by the hair roots. When a criss-cross pattern has been formed in this way (**3b**), extra hairs are sewn, tied or cemented into the web, so forming a semipermanent hairpiece (**3c**). The disadvantages of the system are that the anchor hair inevitably grows, which causes the whole hairpiece to loosen. Because of this the web needs to be tightened every month or two. Also, the stretching of the web can sometimes put such strain on the roots of the anchor hairs that they weaken and fall out.

Face

Since blemishes on the face are so easily seen by others and so difficult to disguise effectively, problems with the face can cause very severe distress to the sufferer. The troubles may range from birthmarks through infections to problems that arise from poor skin care. The state of the skin, particularly that on the face, often reflects the state of health of the rest of the body, so a poor diet, inadequate exercise, insufficient sleep, and overwork can all have adverse effects on the condition and appearance of your face. On these pages we look at some of the common face problems that can be prevented, alleviated, or cured by careful attention to whole body health and to facial hygiene in particular.

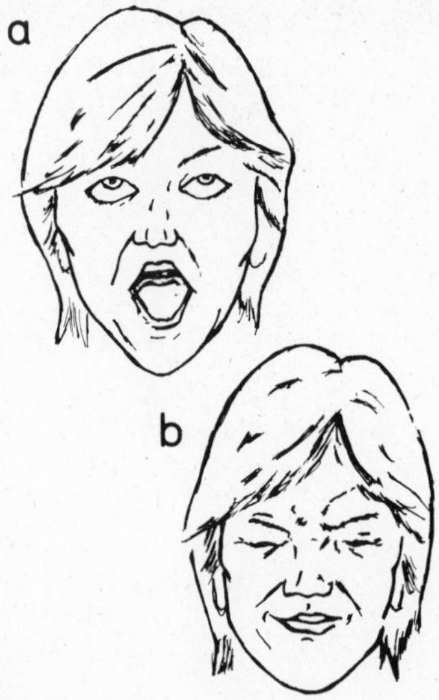

Exercises for the face
Isometric exercises help to keep the muscles of the face supple and in good condition. Isometric exercises are quite strenuous for the muscles concerned, so only do each exercise once a day and maintain the position for a maximum of only six seconds.
a Open your mouth and eyes wide so that your facial muscles are as fully stretched as possible; hold this position.
b Screw up your eyes and mouth and wrinkle your nose so that your facial muscles are contracted; hold this position.

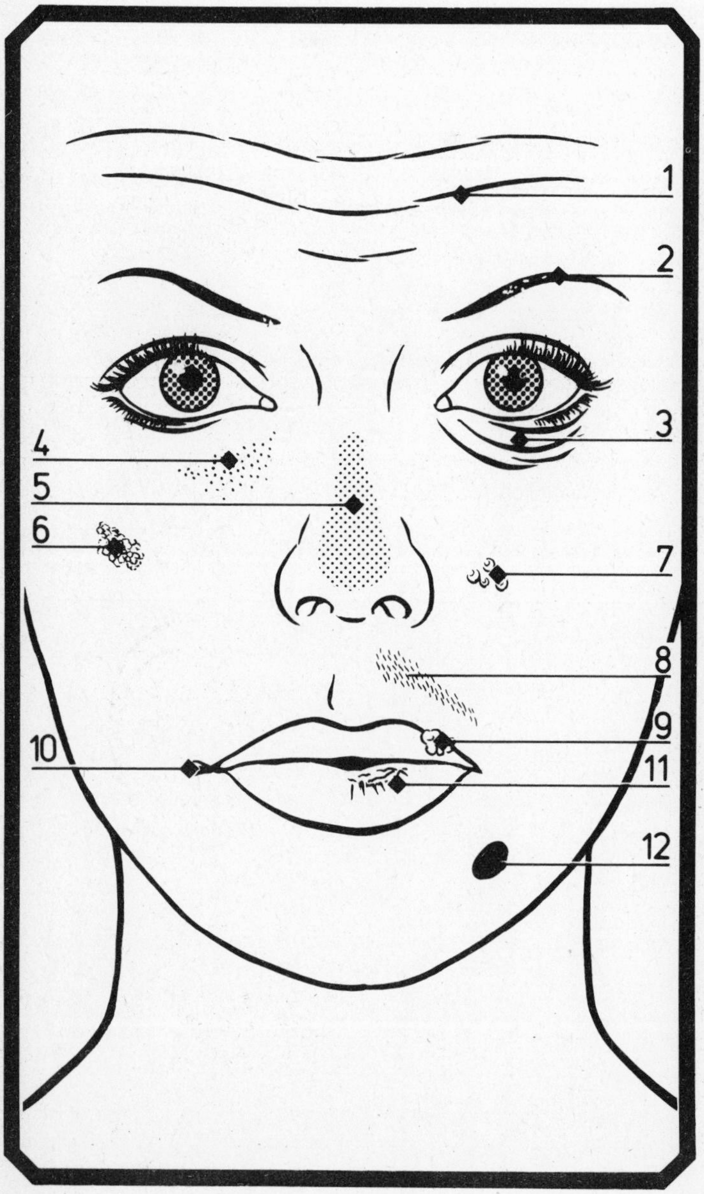

Common face and skin problems
The illustration *left* shows some of the face and skin problems that are to some extent under your own control. If you have a severe infection, see your doctor.
1 Wrinkles; these occur as an inevitable part of the aging process, but if you keep your skin moisturized and clean they may not appear so early.
2 Dandruff of the eyebrows; this is a very unpleasant condition that can be minimized by washing the eyebrows with a medicated soap.
3 Bags under the eyes; these are frequently the result of insufficient sleep, and are also an intrinsic part of the aging process.
4 Blackheads and open pores; thorough cleansing and the use of an astringent lotion will help prevent this condition.
5 Sunburn; the nose is especially susceptible to sunburn, but all of the face (if your skin is fair) should be protected with a sun cream before exposure to hot sun.
6 Dry skin; this often occurs naturally but is alleviated by the use of a moisturizer.
7 Acne; this condition often occurs on oily skin, and can be alleviated to some extent by thorough cleansing of the face several times a day.
8 Unwanted hair; this can be removed temporarily by shaving or plucking, or permanently by electrolysis.
9 Viral infections, such as herpes and dermatitis of the lips; these conditions may be relieved by the use of antihistamine creams and surgical spirit, but are usually best left alone.
10 Corner cracks on the lips; these may be caused by ill-fitting dentures, by fungal infection, or by vitamin deficiency. The lips should be kept dry to enable the cracks to heal.
11 Chapped lips; these are often the result of exposure to wind, and can be alleviated or avoided by using a lip salve.
12 Birthmarks; even very severe birthmarks can be camouflaged by carefully applied cosmetics. Beauty therapists often specialize in this problem.

Acne
Acne vulgaris is a particular plague of the teenage years, and can cause a great deal of embarrassment. If neglected the condition will cause disfiguring scars, so it is worth making the effort to prevent it or to treat it as early as possible. The skin should be kept scrupulously clean; wash your face several times a day and pat it dry. Brush your hair off your face, and do not pick at or squeeze the spots as this will spread the infection. Ultraviolet light inhibits the spread of acne, so sunbathe often or use a sun-lamp as frequently as safety instructions allow.

Unwanted hair
Many women feel that growths of dark or strong hair on the face are unsightly. The most common places for the problem to occur are between the eyebrows, on the upper lip, and on the chin. The only permanent method of removal is electrolysis, which involves killing the hair root with a small electric current, but this is a lengthy and expensive procedure. Shaving causes stubbly regrowth; plucking can be painful and may lead to follicle damage. Waxing and depilatories are messy, and may leave the skin sore. A good temporary measure is to bleach the hairs with a mild cosmetic bleach.

Wrinkles
Wrinkles are folds of skin formed when the skin dries out and loses its elasticity. Although they are inevitable in old age, some skins wrinkle more easily than others, and various factors may hasten their arrival. Avoid overexposure to sun and wind, as these dry out the skin. Make sure that your diet contains plenty of vitamins (see p.23), and avoid exposure to cigarette smoke. Cleanse your face regularly as this will keep the skin well conditioned, but avoid harsh soaps as these, too, have a drying effect on the skin. Keep your face well moisturized during the day and the night.

Shaving
The facial skin of many men is affected by their method of shaving. If you tend to get razor burn or frequent razor nicks, it is probably because you do not soften your beard sufficiently before shaving. Spread lots of foam on your beard and let it soak in for a few minutes, then use a wet razor and rinse it frequently in hot water so that the blade does not become clogged. If you use an electric shaver, make sure that it gives you a good, clean, close shave. If you have an outbreak of acne it is best to grow a beard temporarily rather than to increase tenderness and spread the infection by a daily shave.

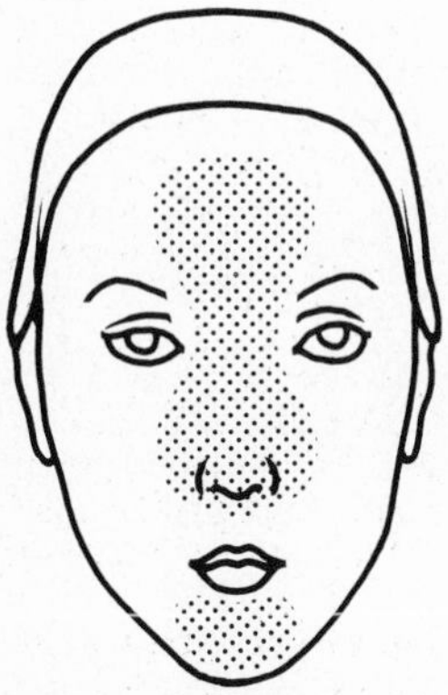

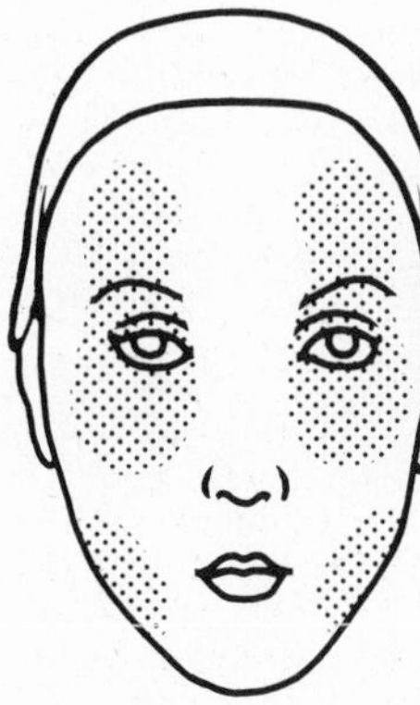

Oily skin
This generally occurs in a panel down the center of the face, as shown *above;* the areas most likely to be oily are the forehead, nose and chin. In addition, the oily panel may spread down to the neck and the top of the chest. Oily skin is difficult to keep clean as it attracts dirt and the pores tend to become blocked and infected. The skin should be washed several times a day with mild soap and then splashed with astringent lotion to remove the last traces of oil and to tone up the pores. Oily cosmetics, especially greasy foundations, will aggravate the problem, but regular washing with antiseptic soap will improve the skin's condition.

Dry skin
Dry skin tends to be most troublesome in the areas shown *above;* the eyes and cheeks in particular may need careful attention. The skin should only be washed with soap and water occasionally; the rest of the time dirt should be removed with a cleansing lotion. If a moisturizer is used every day the skin will be prevented from drying out too much. Cold, windy weather and hot, arid weather will make the condition worse; protect your skin with a barrier cream against extremes of temperature. If you have a "combination" skin, with both oily and dry patches, use soap only on the oily parts and apply moisturizer to the dry patches.

Giving yourself a facial
A facial is a complete cleansing program for your face. There is no need to go to a salon for a facial; a home facial is just as effective as a professional one and considerably cheaper. Facials are equally beneficial to men and women — maintaining a clean and healthy face should be the concern of both sexes.
a Wash your face thoroughly in mild soap and water, and then pat it dry with a soft towel so that the surface is not abraded.
b Cleanse your face with pads of cotton dipped in cleansing lotion; this will remove any stubborn traces of make-up and dirt, and will also clean dirt from deep down in the pores.
c Apply a face pack suited to your skin type. The pack may be in the form of a liquid, a cream or a gel, but any type will dry out excess oil, moisturize and soften the skin, and clean out impurities from the pores. The pack should be removed after the specified time, either by splashing the face with water or by peeling off the mask that has formed.
d Apply a gentle astringent lotion to your face to close and condition the pores. Your skin will feel fresher, smoother and healthier than before.

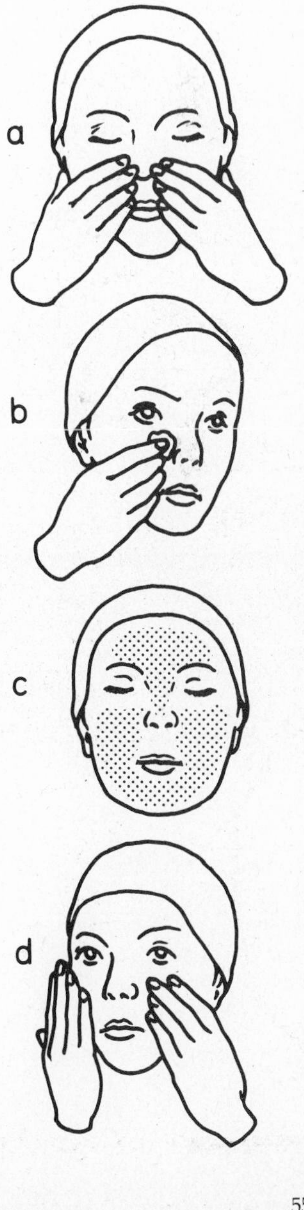

Eyes 1

Healthy eyes sparkle and are free from discoloration and swelling. They can see clearly, are not tender, do not tire easily, and do not itch or water. Most people, however, are troubled with minor eye problems at some time during their lives. On these pages we look at the ways in which you can help your eyes toward better health, by treating them gently and by dealing with minor problems before they become serious. Any pain in the eye or loss of vision is serious, and an ophthalmologist or doctor should be seen at once.

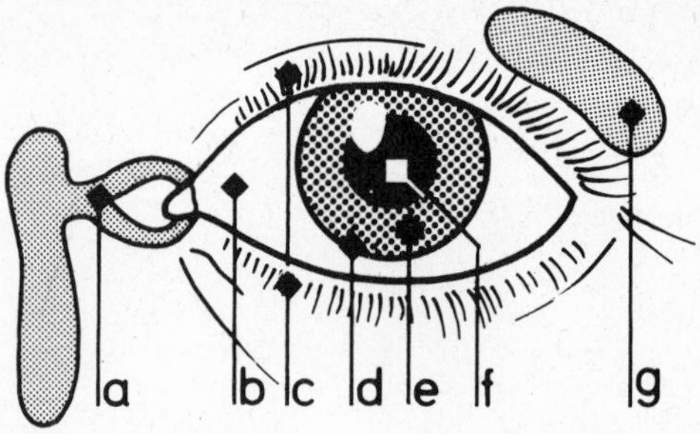

Parts of the eye
a Tear ducts and sac; a tiny opening can be seen at the nasal end of the eye.
b Sclera or white of the eye, covered with the conjunctiva, a clear membrane.
c Eyelids, two protective flaps of skin.
d Cornea, the transparent "window" of the eye.
e Iris, the muscular colored portion of the eye.
f Pupil; this part of the eye alters in size as the light changes.
g Tear gland; this gland secretes the perfect solution for bathing eyes. Blinking washes tears down over the eye, and they then drain away via the tear ducts.

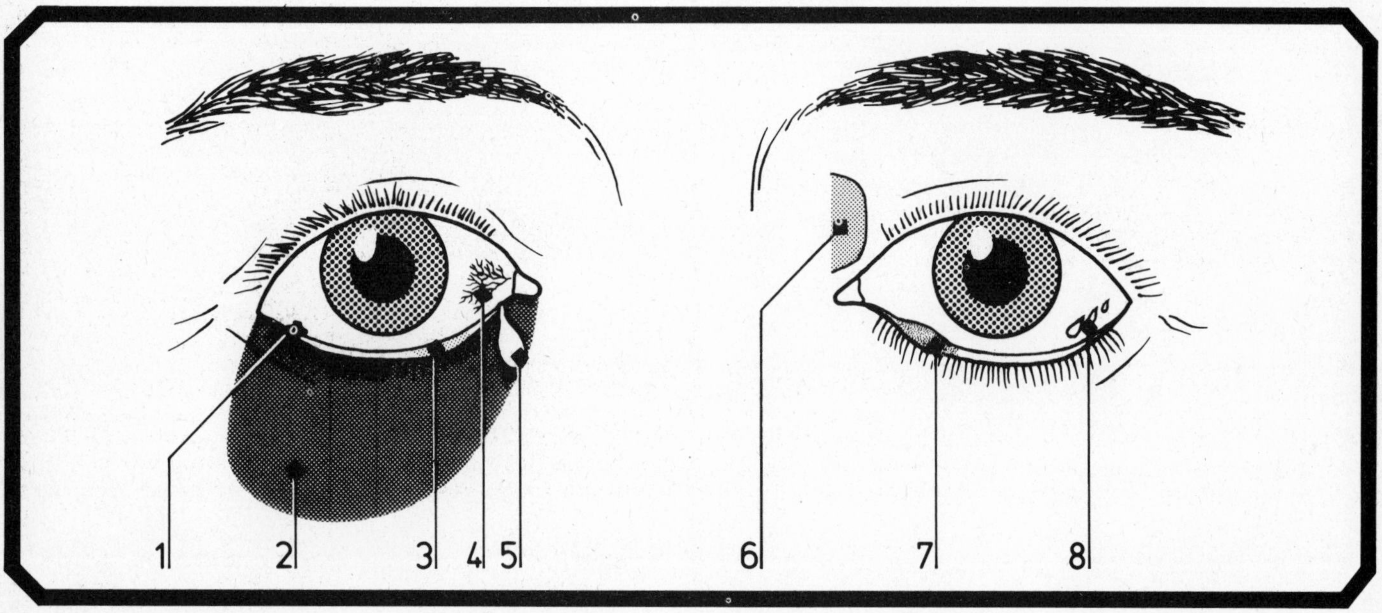

Common eye problems
The diagram *above* illustrates some of the common problems that manifest themselves in or around the eyes. Most of these problems can be treated at home, but if any eye problem or infection persists then you should see your doctor.
1 Foreign body in the eye; removal of specks of dirt etc that have become lodged under the eyelid is imperative for if they remain they may scratch the eyeball. Generally it is better to wash the object out of the eye than to try to remove it manually (see p. 57). If the object is not removed easily, or if any soreness persists after removal, see a doctor.
2 Black eye; this is usually caused by a blow to the eye. The bruising may be eased by several applications of a cold, wet washcloth. If the vision is disturbed see a doctor urgently, and take all children with black eyes to a doctor as they may not report vision disturbance.
3 Inflamed eyelids; these are often the results of allergies, but if yellow crusts are present the cause is an infection.
4 Conjunctivitis or pinkeye; this is reddening of the inner eyelids and the conjunctiva over the white of the eye (see p. 57).
5 Watering of the eyes is common in young babies, and almost always disappears as the baby grows. It is often noticeable also in older people, and in these cases is caused by loose skin around the eyes. Ask your doctor for advice if you have troublesome watering, or if you have any discomfort or discharge.
6 Cyst; benign cysts often occur around the eyes. They usually disappear of their own accord eventually, but will require medical attention if they become infected.
7 Sty; a sty is a boil that generally has formed in one of the hair follicles of the eyelashes. The sty usually reaches a head after several days and will then burst. When this has occurred the eyelid should be wiped frequently with cotton swabs dipped in clean warm water; this will prevent the infection from spreading to other follicles. If sties are recurrent see your doctor, as other follicles may be harboring infection, requiring antibiotic treatment.
8 Splashes of chemicals. Most chemicals can irritate the eye if they come into direct contact. Wash the eye at once with plenty of water, and see a doctor quickly with a note of the chemical that caused the problem. Always wear protective goggles if you are handling strong chemicals that may splash.

Eye strain
Eye strain is caused by using the eyes too much in unfavorable conditions, such as poor light, a smoky atmosphere, or late at night when the eyes are already tired. Excessive reading can also produce eye strain, because it causes the eyes to remain focused at the same distance for an unnaturally long time. All reading should be done in a good light, and you should look up every 30 minutes or so and refocus your eyes on a distant object before returning to your reading. All detailed work should be done in a good light, and if your eyes start to tire you should rest them briefly before resuming the work.

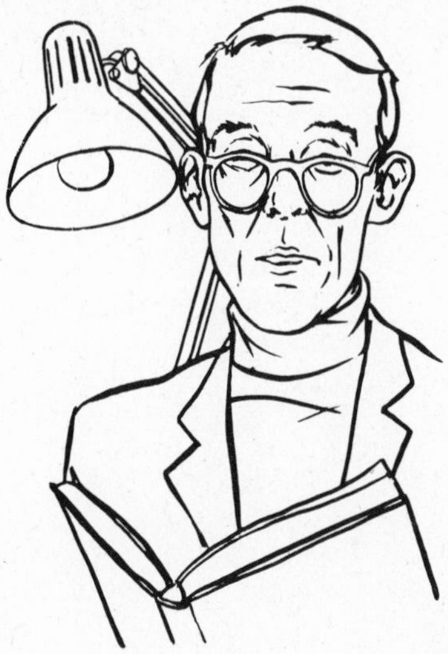

Allergies
Many common allergens cause symptoms in the eyes of sensitized people, usually taking the form of red, sore eyelids. Itching is also a frequent reaction. Common culprits include make-up, dust and chemicals; avoid these as much as possible by using hypo-allergenic cosmetics and by avoiding touching the eyes and their surroundings if your hands are dirty. If you do develop an allergic reaction, bathe your eyelids carefully with warm water and clean cotton or a paper tissue. If this does not resolve the problem rapidly see your doctor.

Conjunctivitis
Conjunctivitis may be a complication of a nose or throat infection or may be independent. There is often a sore, gritty feeling in the eyes, and a yellow discharge that may stick the eyelashes together. Conjunctivitis is very contagious, and can rapidly be passed on through dirty towels, handkerchiefs, washcloths and hands. Destroy all tissues and cotton used for bathing the eye, and boil any linen; disinfect the washbasin after washing your face, and do not use public swimming pools or showers while the infection persists. Do not cover the eye with a protective patch, as this encourages the germs to multiply.

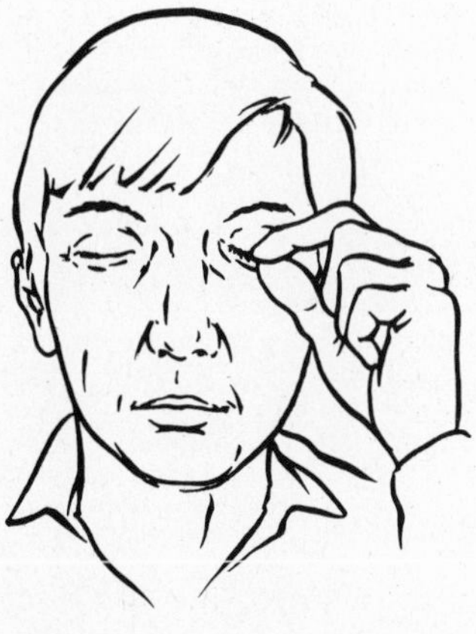

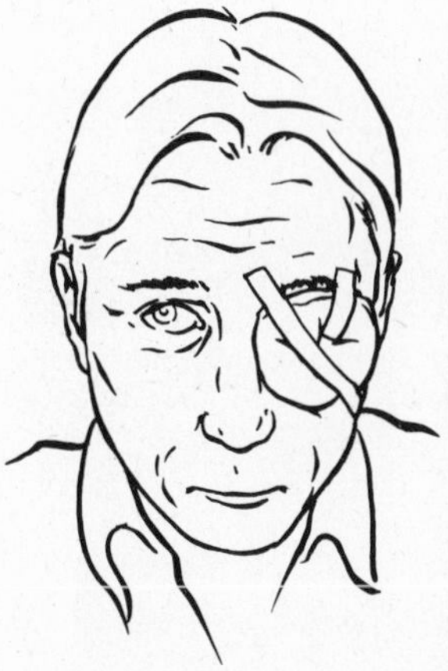

Removing a foreign body
It is quite common for dirt, fibers, eyelashes or small insects to become trapped under the eyelid, and because the eye is so sensitive they usually cause great discomfort. To remedy the problem, first rinse the eye in an eyebath or a handful of water. If this doesn't dislodge the source of the trouble, lift your upper eyelid by the edge and pull it out and down over the lower lid, as shown *above*. If this measure also fails, it is probably best to see a doctor; never try to use tweezers, cotton tips etc, as they might easily damage the eye.

Compresses
Compresses can be cool, to soothe swelling and bruising, or warm to speed up the course of an infection. For a black eye, a cold compress should be held or lightly taped against the eye as shown *above;* this reduces the swelling and helps the blood to clot so that the bruising is minimized. The traditional remedy of applying a raw steak is based on the fact that the meat is moist and cool. A warm compress can be used to encourage a sty to come to a head and burst as quickly as possible. The compress need not be held against the eye all the time; warm bathing at intervals will be equally effective.

Do
- Treat your eyes gently at all times, remembering that most damage to the eyes is irreversible.
- Rest your eyes when they are tired or sore.
- Avoid substances to which you know you are allergic.
- Use a good light when reading.
- Look up and refocus your eyes regularly when reading.
- Do all detailed work in a good light.
- Make sure that you have sufficient sleep each night.
- Make sure that any foreign body that becomes trapped in your eye is removed before it can damage the eyeball.
- See your doctor if your eyeball is accidentally scratched.
- Use hypoallergenic cosmetics if your eyes become irritated when wearing make-up.
- Remove all make-up, especially mascara, from your eyes before you go to bed.
- Burn or boil all handkerchiefs, washcloths etc that have been used by someone with sties or conjunctivitis, as both these conditions are very contagious.

Don't
- Read or do detailed work in a poor or indirect light; the eyes have to strain unnaturally to focus under such conditions.
- Try to poke out objects that are lodged under your eyelids; wash them out instead.
- Watch television in a darkened room; this causes great strain to the eyes because of the contrast between the bright light and the dark background.
- Paint eyeliner or color on the part of the eyelid visible inside the eyelashes; particles of make-up are certain to float onto the eye itself and will cause problems.
- Ignore persistent eye problems; always see a doctor or ophthalmologist if you are constantly having trouble with your eyes.
- Allow pus or dried eye secretions to remain in or around your eye as they can easily cause reinfection.

Eyes 2

Vision
Vision is the ability of the eyes to receive light waves, bending them through the cornea, pupil and lens to focus on the retina, a thin membrane at the back of the eyeball (**a**). Impulses from the light-sensitive retina travel up the optic nerve from each eye and cause a three-dimensional picture to be seen in the brain. Eyeballs vary in length from person to person. Longer than average eyes have the point of focus in front of the retina (**b**); this is near-sightedness, in which only near objects are seen clearly. If the eyeball is shorter than usual, the point of focus is behind the retina (**c**); this is far-sightedness, in which only distant objects are seen clearly. Other vision problems include presbyopia, astigmatism and squint. Presbyopia, or aging sight, is a progressive loss of elasticity that may occur in old age, causing difficulty in focusing. Astigmatism is an uneven bending of the light rays through the cornea or lens, causing blurred vision. Squint, or strabismus, is an imbalance of the eye muscles, causing one eye to turn inward or outward. Any baby or small child with a tendency toward "crossed eyes" should be taken to an eye specialist as soon as possible, as sight may not develop normally in the affected eye.

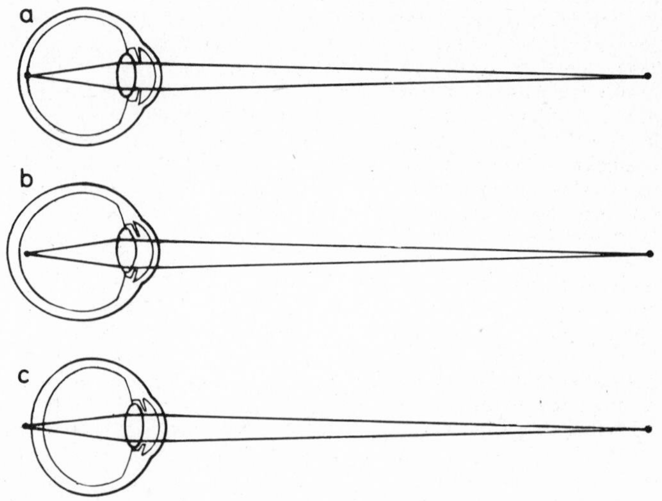

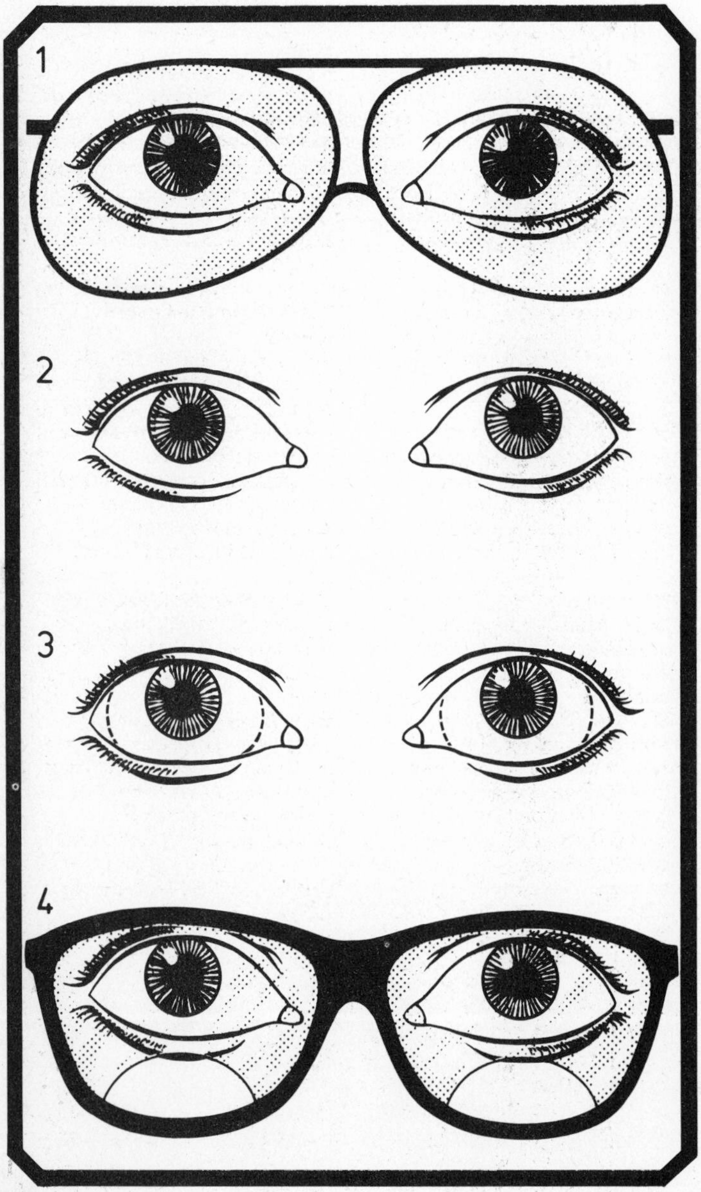

Corrective aids
Lenses of various kinds are the most common aids for defects that arise from focusing problems. Lenses are made from polished glass or plastic, and are shaped or treated so that they correct the defect by changing the direction of the light waves that pass through them. Corrective lenses may be prescribed for only one eye if the vision in the other is normal; in this case the person may wear a pair of eyeglasses in which one lens is plain glass, or may use only one contact lens.
1 Eyeglasses; these consist of a pair of lenses, prescribed individually for each eye, connected by a frame that goes over the bridge of the nose.
2 Hard contact lenses; these are small lenses of rigid glass or plastic that are floated over the top of the eyeball and held there by the suction of the eye's natural fluids. The lenses usually cover only the center of the eyeball, but in rare cases may be larger.
3 Soft contact lenses; these are larger than most of their hard counterparts, and are gelatinous in form. Many people find them easier to wear than the hard lenses, and some do not even need to be taken out at night.
4 Bifocals; these are glasses for people who need a weak lens for ordinary vision and a stronger lens for reading or detailed work. The bottoms of the lenses contain arcs of a more powerful refraction, and as the eyes look downward the beams of light they receive are those that have passed through the stronger lenses.
It is important to remember that the very old and the very young frequently will not complain about eye problems, so those who are caring for them must be extra vigilant in noticing anything unusual that may be a result of vision problems. Warning signs may include frequently rubbing the eyes (this may happen if the vision has become blurred), or constantly tripping over or bumping into objects.

Professional eye care
It is important to have your eyes checked regularly so that you can be sure that they are in good health. If you have any overt defects in vision the correct lenses will be prescribed for you or surgery arranged, and the specialist will also be able to spot many signs of latent eye trouble such as the warning symptoms of glaucoma or detached retina. You should also make an extra visit to the ophthalmologist if you suffer from persistent unexplained headaches, especially after reading, or if you have sustained an eye injury.

Glasses
Glasses should be chosen for fit, comfort and appearance; if they are unsatisfactory in any of these respects you will soon become reluctant to wear them regularly. Glasses are readily available and easy to fit, and tend to be cheaper than contact lenses; they are also easier to clean and maintain, and are not so easily mislaid. You will usually be able to choose from many frame styles, such as those shown here; the frame should rest on the bridge of your nose and not slip down, and the earpieces should not chafe. Wear your glasses as often as your ophthalmologist recommends.

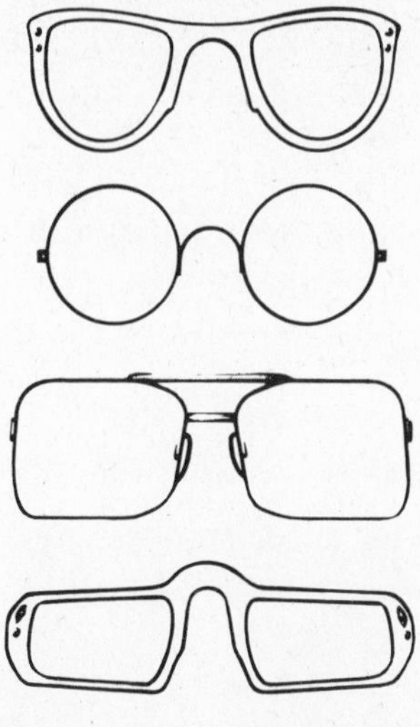

Contact lenses
Contact lenses are of two basic types: hard and soft. Soft lenses are more easy to adjust to and can generally be worn for longer periods than the hard type, but are more expensive and have a shorter life. Hard lenses are easier to keep clean, and easier to alter to suit changing eye needs, but many people experience difficulty in accustoming the eyes to wearing the lenses. Contact lenses are more difficult to fit than glasses, and may require many visits to the ophthalmologist; they are not suitable for all people's eyes, and can cause harm if they are not used correctly.

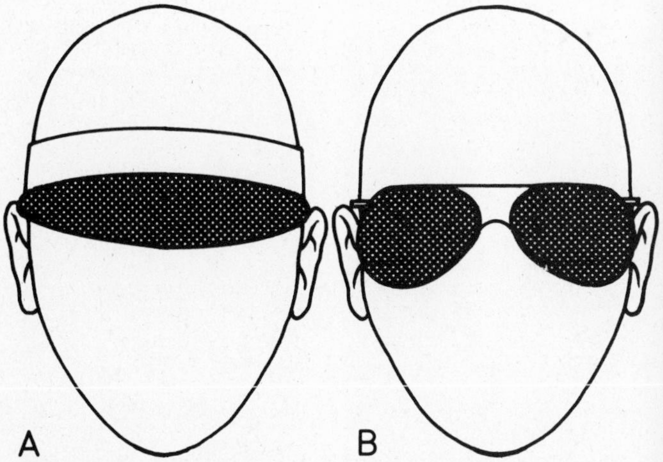

Protection against glare
Strong sunlight can cause eyesight problems ranging from discomfort and glare to permanent blindness if the bright sun is viewed directly. The glare caused by the sun is heightened when it is reflected off snow or water, so special care should be taken when sailing or skiing. The most common way of protecting the eyes from glare is to use dark glass or plastic, worn either as a one-piece shade on a headband (**A**) or as a pair of sunglasses (**B**). Cheap sunglasses contain lenses that are merely colored; more sophisticated versions include those with polarized lenses that reduce glare and those with photochromatic lenses that increase their protection automatically as you move into stronger sunlight. For those who wear ordinary glasses it is possible to have their prescribed lenses tinted or to buy dark lenses that clip onto the glasses frame over the usual lenses. Even the strongest sunglasses, however, are not sufficient protection for looking directly at the sun, even when watching an eclipse, and the sun should never be looked at through a telescope as the rays can burn severely.

Do
- Ensure that your child's vision is tested early in life.
- Visit your optician or ophthalmologist regularly.
- Choose glasses that are comfortable and well-fitting so that they do not chafe no matter how long you have to wear them.
- Choose a style of eyeglass frame that suits your face, so that you do not feel self-conscious when wearing them.
- Wear your glasses or lenses as often as recommended.
- Maintain strict hygiene if you use soft contact lenses in particular.
- Keep glasses and lenses in their cases when not in use.
- Protect your eyes adequately from glare.
- Take extra precautions against glare if you are near water or snow in bright sunlight.
- Seek professional advice if you have unexplained headaches or if you experience problems with your vision.
- Wear your prescribed lenses for tasks that require good eyesight for safety reasons, such as driving, operating machinery, using sharp tools.
- Remove hard contact lenses at night.
- Tell your optician and ophthalmologist if you are diabetic or if you have high blood pressure.
- Wear protective goggles or shields if your work or hobby requires it.

Don't
- Wear glasses that slip down the bridge of your nose or rest on your cheekbones.
- Fiddle with glasses when you are not wearing them; this may loosen the screws and affect the fit.
- Insert contact lenses with dirty hands.
- Insert contact lenses without bathing them first with lens solution.
- Continue to wear a contact lens that has dirt or dust lodged behind it; take it out, clean the lens and bathe your eye before reinserting the lens.
- Sleep, even briefly, with hard contact lenses in position.
- Leave contact lenses in position if your eyes become sore.
- Borrow someone else's glasses; you should only wear lenses that have been specifically prescribed for your eyes.
- Use glasses or contact lenses that have been scratched or damaged; take them to your optician and have them repolished or replaced.
- Wear glasses that will break easily when taking part in sports activities; extra-durable types can be bought for this purpose.

Ears

In addition to their hearing function, the ears are important in the sensation of balance. The outer ear comprises the ear flap (pinna) and the canal leading inward from the pinna. The middle ear includes the eardrum and a chamber that is crossed by three tiny bones; the Eustachian tube leads from the middle ear to the pharynx. The inner ear contains complex mechanisms that convert sound vibrations into impulses for transmission to the brain. Other mechanisms in the inner ear are sensitive to changes in the position of the head and so provide information used in balancing the body. Because of the delicacy of the ear mechanism, ear problems can be both painful and disturbing; here we look at some of the common ear problems and suggest ways to avoid or alleviate them.

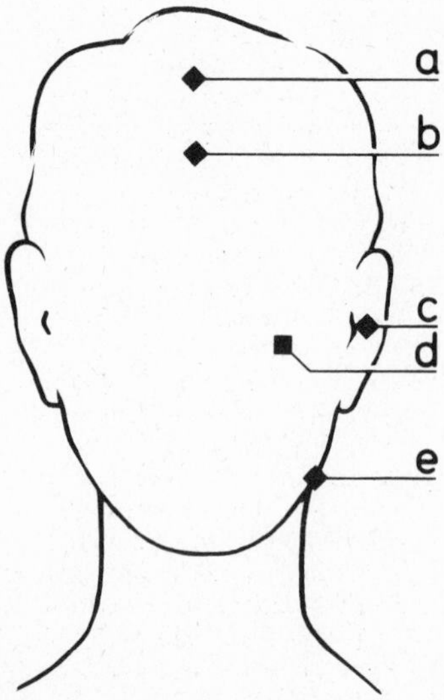

Complications of ear problems
The diagram shows the sites of some of the common complications of ear problems.
a Headache; this may occur during infection because of bacterial poisons and subsequent inflammation.
b Vertigo is caused by a disturbance of the balance center in the inner ear.
c Temporary or permanent deafness may result from ear infection or damage.
d Blocked Eustachian tubes; these occur when an infection reaches the tubes linking the ear to the nose.
e Swollen lymph nodes; these may occur in the neck when the ear is infected.

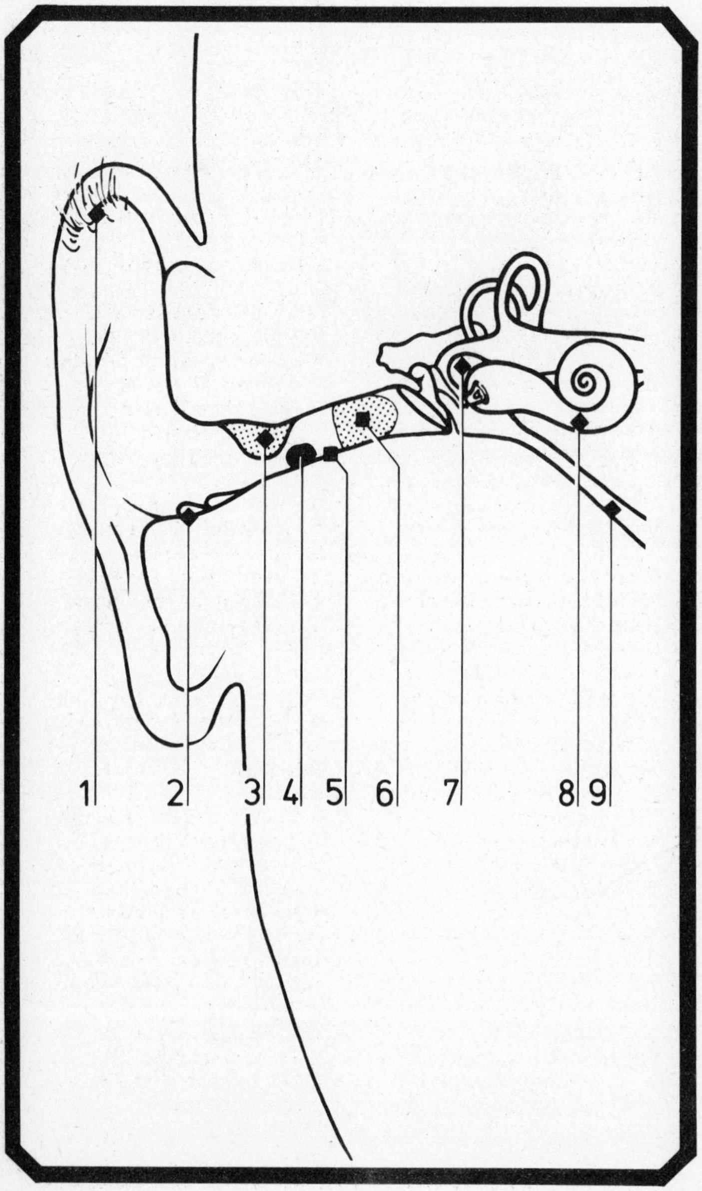

Common ear problems
The illustration *left* shows some of the common problems that may develop in the ear.
1 Hairy ears; these occur particularly in men, and a tendency toward them may be hereditary. The easiest and safest way to control the problem is to clip the hairs closely every two or three days with nailscissors.
2 Discharging ear; this is always a sign that something is wrong with the ear. The only material that the ear naturally secretes is wax; if the ear has a watery, bloody or infected discharge, see your doctor. Never plug a discharging ear as this may drive the infection deeper.
3 Boil inside the ear; this condition is often the result of scratching the ear with a dirty fingernail, hairpin etc, and can be very painful. A warm compress may ease the pain, but you should seek a doctor's advice so that the infection does not spread.
4 Foreign body inside the ear; children are especially prone to pushing peanuts, beads etc into their ears, and the objects often become lodged. Take the child to a doctor; attempts to remove the object yourself may well force it further into the ear.
5 Otitis externa; this is an infection of the outer ear. Ear infections that develop after swimming, perhaps as a result of inadequate drying, are usually otitis externa.
6 Impacted wax; the ear usually cleans itself of its natural wax through the movements of chewing and talking, but occasionally wax becomes impacted. Contributing factors in this problem may include dust, dry air, and probing in the ears with the fingers. The ear needs to be syringed with warm water to dislodge the obstruction, but this should be done by a doctor rather than at home.
7 Otitis media, an infection of the middle ear. This condition is very painful, and requires a doctor's attention as there is a severe risk of the eardrum being perforated if the infection continues unchecked.
8 Inner ear infection; this also is an excruciatingly painful and potentially serious condition. When the inner ear cavity, or labyrinth, is inflamed, deafness, disturbance of balance and vomiting occur; the hearing impairment and balance disturbance may become permanent if the condition is not treated.
9 Eustachian tube infection; bacteria found here may have traveled down from the ear or up from the nose; in either case the ear will be affected and pain will result as the pressure behind the eardrum is altered.

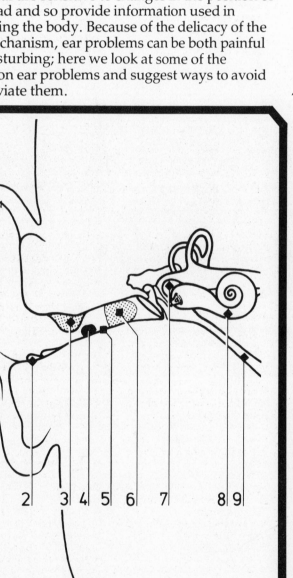

Earache
Earache is a very painful condition that often arises from an infection. The infection may be the result of a scratch or boil in the external canal of the ear, or a bacterial invasion of the middle ear, the drum, or the Eustachian tubes. Infected adenoids, a head cold, allergies and even toothache may also cause earache. Aspirin, acetaminophen or a warm pad or compress may ease the pain, but if the ache persists see a doctor; the neglect of an ear infection may result in perforation of the eardrum, which could produce permanent deafness. Earache is particularly common in children, and should always be taken seriously.

Noise
Noise is one of the most widespread but least recognized hazards of the modern world, and can cause permanent deafness. Industrial noise is controlled by law, but if you feel that these laws are not being enforced where you work or that your hearing is being impaired at work, ask to have the noise level assessed. Industrial earmuffs should be provided and worn if the noise level is higher than recommended. Music is often an unsuspected source of ear damage; avoid too-frequent exposure to loud disco music, and do not turn the volume up excessively when listening through headphones.

Swimming
One of the most common ear problems associated with swimming is swimmer's ear, an infection of the outer ear that relies on a moist surface to develop. If you are prone to swimmer's ear, wear earplugs made of waxed lambswool or a similar material while in the water. Dry your ears thoroughly with a soft towel after swimming; if water is trapped in your ear, lie on your side until the water runs out. Other common ear problems for swimmers are usually related to changes in pressure when underwater.

Pressure
The ears are very sensitive to changes in pressure, such as those experienced when going up or down in an elevator or airplane. The discomfort caused in these circumstances, which makes the ears feel as though they are blocked, can often be relieved by yawning or by swallowing (helped by sucking candy). Pressure on the ears underwater can sometimes be painful; if you are diving in from the surface you should avoid going too deep, and if you are scuba diving you should follow the correct drills for slowly adjusting the pressure in your ears.

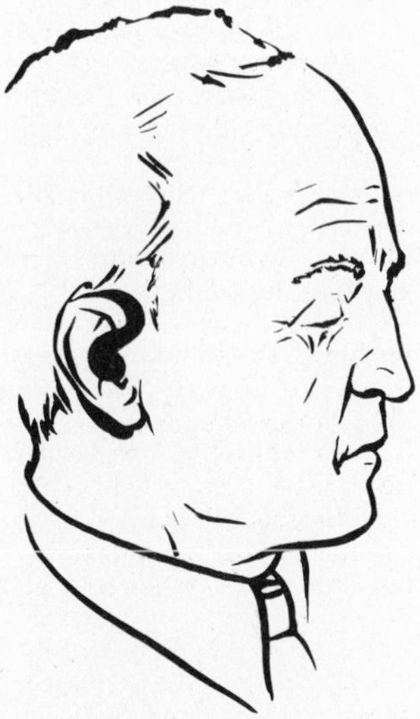

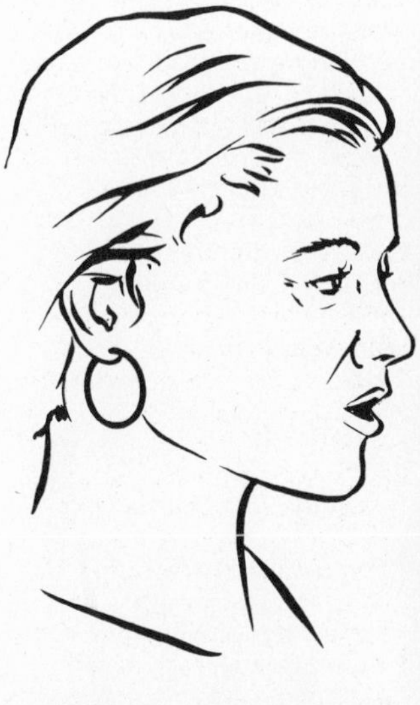

Hearing aids
Partial loss of hearing is often a natural result of the aging process, or may occur after a severe illness that has affected the ear or the surrounding bone. Partial deafness can frequently be alleviated by a hearing aid, which magnifies the sound waves reaching the ear to a level at which the damaged hearing mechanism can pick them up. Unfortunately one common effect of aging on the hearing mechanism is distortion of the sound waves rather than simple attenuation, and in these cases hearing aids often increase the problem. Of course, if deafness becomes total a hearing aid will not help at all.

Earrings
The earlobes can be pierced to enable you to wear earrings that pass through the lobes and are secured by a metal guard at the back. Piercing should always be done professionally, and for about two weeks afterward the lobes should be swabbed daily with antiseptic to avoid infection. The training rings or studs should be turned three times a day to prevent the holes from healing up over them. Always use earrings with shafts of silver, gold or hypo-allergenic metal, and do not push the guards too far up the shafts. Never wear hooped or dangling earrings during sports or dancing as they may catch on something and tear your ear.

Do
- Clean your ears gently with a warm washcloth daily.
- Visit your doctor if you have a discharge of any kind from your ear, or if you have an object lodged in your ear canal.
- Wear earplugs while swimming if you suffer from ear problems.
- Dry your ears thoroughly after swimming, and drain out any water lodged deeper in the ear.
- Have your hearing tested regularly.
- Visit your doctor as soon as possible if you feel that your hearing is impaired in any way.
- Wear industrial earmuffs if you work in a place with a high noise level.
- Try a warm compress on your ear to ease earache; in many cases this will be effective.
- See your doctor if you have a severe earache or one that has persisted for more than a few hours.
- Watch for warning signs of ear trouble if you have sinusitis, a head cold or severe allergy symptoms.
- Have your ear fitted for a hearing aid if you suffer from partial deafness.

Don't
- Poke dirty fingers, pencils, hairpins or any other objects into your ear canals.
- Clean your ears by forcing cotton tips or a washcloth down the ear canals.
- Try to swab out a discharging or infected ear.
- Syringe out impacted wax at home.
- Allow water to remain in your ear canals after swimming.
- Put your head underwater if you have a blocked nose; the changes in pressure may cause considerable pain.
- Dive deeply into water from the surface.
- Neglect de-pressurizing routines when scuba diving.
- Expose yourself too frequently to loud music.
- Work without ear protection in an environment where you find the noise level uncomfortable.
- Turn up the volume of music beyond the normal level when listening through headphones.
- Neglect an ear infection or earache.
- Blow your nose vigorously; anything other than gentle blowing may force bacteria up the Eustachian tubes.
- Resist being fitted for a hearing aid from reasons of vanity or because you think it will age you; it is far more aging to appear deaf.
- Buy a hearing aid on the recommendation of advertisements; always seek professional advice.

Nose and mouth

The nose and mouth tend to be particularly susceptible to viral and bacterial infections. Airborne and food-borne infectious organisms have easy access, and the warm, moist mucous membranes lining the nose and mouth encourage the culture of these organisms. Bacterial infections such as tonsillitis and strep-throat can usually be cured with antibiotics; viral infections, such as colds, cannot be cured by drugs although the troublesome symptoms may be relieved. On these pages we look at some of the infections and other problems that affect the nose and mouth and describe some of the ways in which you can help yourself toward better health by preventing such problems or minimizing their effects.

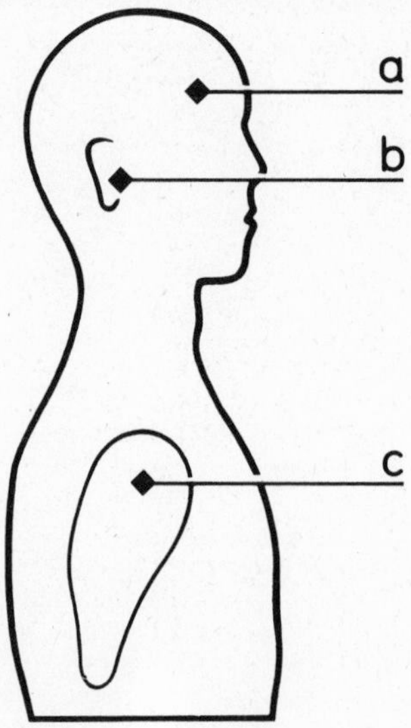

Side-effects
The diagram here shows some of the other parts of the body that may be affected by nose and mouth problems.
a Head; infections of the nose and sinuses may lead to headaches.
b Ears; temporary deafness is a frequent side-effect of many nose and throat infections.
c Lungs; mucus and phlegm from nose and throat infections may travel down into the lungs and cause coughing, or in severe cases lung infection.

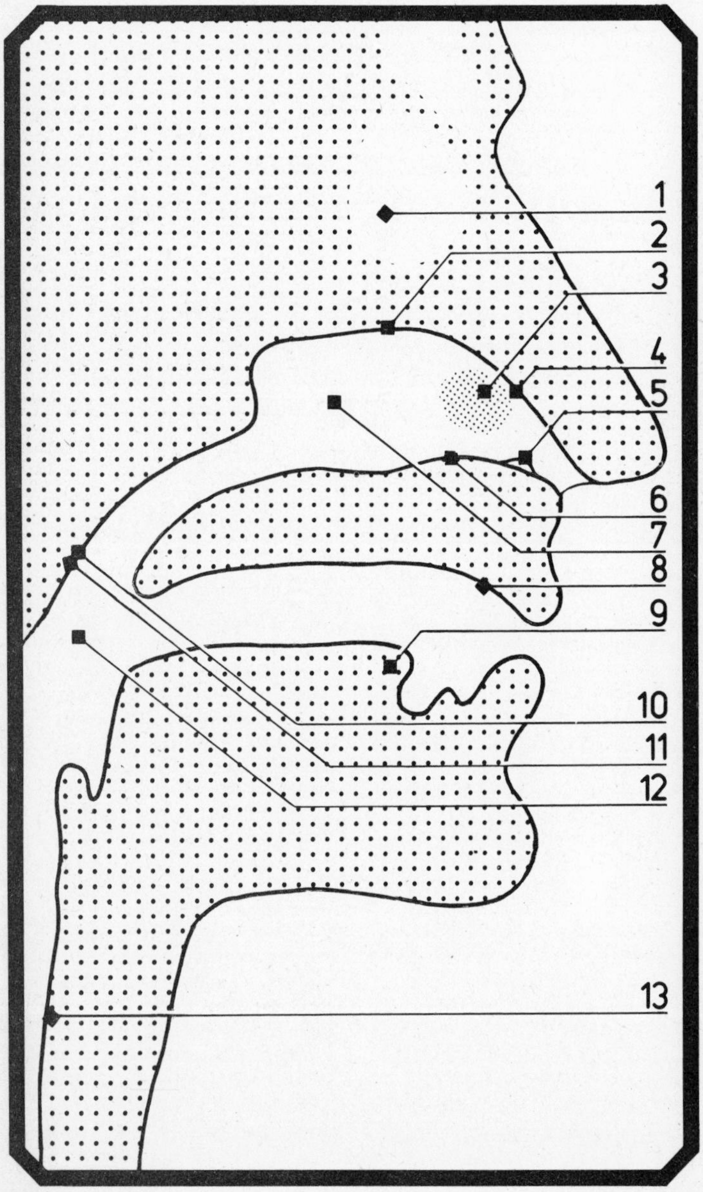

Common nose and mouth problems
The diagram plots the location of some of the most common problems in these areas.
1 Sinusitis; this condition often occurs when bacteria from a nose infection spread into the sinuses. It produces a purulent discharge from the nose. Sinusitis pain may be relieved by aspirin or acetaminophen, and by applying heat to the affected area.
2 Inflamed nasal membranes; this condition is frequently a result of an allergic reaction.
3 Foreign body in the nose; if a child has a blockage and discharge in only one nostril, suspect a small object lodged there and take him to a doctor. Don't try to remove the object yourself.
4 Nosebleed; this condition is caused by the rupture of one of the many tiny blood vessels that line the nose.
5 Boil in the nose; this very painful condition is often caused by scratching the lining of the nostril with a dirty fingernail, pencil etc. The boil should be bathed several times daily with twists of cotton dipped in hot antiseptic solution, and it is wise to seek a doctor's advice.
6 Dry mucous membranes; this condition may be caused by a lack of humidity in a centrally heated home, or by an infection and fever. You can increase the humidity in your home by placing a dish of water in every room.
7 Cold in the nose; this is one of the most enigmatic and bothersome of all common infections; no cure has yet been found.
8 Thrush; this condition is an infection of the mouth by the Candida albicans fungus, causing curdy patches. Mild solutions of gentian violet painted on the mouth lining may cure the condition.
9 Virus blisters; these occur on the cheeks and tongue, but generally disappear of their own accord.
10 Tonsillitis; this is the infection and inflammation of the tonsils.
11 Quinsy; this very painful condition is caused by an abscess around the tonsils.
12 Sore throat; a sore throat can be a complication of many bacterial or viral infections.
13 Laryngitis; this is inflammation of the voice box. Where the vocal cords are affected, hoarseness results. Causes include infection, excessive shouting and other overuses of the voice. Treatment comprises the inhalation of steam and complete voice rest for 48 hours.

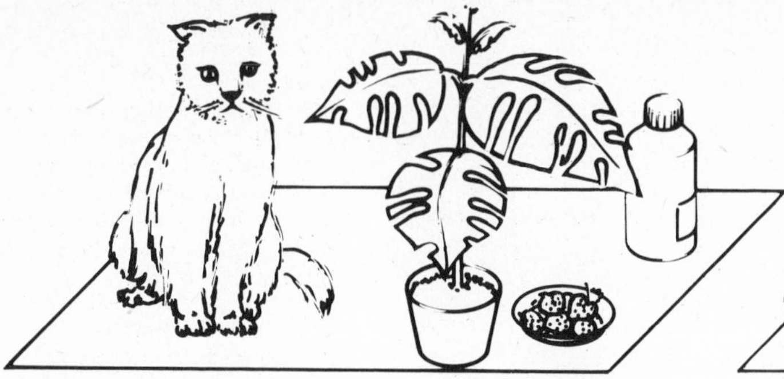

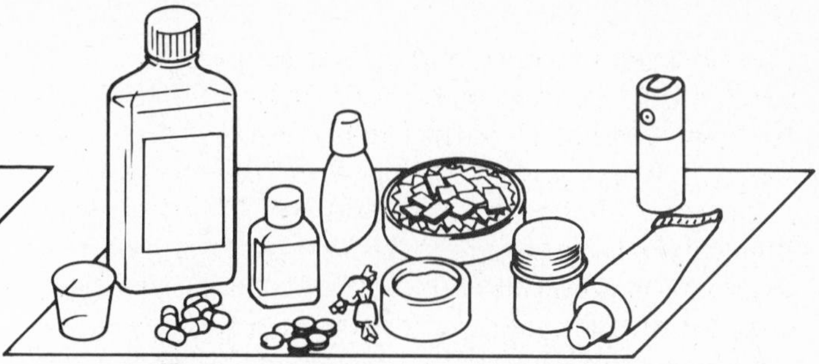

Allergies
Very common substances can cause distressing allergic reactions in sensitized people. The symptoms often include watery eyes, a runny nose, and inflamed membranes of the eyes, nose and throat. Causes of allergies may include pollen, house dust, animal fur, chemicals, certain foods or particular plants. The main control of allergies consists of identifying the source of the reaction and avoiding it as much as possible. When this is not possible, prescribed medication may help to alleviate the symptoms.

Medications
The range of medications designed to cure or relieve nose, mouth and throat problems is enormous, and constitutes a major portion of the over-the-counter medicine consumed. Some examples are cough medicines, lozenges, decongestants, menthol inhalants and rubs, antiseptic sprays, painkillers, catarrh remedies and patent "cold cures." In general the fancy brand names only contain substances that you can obtain much more cheaply in their plain form, such as aspirin, acetaminophen, menthol, caffeine and glucose.

Communicable diseases
The chart *right* illustrates the percentage of the population in the Western world likely to be ill from communicable diseases at any one time, based on figures from general practices. The total percentage, that is those ill from any communicable disease, is 8.5% of the population (**A**). The second part of the diagram (**B**) shows the percentage likely to be ill from various nose and throat infections: 4.7%, or over half the total, are those suffering fom colds, influenza, tonsillitis, sinusitis, laryngitis or tracheitis.

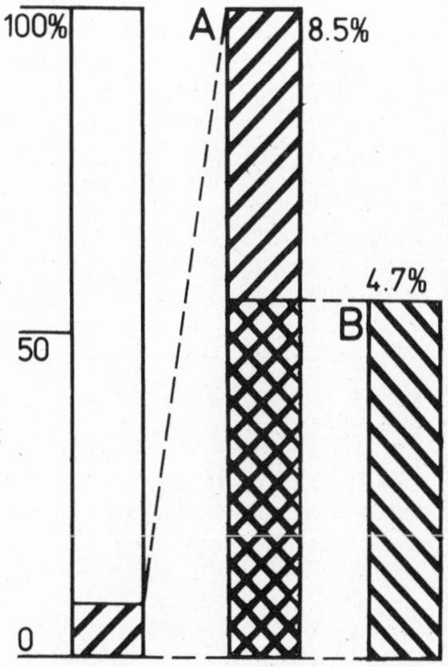

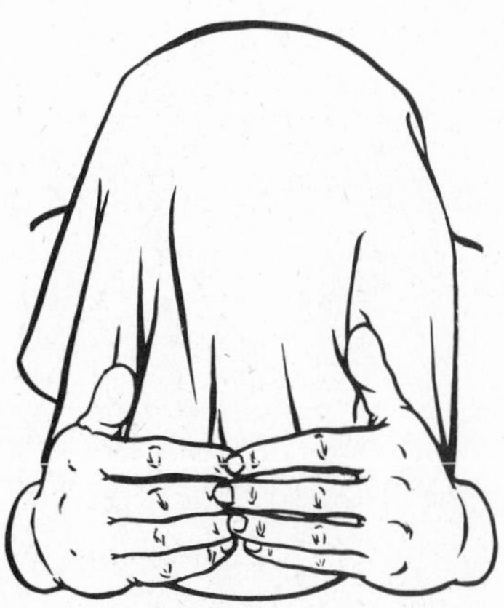

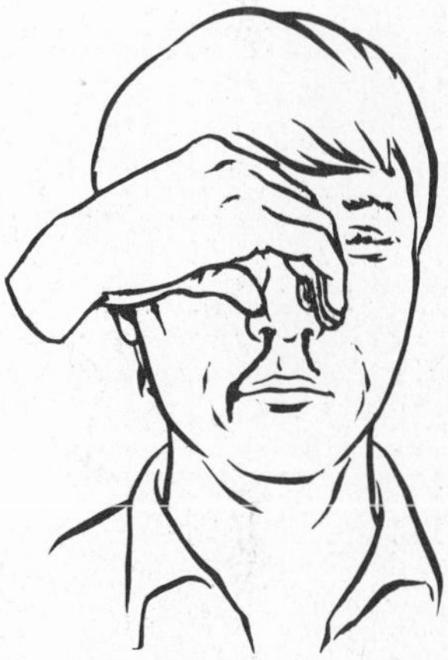

Colds
Although much time and money have been spent in trying to find a prevention or a cure for the common cold, neither has yet been done effectively. The main factor that will predispose you to a cold is low resistance. A cold is best left untreated and will normally be self-limiting in about 7 days. So-called cold "treatments" may prolong the symptoms or produce side-effects. Inhalations to clear a blocked nose, and aspirin or acetaminophen to relieve pain, may help to reduce the worst discomfort of a cold, but limit your medications to these. Hot drinks may have a soothing effect.

Sore throats
One of the best methods of soothing a sore throat temporarily is by gargling with a mouthwash; this washes the surface of the throat, but does not remove the cause of the trouble. Mix the liquid as directed, then take a mouthful; swish the liquid around your mouth, then tip your head back and gargle. Spit out the liquid and repeat the process several times with fresh mouthfuls of solution. Aspirin dissolved in water may be cheaper then brand-name mouthwashes. Mild local anesthetics can be bought in lozenge form to relieve sore throats.

Stuffy noses
The misery of a blocked nose, with its likely side-effects of headache, partial deafness and nasal speech, may be relieved by inhaling steam. The warmth of the steam soothes the nose and helps to clear the airways, and if medication such as menthol is added the benefits are increased. Special vaporizers can be bought that produce steam for several hours; these are good for relieving bronchitis as well as stuffy noses. Alternatively you can pour boiling water onto menthol or any other over-the-counter inhalant and inhale the steam; putting a towel over your head as shown *above* helps to concentrate the steam.

Nosebleeds
The lining of the nose is rich in tiny blood vessels that are very near the surface, and these may easily be broken by scratching the inside of the nose, by blowing the nose too hard, or by being hit on the nose. The result is a nosebleed, sometimes very alarming in appearance as the nose seems to be pouring blood. The most effective way to halt a nosebleed is to pinch the lower part of the nose gently, or to press the thumb against the affected side, as shown *above*. Hold the pressure for about 10 minutes, and do not sniff or blow the nose or you may prevent the blood from clotting.

Teeth and gums 1

In the Western world we have the most comprehensive dental services and public dental health programs, and yet probably have the world's worst teeth. Dental cavities are among the most prevalent medical problems in many Western countries. This condition arises mainly because of the high sugar content of our diet, aggravated by poor personal dental hygiene. Many people have a full set of dentures by middle age, but this can be avoided if the teeth and gums are adequately cared for through childhood and adulthood. Here we look at many of the ways in which you can take care of your teeth, whatever their present state and whatever your age, so that trouble in the future will be minimized.

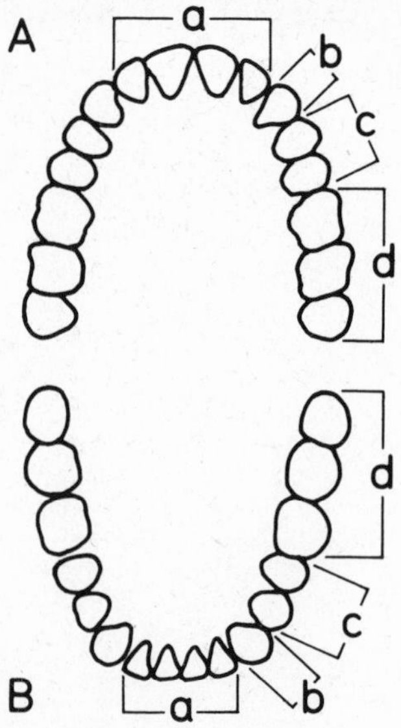

Different types of teeth
The diagrams show the arrangement of the upper (**A**) and lower (**B**) teeth in the complete dentition of an adult.
a Incisors; these are teeth with sharp, flat tops.
b Canines; these are pointed teeth.
c Premolars; these are the small double teeth.
d Molars; these are larger double teeth. The third molars on each side, top and bottom, are known as the wisdom teeth. The primary dentition of children contains only the incisors, canines and premolars; the first permanent molars emerge at about age 6.

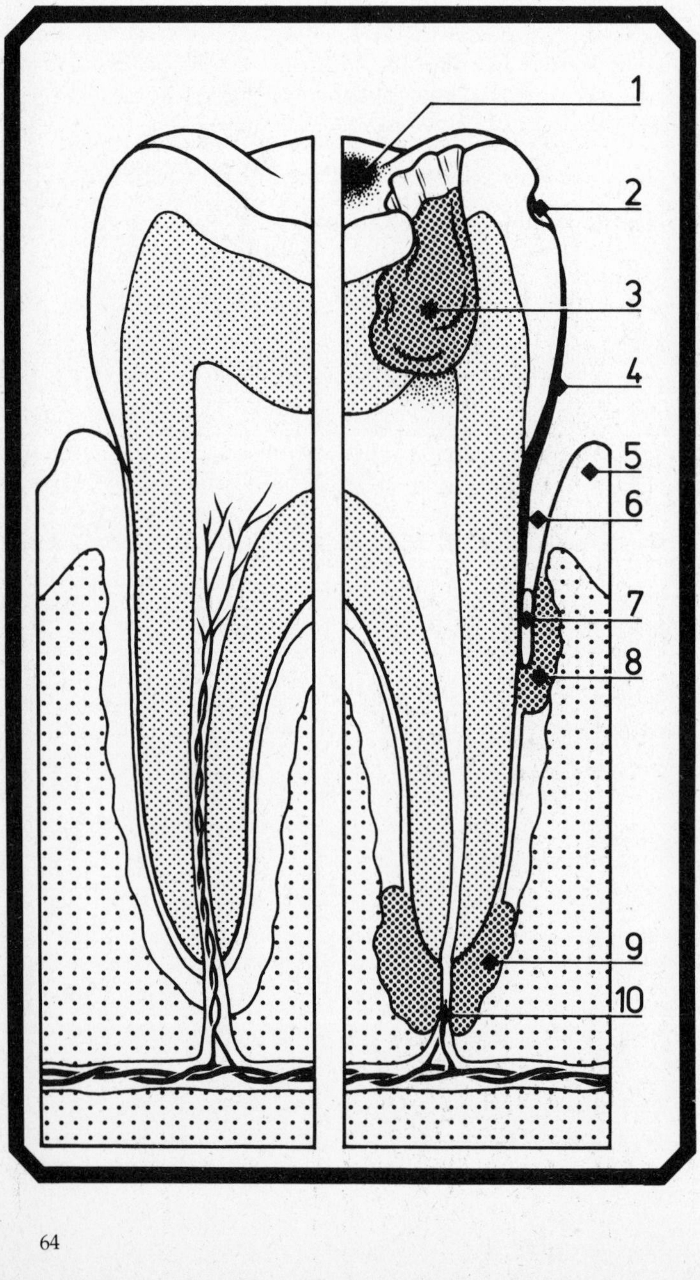

Tooth and gum problems
The illustration shows some of the common problems that may arise as a result of poor dental hygiene.
1 Discoloration of the tooth; this may be a result of excessive smoking, or excessive consumption of tea or coffee, or it may be an indication that the pulp at the center of the tooth is dead. Some drugs may cause permanent discoloration of children's teeth.
2 Small cavity; this cavity, caused by tooth decay, is still confined to the enamel of the tooth and has not yet reached the sensitive dentine and pulp.
3 Large cavity; here the tooth has decayed right down to the central pulp where the nerves of the tooth are found, causing first of all pain and sensitivity and finally death of the pulp.
4 Plaque, a sticky, bacteria-filled film that builds up on the tooth as a result of ineffective cleaning. If plaque is not removed, it hardens into a substance known as calculus or tartar.
5 Gingivitis, an inflammation of the gums caused by plaque accumulation. This problem is aggravated by adverse conditions in the biological balance of the mouth.
6 Periodontal pocket caused by the breakdown of the bone and fibrous attachments holding the tooth in the gum. As more of the periodontal attachments decay, the tooth loosens and finally drops out.
7 Debris, plaque and tartar, collected in the periodontal pocket. Even meticulous cleaning cannot remove debris that is located so far under the gum, and once pockets are formed debris and plaque build up rapidly, leading to foul breath and infection.
8 Gumboil or periodontal abscess caused by the decay of debris in the periodontal pocket and the subsequent infection.
9 Abscess at the base of the tooth, caused by bacteria in the decaying tooth pulp. Since the infection has no escape route, great pain is caused.
10 Loss of blood supply to the tooth causes death of the pulp, which in a healthy tooth has its own blood supply.

Treat your teeth gently
Teeth can be damaged through careless habits or by failing to protect them properly in specific situations. Never open bottles or crack nuts with your teeth as this can permanently damage them by cracking the enamel, and do not bite sewing thread as the edges of the front teeth will be worn away. Do not chew habitually on hard objects such as pens and pencils, and do not bite your nails or grind your teeth. If you're involved in sports such as hockey, boxing or karate, where you are likely to receive blows in the face, wear a gum-shield to protect your teeth.

Brushing instructions
The illustrations show brushing techniques recommended for maximum efficiency in plaque removal.
1 Place the brush against the teeth as shown and move it slightly from side to side so that the bristles reach into the gap between the teeth and the gums.
2 When the bristles are well-positioned, brush away from the gums with a slightly rocking action. Repeat steps 1 and 2 on the insides and outsides of the top and bottom teeth.
3 Brush to and fro across the top surfaces of the teeth.
4 Brush the insides of the front teeth by tilting the brush and brushing away from the gums.

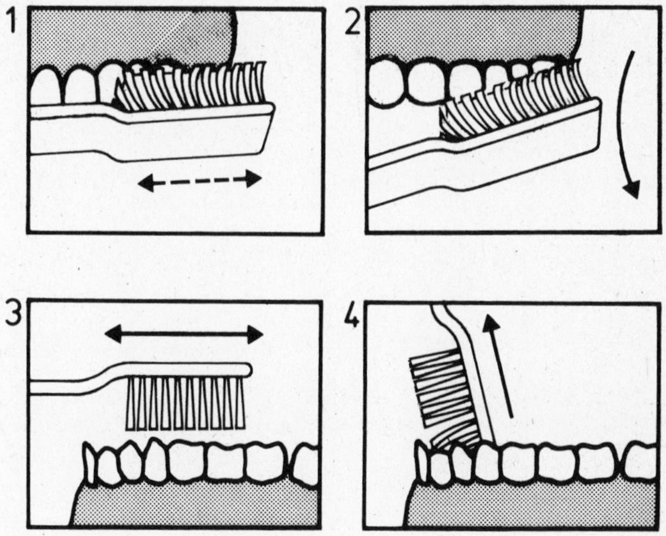

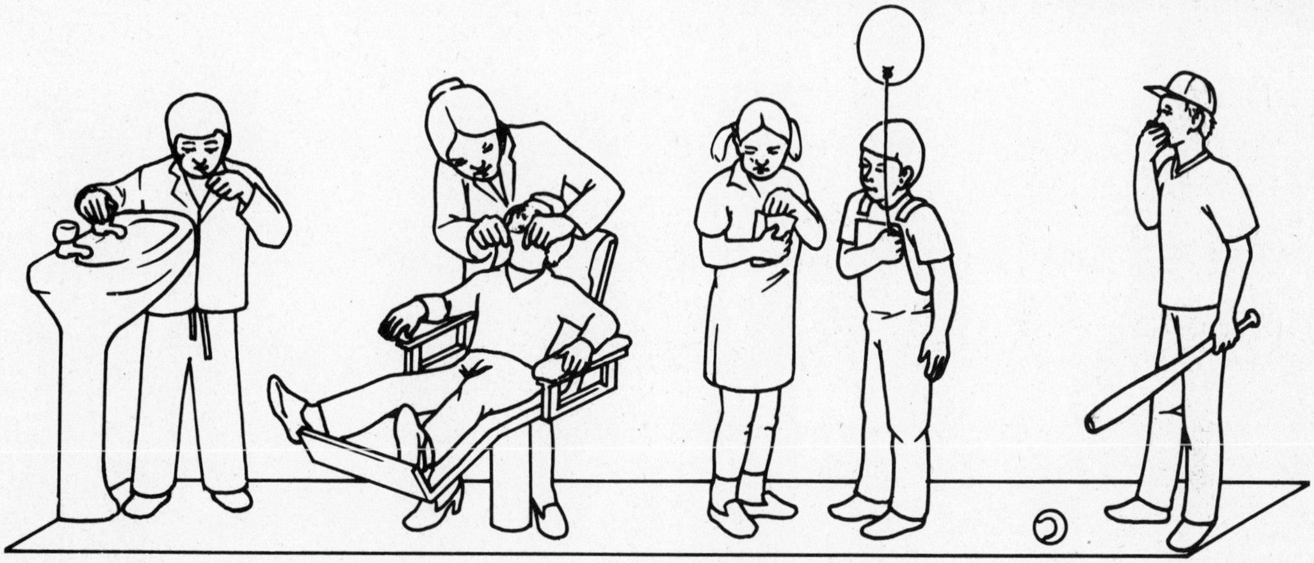

Brushing the teeth
Brushing is one way to fight tooth decay, as it removes most of the plaque and bacteria from the surfaces of the teeth. Your toothbrush should have a small head, with medium-firm multi-tufted nylon bristles; it should be changed as soon as the bristles begin to splay. Teeth should be brushed after every meal, as acid begins to form immediately; plaque collects in a matter of hours. Even babies' and toddlers' teeth should be brushed, and children should be taught good brushing habits as soon as they are old enough to clean their own teeth.

Professional tooth care
Professional tooth care is always worth any expense involved, as you are investing in future good health. The dentist should be seen two or three times a year for a check-up and for oral hygiene advice; he and the dental hygienist will advise you on the best hygiene routine for your teeth and gums, and demonstrate good brushing and flossing techniques. The dentist may help in decay prevention by applying fluorides or fissure sealants to your teeth, and if decay does set in he will be able to arrest its progress with crowns or fillings. Thorough professional cleaning will remove any built-up tartar.

Teeth and your diet
Taking care of your teeth should involve some attention to diet, as sensible eating habits will help protect your teeth from unnecessary disease and decay. Cut down drastically the number of times each day that you eat sweet or starchy food; sugar and starch form acid in your mouth and attack your teeth immediately. Ideally you should only eat sweet foods, including candy and sodas, at mealtimes, and then clean your teeth to remove the sugar from your mouth. If you have snacks between meals, eat nuts or raw vegetables; crisp foods such as carrots or celery also help to remove debris from the teeth. Avoid sugared tea and coffee between meals.

Accidents to your teeth
Even people who take good care of their teeth can suffer mishaps. If you chip your teeth or lose a filling or crown, see a dentist as soon as possible, as decay can set in if the soft dentine of the tooth is left unprotected. If your teeth become sensitive to hot and cold, your dentist will check them for decay; if no decay is present he may recommend a brand of toothpaste specially formulated for sensitive teeth. If you have a tooth knocked out, rinse it in clean water and replace it in the socket, and then rush to the hospital or to a dentist; it may be possible to splint the tooth so that it can reestablish itself in the gum.

Teeth and gums 2

Back-up care
As well as regular brushing, there are a number of other dental aids that will help you to clean your teeth more efficiently. It is very difficult for ordinary toothbrushes to clean adequately between the teeth, and this is where food debris tends to collect, often leading to hidden cavities that only become apparent when they begin to cause pain. The aids shown *right*, used after you have brushed your teeth as thoroughly as possible, will increase the effectiveness of your home dental care.
1 An interdental brush has short, stiff bristles that are particularly effective for brushing between the teeth; the angled head helps you to reach otherwise inaccessible parts of your teeth.
2 Disclosing tablets stain plaque bright red, and will show you the places that you have not cleaned adequately.
3 Dental floss is a twisted thread that should be wound around the two second fingers and moved up and down between the teeth until all plaque is removed from those areas.
4 In particular cases your dentist may prescribe wooden toothpicks as an aid to plaque removal; the toothpick should be held with the flat surface against the gum to avoid traumatizing the skin.

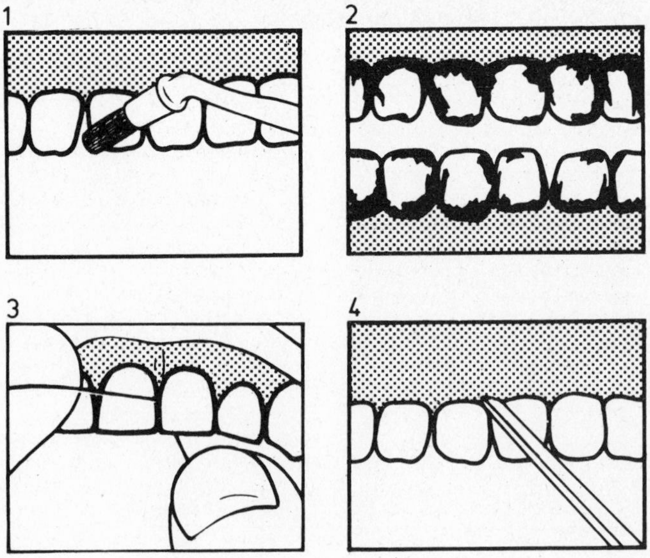

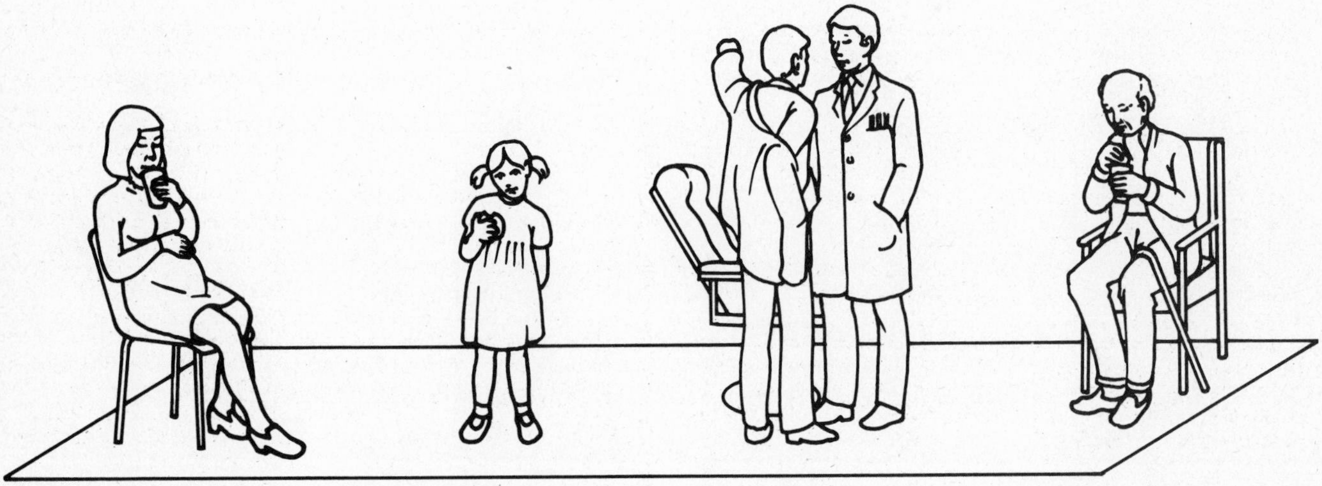

Care during pregnancy
During its development and growth in the uterus the child's first teeth are forming, utilizing calcium from the mother's body. Consequently, if the mother's diet does not include sufficient calcium, her teeth will suffer as the calcium is diverted for the baby's body to utilize. Taking a good supply of calcium in milk, cheese and yoghurt should ensure that the mother's teeth remain healthy, and she should visit the dentist at least once during pregnancy. Although it is not now believed that drinking fluoridated water during pregnancy will benefit the child's teeth, fluoride supplements during infancy will do so.

Care in childhood
Many people neglect to teach their children tooth care, as they argue that the baby teeth are going to drop out anyway. But children should be taught good dental hygiene so that it becomes automatic, and also because the first permanent teeth appear at age six or seven and should be cherished if they are to last a lifetime. Teach your children to brush their teeth after every meal, and to use disclosing tablets so that they know they have done it properly. Don't allow them to eat candies, cookies and sweet drinks between meals; give them crisp vegetables and fruit for school snacks. Above all, try to set a good example.

Care in adulthood
By adulthood, all the permanent teeth are in place, although the wisdom teeth may still be partly submerged by the gums. With good care, there is no reason why these teeth should not see you into old age. Continue to brush your teeth regularly, and visit a dentist immediately if you have any pain. If there is one area of your teeth that you find persistently hard to clean, the dentist will advise you how to tackle it or send you for orthodontic treatment. If your teeth are particularly craggy, he may fill the fissures in your double teeth with sealant, preventing debris from lodging there.

Care in old age
Care of the teeth in the elderly is an important aspect of total health, as bad teeth can make it difficult for the elderly person to eat sufficient roughage and adequately nutritious food. Decreased flexibility may make it harder to clean the teeth effectively, but it is worth persisting. If you have a full or partial denture, it should be removed after every meal and cleaned using a soft brush with soap and water or a recommended cleaner. If the denture is taken out at night, it should always be kept in water or a sterilizing agent. See your dentist regularly in case your denture needs adjusting.

Halitosis
Halitosis, or bad breath, is most often caused by neglect of some part of the dental hygiene routine. If there are untreated cavities in the teeth, the bacteria in these can cause bad breath, and so can the bacteria in decaying food debris or plaque building up around the teeth and gums. Sore throats, sinus problems and digestive troubles can all lead to severe halitosis. If you suffer from bad breath, first of all see a dentist, who will help you to clear up any problems originating from the teeth or gums; if the problem lies elsewhere, a doctor will be able to help. Mouthwashes and gargles will do little to ease the problem as they do not remove the infection at its source.

Mouth ulcers
Although the causes of these vary considerably and are sometimes unidentifiable, they can be caused by various problems relating to the teeth and gums. Inadequate cleaning of the back teeth can lead to a build-up of plaque or debris that will eat away at the gum and form an ulcer. If there is an abrasion such as a chipped tooth, a ragged filling or an ill-fitting denture, constant movement against the cheek may cause an ulcer; see a dentist for the remedy. If an ulcer persists for more than a week or two seek a doctor's advice, as persistent ulcers may be the first signs of cancer.

Gingivitis
This complaint is an infection of the gums caused by their constant contact with plaque that has collected where the teeth meet the gums. The gums become red and inflamed, often painfully, and are prone to bleeding when the teeth are cleaned; this makes correct brushing difficult, and aggravates the problem. To prevent gingivitis, ensure that all plaque is removed from the teeth and gums regularly. Brush the gums as well as the teeth during your dental hygiene routine; this will keep them healthy and help to stimulate their blood supply.

Periodontitis
When infection spreads to the fibrous attachments that hold the teeth in the jaw these are broken down and form a pocket between tooth and gum. Food debris and plaque collect in this pocket, out of the reach of a toothbrush, and perpetuate the problem, leading to foul breath, pus and abscesses; the teeth are loosened by the destruction of still more of the attachments, and eventually fall out. Many perfectly sound teeth are lost in this way. Prompt dental treatment and strict oral hygiene are essential if the course of this unpleasant disease is to be halted.

Diet and the teeth
A great deal of research has been done into the effects of particular foods on the formation of dental caries. One of the most important findings is that a substantial decrease in the sucrose (table sugar) content of the diet leads to a corresponding decrease in the incidence of caries. This is so even when the total carbohydrate balance in the diet is not reduced, which implies that starches are not as cariogenic (caries-causing) as sucrose. Sucrose, which is the commonly-used sweetening agent in home cooking and in beverages, is far more cariogenic than the sugars fructose (found in fruit) and glucose. Sugars are particularly likely to cause caries if they are ingested in a sticky form that can easily remain on the teeth, for instance when they are eaten as honey, molasses, syrup or soft candy. The longer the sugar remains in the saliva, the more the teeth are damaged; this underlines the need for cleaning the teeth after meals. Research is still being done into the cariogenicity of non-sugar sweeteners.

Foods for healthy teeth
Foods that are high in sugar should be drastically reduced in your diet to ensure healthy teeth and gums. There is a great deal of sugar in candy, cakes, soft drinks, chocolate drinks, pastries and jelly; sugar is also a common "hidden ingredient" in such foods as hamburgers, salad dressings and mayonnaise. All these foods should only be eaten at mealtimes, when the teeth are going to be cleaned directly afterward. Fresh fruit and vegetables are generally very good for the teeth, especially if they are crisp and are eaten raw, but some, particularly apples, are high in sugar. Starch is converted into sugar by the saliva, and then forms acid in the mouth in the same way; although starches have not been implicated in dental caries as seriously as sugars, they should not be eaten in excessive quantities. Foods containing a great deal of starch include cookies, pastries, bread, crackers, french fries and potato chips. Foods that contain little sugar and starch, and which will help to promote healthy teeth, include carrots, tomatoes, rhubarb, mushrooms, green vegetables, cucumbers, marrows and squashes.

Do
- Cut down the sugar and starch in your diet.
- Eat crisp fruit and raw vegetables.
- Clean your teeth after every meal.
- Use the correct brushing action.
- Use back-up techniques such as dental floss, interdental brushing and gum massage.
- Give an infant or toddler prescribed fluoride supplements if you live in an area without fluoridated water.
- Ensure that your daily diet contains a pint of milk or its equivalent in yoghurt or cheese if you are pregnant.
- Visit the dentist regularly.
- Wash dentures after every meal.
- Have any dentures checked regularly for fit.
- Visit your dentist at the first sign of gingivitis or tooth damage.

Don't
- Eat a diet high in sugar and starch.
- Eat sweet or starchy foods between meals.
- Constantly chew gum or candy.
- Allow food debris to remain on your teeth after a meal.
- Neglect the spaces between your teeth when removing plaque.
- Try to cover bad breath with mouthwashes or gargles.
- Use an old or splayed toothbrush.
- Use anyone else's toothbrush.
- Use a toothbrush that is too hard or too soft.
- Scrub at your teeth so that bacteria are driven under the gums.
- Open bottles or hair pins, crack nuts or break thread with your teeth.

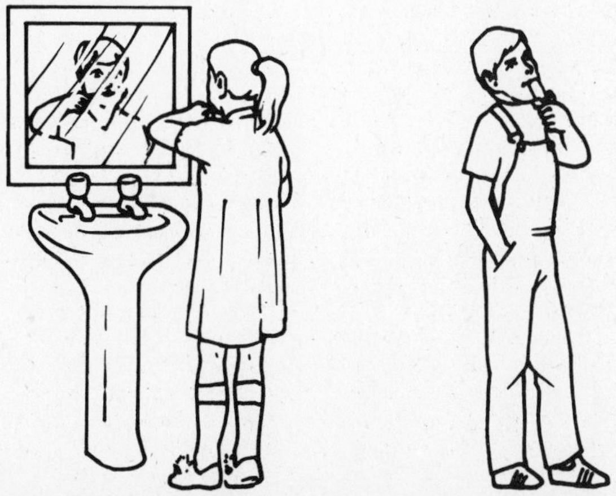

Bones and joints 1

There are more than 250 bones inside a human body that serve as shields, struts and levers. They help to produce blood, store valuable minerals, and protect the vital organs. Each type of bone is designed to serve a special purpose. Flat bones like the hip bones, breastbone, shoulder blades and skull shield or cradle vulnerable organs. Long bones like those of limbs and ribs act as levers; these use tough elastic linkages called ligaments, soft cartilage buffers at bone ends, and lubricating fluid produced by the synovial membrane that lines joints at such places as ankle, elbow and shoulder. Disease and accident may damage bones or the accessories that keep them working, but dislocation, sprain, fracture and even potentially disabling arthritis are treatable.

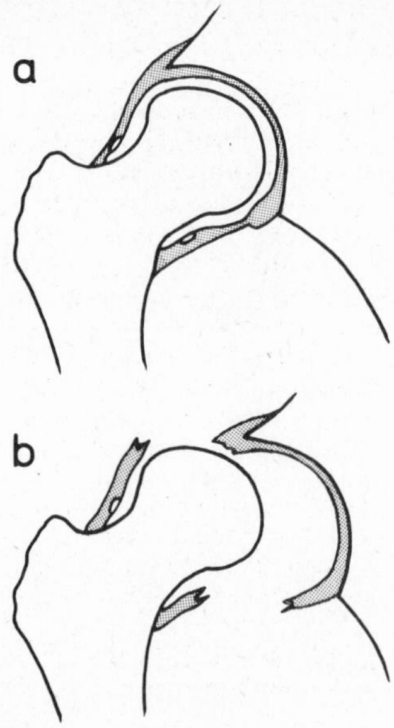

Dislocations
The finger, thumb, shoulder and jaw are the most common dislocation sites, followed by the hip and knee. A joint (**a**) is dislocated when an injury tears ligaments that keep two bone surfaces in place (**b**). There will be swelling, pain and stiffness, possibly even an undiscovered fracture. Never try to push the separated bones together; you could make the damage worse. Instead, simply support the damaged joint in the position where it feels most comfortable and seek medical attention. Doctors will manipulate the joint to return it to the right position. Full joint recovery can take several weeks.

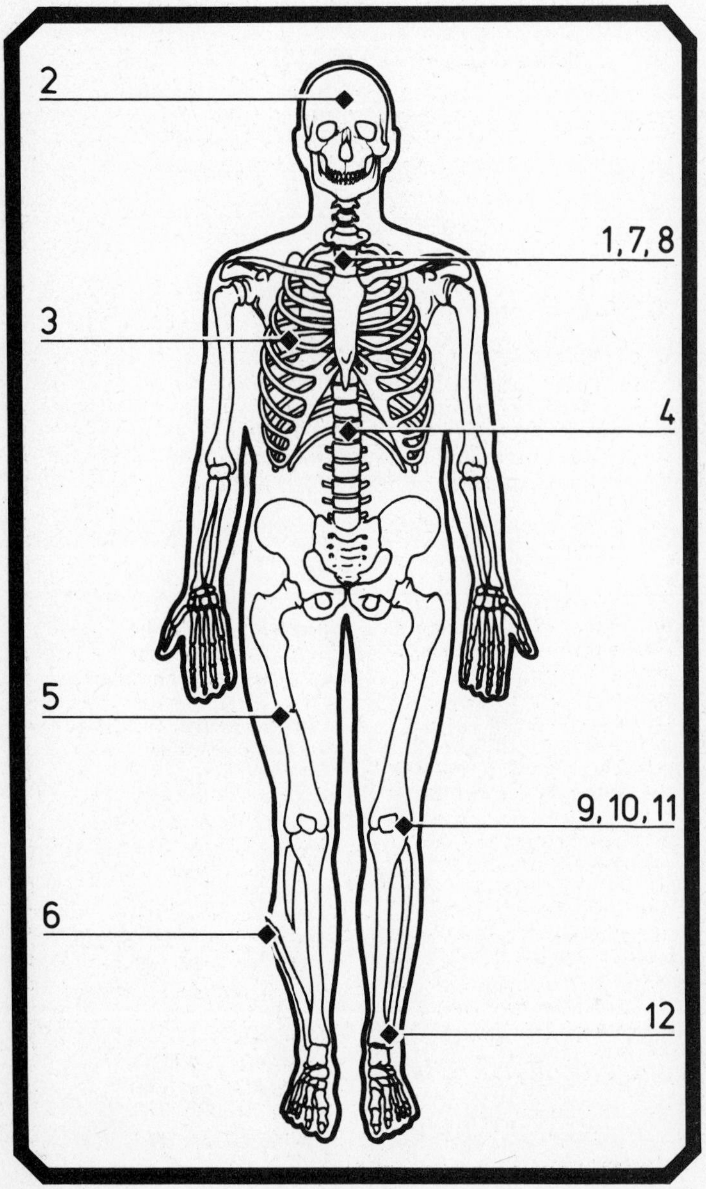

Bone and joint problems
1 Osteoporosis; abnormal thinning of bone makes it brittle and a slight jolt may cause a fracture, for instance of vertebrae. Occurring in post-menopausal women and the old, osteoporosis may be treated by the drug calcitonin. Old people should take extra care to avoid falling.
2 Skull fracture is suggested if head injury is followed by loss of blood or watery fluid from ear or nose, or if the eyes grow bloodshot. Place a sterile dressing over the affected ear or nostril, lay the patient on the affected side, and get him to a hospital.
3 Rib fracture is suggested after a chest injury if there is pain on deep breathing, perhaps with coughed up blood or a sucking noise from a chest wound. Loosen tight neck, chest, and waist clothing, and lay the patient down with his back and head propped up; seal any wound, especially a sucking one, with a dressing, and call an ambulance.
4 Pelvic and spinal fractures are likely if injury causes back or pelvic pain, the patient cannot stand, and his lower body feels numb. Keep him still and warm (with a coat or blanket) and call an ambulance.
5 Greenstick fracture involves splintering of a bone's outer surface. As in many fractures there is pain, swelling and loss of use of the limb or part of the limb.
6 Compound fracture; a broken bone pierces the skin and there may be much bleeding.
7 Whiplash injury; ligaments and muscles around the fifth cervical vertabra are torn by sudden head movement, often in an automobile crash. Treatment involves wearing a sponge rubber collar for some weeks.
8 Slipped disk; this involves the pulpy center of one of the semi-cartilaginous disks between the vertebrae poking out through a torn ligament. There is dull, aching back pain worsened by jolting or coughing.
9 Osteoarthritis occurs when the cartilage of weightbearing joints degenerates, producing audible creaking of bones and stiff, aching joints.
10 Rheumatoid arthritis is inflammation of tissues lining joints, producing swollen, stiff joints: it is very painful, and may eventually produce deformities and immobility.
11 Bursitis – inflammation of lubricant sacs between bones, tendons and muscles – produces local tenderness and swelling. Housemaid's knee and bunions are examples of bursitis.
12 Sprains are caused by damage to ligaments connecting joints such as those in the ankle, back and wrist.

Slipped disk
Many people wrongly blame minor back troubles on a slipped (or ruptured) intervertebral disk. But if doctors diagnose this trouble the treatment takes several weeks. The patient must spend the time lying on a firm bed; if the mattress is soft, a board should be placed under it. Moist heat applied as hot packs can help, but most patients need analgesics to relieve pain. Doctors may advise wearing a lumbar corset or undergoing traction. Surgery to remove the ruptured piece of disk is a last resort. Anyone with a history of slipped disk trouble should seek medical advice before starting on a program of exercises.

Arthritis
Dieting helps overweight people to reduce the stress suffered by osteoarthritic joints. Other aids include improving poor posture; a walking stick held in the hand opposite the worst-affected hip, knee or ankle joint; and non-weight-bearing exercises (such as swimming) that rebuild wasted muscles without stressing the affected joints. A surgeon may replace severely damaged joints with artificial ones. Painkillers and anti-inflammatory drugs help this and rheumatoid arthritis; sufferers of the latter also benefit from physiotherapy and rest. Often rheumatoid arthritis becomes inactive before serious damage occurs.

Bursitis
Inflammation of a bursa (a sac containing lubricating fluid to protect the end of a bone) is best controlled by resting the joint and avoiding the activity that caused the trouble. Thus the type of bursa called a bunion improves if the patient wears well-fitting shoes (see pp. 122–123). As another example, a baseball pitcher may suffer bursitis in the shoulder, which will be relieved by resting the pitching arm. Aspirin and locally applied heat are other aids. If bursitis persists, the joint may need splinting to immobilize it. Sometimes doctors relieve symptoms by injecting steroid drugs into the affected part.

Osteopaths and others
When orthodox medicine yields no relief for sufferers of back pain and similar conditions many people try osteopathy, chiropractic or acupuncture. Osteopaths treat dislocations and some other conditions by manipulating joints or muscles. Chiropractors manipulate the spine because they think that displaced vertebrae pressing on the spinal cord cause disease. Acupuncturists treat diseases by inserting needles into so-called vital points in the body. Orthodox medical experts argue that such treatments are ill founded, but many admit that sometimes they seem to work.

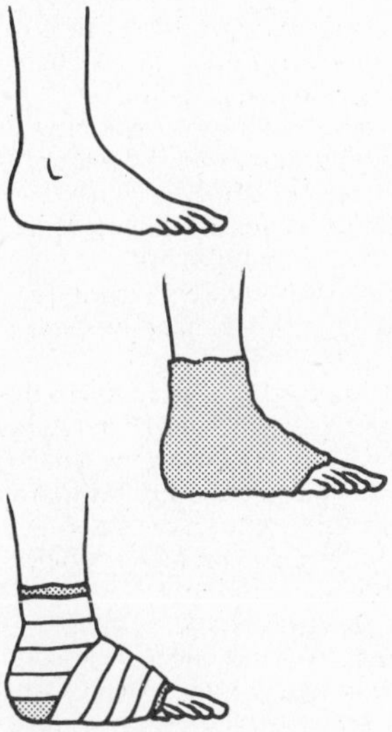

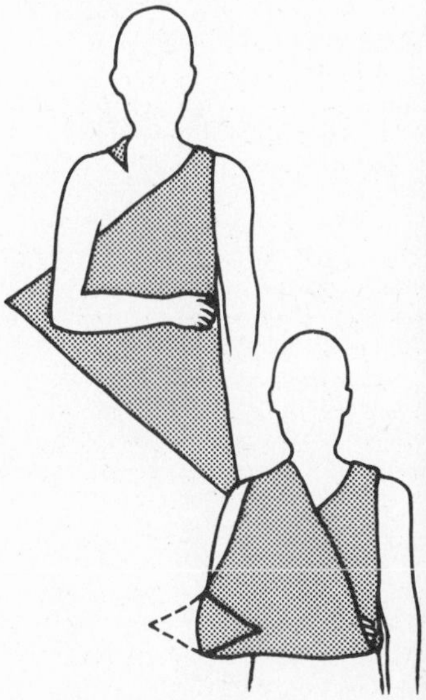

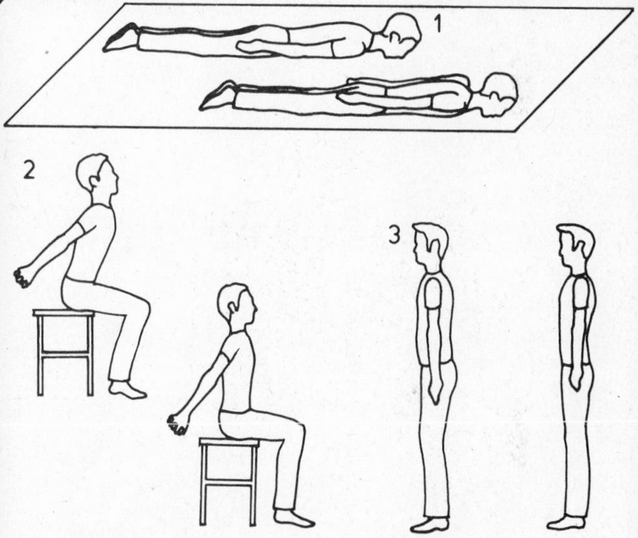

Sprains
Treat torn or bruised ligaments (for instance in a knee or an ankle) by resting the injured part. With firm support and gentle use a sprained ankle may recover in only a few days. A cold compress is useful for first aid; treatment is by deep massage to disperse blood and fluid that has collected round the injury, and the application of a firm elastic bandage. The diagrams *above* show the procedure for a sprained ankle. First, lay a thick layer of cotton over the ankle, then firmly fix in place by bandaging. You may need to add a second layer of cotton covered with a second bandage. If the sprain is still painful take mild analgesics. If you suspect there may be a fracture seek medical advice.

Fractures
Immobilize any part of the body with a suspected fracture until you can get medical attention. For an arm make a sling, as shown *above*, by folding a headscarf or dish towel into a triangle. Support the arm across the chest. If the fracture is near the elbow, bandage the straight arm to the body; if necessary, for instance for a fractured clavicle, place a pad in the armpit or between arm and body. Bandage a fractured leg to the good leg above the knee and around the feet, avoiding the fractured area. You can similarly bind a broken finger to its neighbor. If broken bone pokes through the skin, first cover with a sterile dressing.

Advice for backache sufferers
Unless advised otherwise by a doctor, sit on hard, straight-backed chairs; sleep on a firm mattress; and organize work surfaces so that you do not have to lean forward. To get into bed, face the bed, placing both hands on it for support. Raise one knee at a time onto the bed. Crawl into position and roll onto your side, using a pillow to keep your head and spine in line. To get out of bed point your feet toward the foot of the bed; ease one leg over the edge of the bed as you half rise, then lower the second leg to the floor, supporting your trunk with both hands. Stand slowly.

Exercises for backache
Unless doctors advise otherwise, backache sufferers (other than those with slipped disks) may benefit from these exercises; do each exercise twice daily.
1 Lie face down with your arms at your sides; contract your abdomen and buttocks and bring your shoulder blades together.
2 With your hands clasped behind you, bend forward as you lift your head and bring your shoulder blades together. Pull both hands down and back, and sit upright.
3 Stand erect, and hold your head up as you contract your abdomen and buttocks. Hold this position for five seconds.

Bones and joints 2

Keeping the various parts of the musculoskeletal system in balanced relationship with one another – in other words cultivating good posture – can play a vital role in preventing or treating backache and certain other ailments. Maintaining correct posture reduces the risk of accidents in everyday living and working, as well as in play and sport. It also delays or prevents onset of osteoarthritis due to injury. On the other hand, bad posture produces poor muscle coordination and hampers circulation, thus handicapping would-be sportsmen and leaving anyone less energy at the day's end for active recreation. Back strain risks increase if you have poor posture, if you bend or lift incorrectly, if you wear wedge or platform shoes, or if you are pregnant or obese.

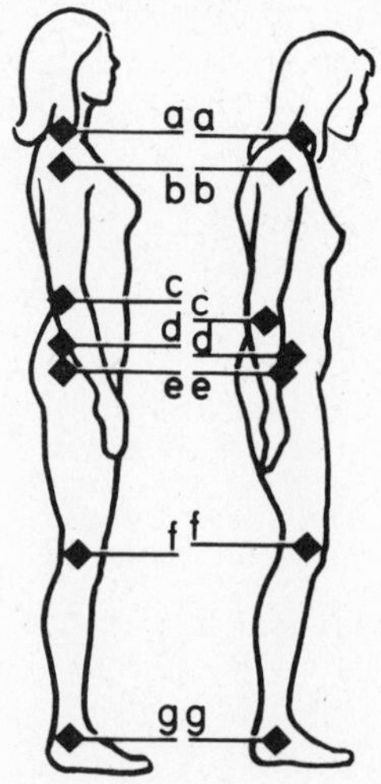

Posture and alignment
People with good posture stand so you could draw a vertical line through certain key points of the body. Check your posture against the key points listed here, standing sideways to a full-length mirror. Pull your head up, shoulders back, chest out. Keep your back straight, arms loosely at the sides, buttocks relaxed, knees slightly bent, weight evenly distributed. But avoid a tense posture; be relaxed.

a Neck.
b Shoulders.
c Lower back.
d Pelvis.
e Hip joints.
f Knee joints.
g Ankle joints.

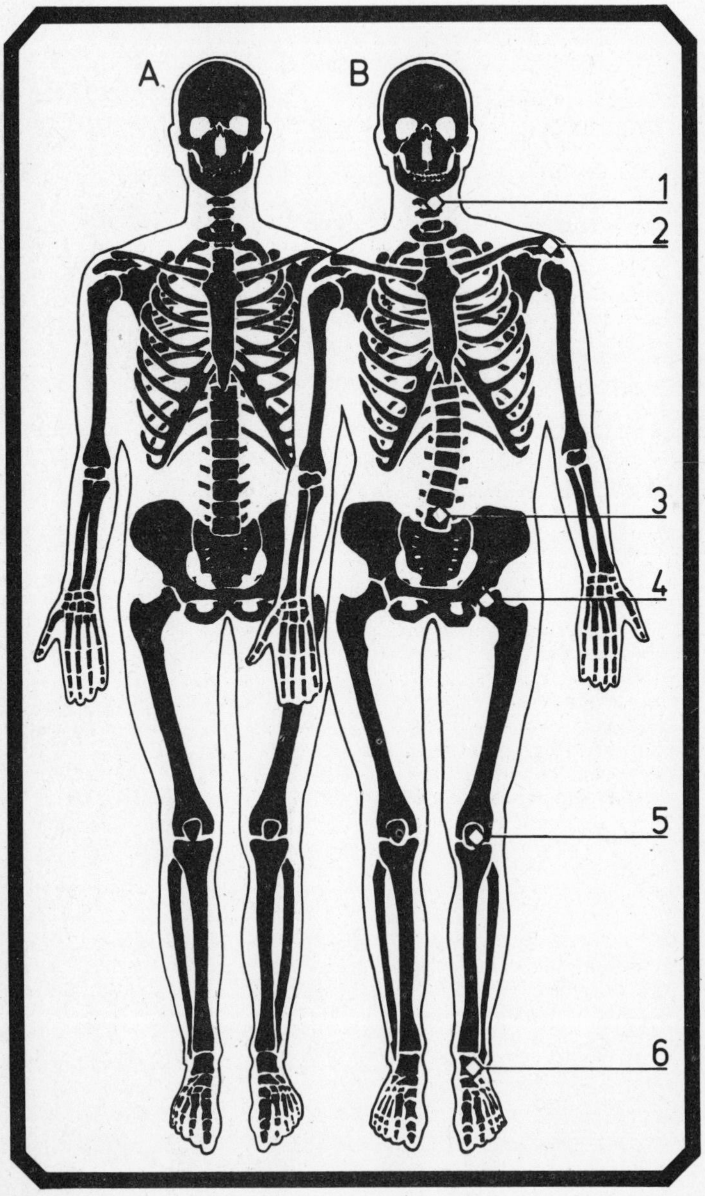

Postural problems
Two bodies *left* show how posture affects alignments in the skeleton. Body **A** stands correctly balanced so that the spine (seen from the front) is vertical, and the bones of both shoulders, both hips, and both hands are horizontally aligned. Body **B** adopts an awkwardly unbalanced posture in which the spine curves to one side and the body's symmetry has been destroyed so that shoulders, hips and hands are tilted. Poor postural control means that key sections of the body are supported by unbalanced sets of muscles and ligaments, and the following troubles may be caused.

1 Head-neck junction:
Headaches.
Muscle pain in neck and upper back.
Disk degeneration.

2 Shoulder girdles:
Painful shoulder muscles.
Capsulitis.
Pinched nerve.

3 Lumbo-sacral articulations:
Low-back pain.
Disk degeneration.
Sciatica.

4 Hip joints:
Muscle strain affecting buttocks and hamstrings.

5 Knee joints:
Strained ligaments.
Strained tendons.
Osteoarthritis.

6 Feet and ankles:
Strained and painful muscles in foot and leg.
Painful knee, hip and ankle joints.
Stress fractures likely.
Varicose veins.

The Alexander principle
Frederick Matthias Alexander of Tasmania proposed one of the most influential of several theories suggesting that a wide range of ailments is triggered by skeletal distortion due to habitual poor posture.
Many of the remedial guidelines recommended by medical practitioners today are based on Alexander's methods for correcting bad posture and poor body use. Alexander argued that after childhood people adopt an easy slumping posture. This often means that the neck is slanted sideways, forward or backward – distortion compensated for by misalignment lower in the spine. He urged re-education of bone and muscle in action and at rest to create a body in balance around the spinal cord. Alexander recommended realigning the vertebrae to loosen the spine and correct its misalignment. He proposed bringing shoulders out forward; tucking in the abdomen; and tilting the pelvis slightly up and forward. (All this is easier if the knees are slightly bent.) At the same time people should avoid "unhealthy" muscular reactions to stress or physical constraints. Alexander believed physical re-education only works if the individual is constantly aware of how he holds himself. The rewards, so Alexander held, are twofold: not just improved physical wellbeing, but also better mental health.

Spinal disorders
These include scoliosis, where the spine curves to one side, and lordosis, where the spine's lumbar vertebrae curve inward. Some such spinal conditions are progressive; others are less serious and respond better to exercises. If doctors approve, scoliosis sufferers can try these exercises.
1 Kneel with arms above your head, then bend forward from the hips and touch the floor. Walking on your knees, pivot right then left around your hands.
2 Kneeling on one knee propped by the opposite arm, lift and extend the other arm and leg in line with the body; repeat with opposite limbs.

1

2
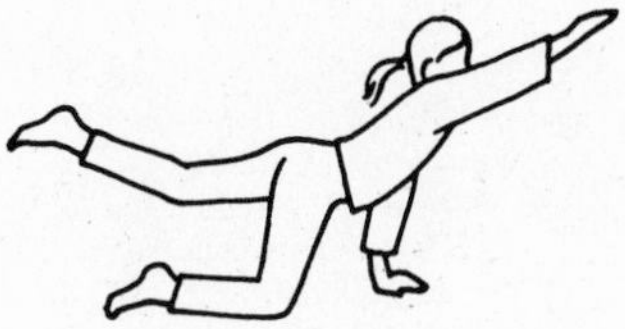

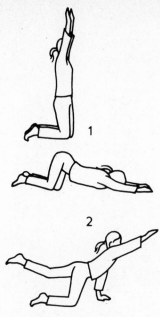

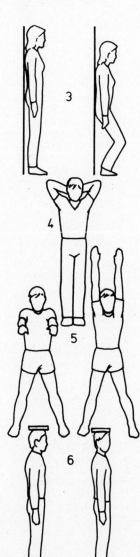

Posture and daily activity
Using the body correctly to perform daily chores can help to prevent straining the back and so avoid back injuries. Keep your back as straight as you can to lift a load from the floor: kneel or squat, do not bend. Open a drawer or put food in the oven in the same way. If kneeling to clean a floor, raise your buttocks so that hips and shoulders support the spine. When carrying a load in one hand, balance it with a load in the other, or half support it on a hip. Sit with the pelvis touching the back of the chair and keep a slight spinal curve. Aim to keep the body's local centers of gravity aligned directly above its base.

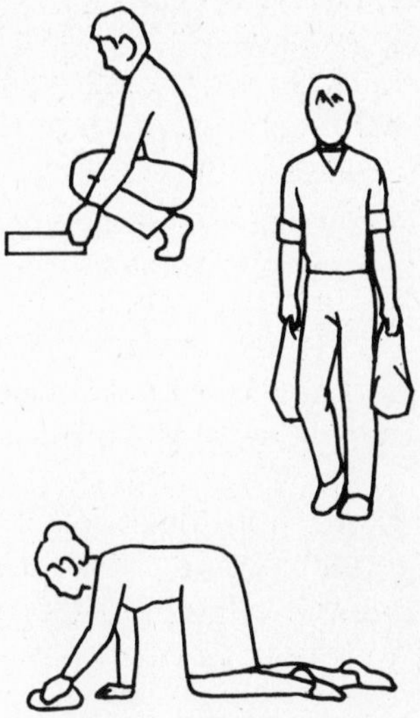

Posture exercises
Some simple exercises help to relieve aches and pains caused by maintaining a position for some time without moving. Rotate the shoulders, neck, trunk or any other joint that feels stiff. Rotating the affected joint helps relax muscles. Habitually bad posture may be improved by regularly practicing the following exercises. Relax your body apart from the muscles involved in exercising.
3 Stand with your back against a wall. Slightly bend the knees, tilt the pelvis upward, lower the head and broaden the shoulders.
4 Stand with correct posture. Clasp your hands behind your neck; pull the elbows back and up and hold for 5 seconds.
5 Stand with feet well apart, and holding your arms straight raise them forward then up so that your shoulders brush your ears. Continue moving your arms to complete a backward circle. Try this exercise 5 – 10 times.
6 Stand with correct posture and balance a book on your head. Turn your head right then left, counting 5 in each position. Pointing one foot forward, rise on the toes of the other foot. Count 5 then try the other leg, still balancing your book. Now bend your knees and count 5, then straighten. Repeat 5 times.

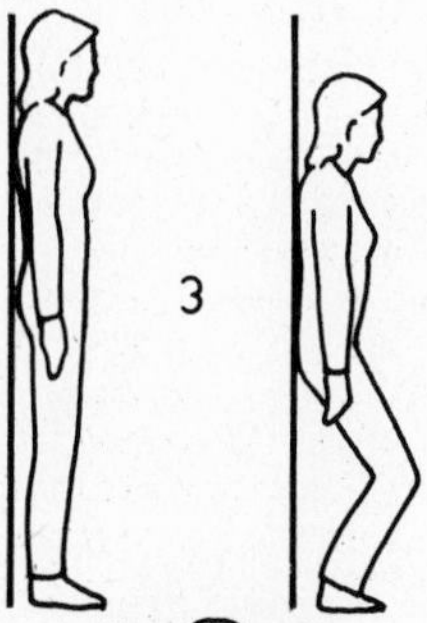
3

4
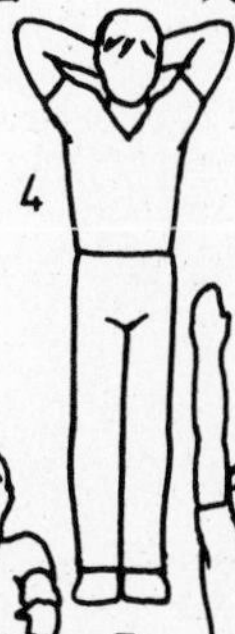

5

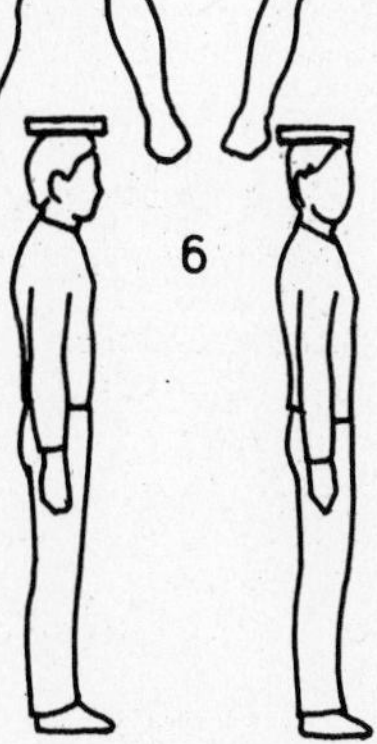
6

7 As you sit down make sure your neck and spine are aligned, and, keeping your back straight, bend at the hips and knees. Once seated avoid slumping.
8 Sitting upright against a straight-backed chair bring both arms together behind your head so that each hand can touch the elbow of the other arm. Count 5. Repeat 3 times. A variant of this is clasping forearms behind the chair and pulling your shoulders back. Hold the position for 10 seconds.
9 Sitting with your hands on your hips bend your body to the left and hold it there, counting 5. Then bend your body to the right. Repeat 3 times for each side.
10 Lie flat on your back on the floor. Place your arms out at the sides, with palms downward. Bring both knees up and arch your back without lifting your buttocks off the floor. Next, flatten your spine against the floor. Then tighten buttocks and lift them. Meanwhile keep shoulders and arms on the floor. Repeat all this three times.

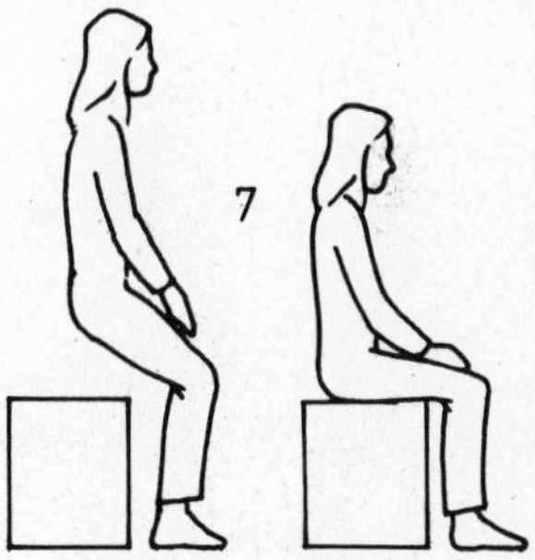
7

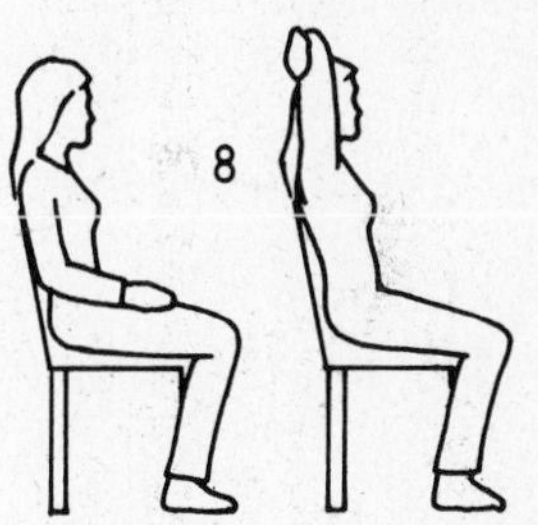
8

9
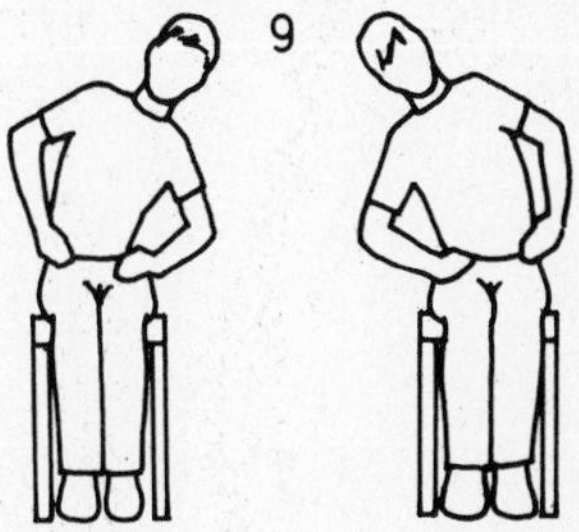

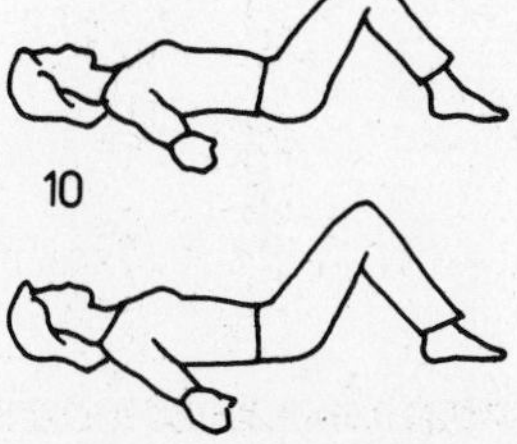
10

Muscles 1

Muscle is strong, elastic tissue that moves limbs, pumps blood and nutrients round the body, controls air movement in and out of the lungs, and drives food through the esophagus and intestines. Muscles are basically bundles of fibers activated by nerve cells. A nerve stimulus makes a muscle contract. When the stimulus stops, the muscle relaxes and lengthens. Many muscles are joined to bones, directly or by tough white cords called tendons. Muscles working as opposing pairs operate each limb. When one muscle in a pair contracts the other relaxes, and vice versa. By coordinating their activities, opposing muscles make it possible to move the limbs. Exercise helps to keep muscles fully functional. Many muscle problems stem from underused, fatigued, torn, or strained muscle fibers and tendons.

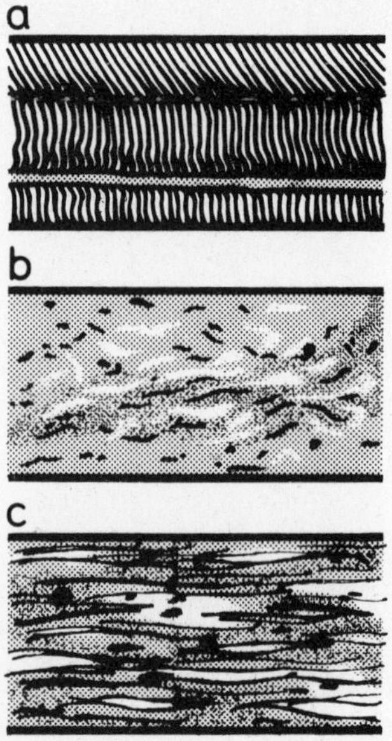

Muscle types
There are three main types of muscle in the body.
a Voluntary (also called skeletal or striped) muscle comprises parallel bundles of fibers that look striped when seen under a microscope. We can consciously control these muscles, which make up much of the arms, legs, face, neck, chest and abdomen.
b Involuntary (or smooth) muscle contracts in a slower, more rhythmic, way than striped muscle, and is made somewhat differently. It occurs in the walls of stomach and intestines and works automatically.
c Cardiac (heart) muscle is striped rather like voluntary muscle but works automatically.

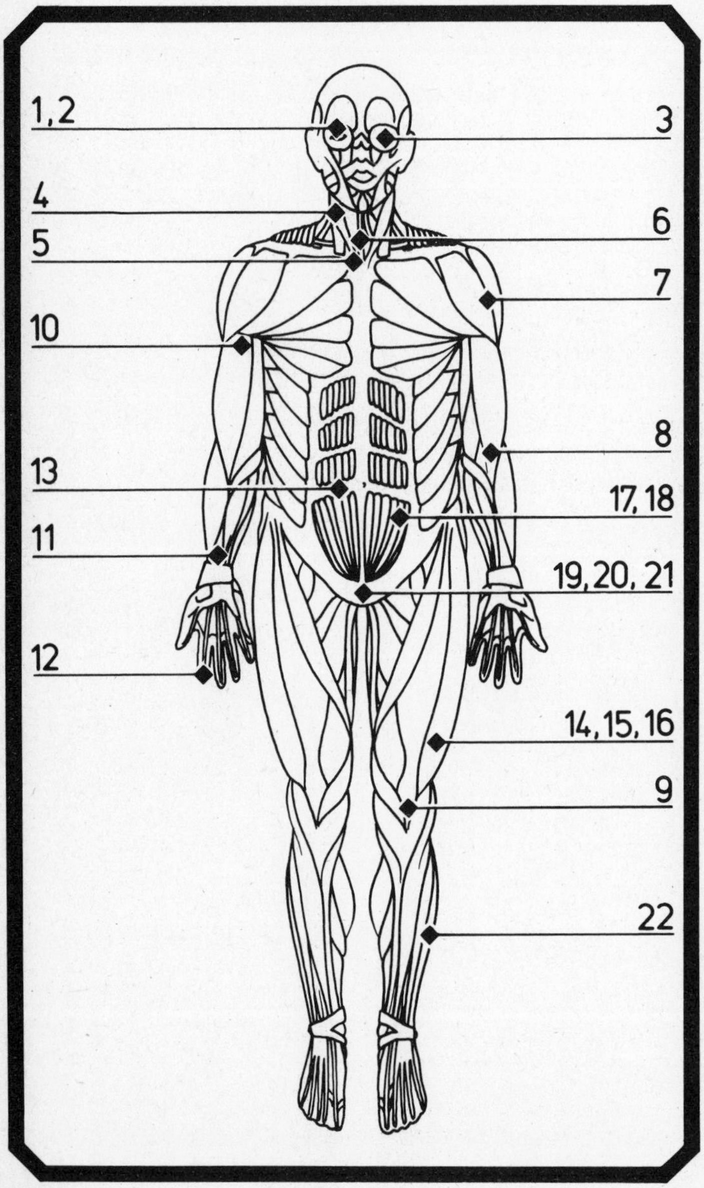

Sites of problems
The following troubles show up in muscles or tendons but some are rooted in disorders of the nerves that operate them.
1 Tics: blinking, mouth-twitching, nose-wrinkling and head-shaking are typical habit spasms; a non-critical attitude toward the person affected is helpful.
2 Bell's palsy is paralysis of the facial nerve affecting one eyelid and one side of the forehead and mouth. It is usually only temporary.
3 Crossed eyes (strabismus): the eyes are unable to work as a pair because muscles that control eyeball movements are imbalanced.
4 Stiff neck: this is often a mild disorder caused by muscle cramp due to sudden twisting, sleeping uncomfortably, or chill.
5 Spasm of involuntary muscle affecting the bronchial tubes produces asthma symptoms.
6 Choking is often triggered by swallowing a foreign body, aggravated by muscle spasm (see also p. 96).
7 Tenosynovitis (inflammation of the lubricating sheath around a tendon) may affect shoulder, elbow, wrist, hip, thigh, knee, or ankle.
8 Bursitis (inflammation of a sac lubricating a joint) can be caused by a calcium deposit on a tendon. A painful shoulder, elbow, or knee results.
9 Torn tendons often occur at joints where strong forces act, for instance the knee and ankle.
10 Ruptured biceps (at upper end) may occur in middle-aged people who lift or pull heavy weights.
11 Wrist ganglion is a painless lump in the wrist produced by a cyst affecting a tendon (see p.116).
12 Raynaud's disease (see p.88) involves spasm affecting blood vessels in the fingers.
13 Stitch is a spasm of the diaphragm that may be caused by poor breathing in exercise.
14 Cerebral palsy can produce twitching limbs and partial facial paralysis.
15 Poliomyelitis is a viral disease that may paralyze limbs. Oral vaccine prevents it.
16 Muscular dystrophy involves wasting and loss of use of muscles. Many forms tend to be inherited; tests before birth can detect the disease in a fetus.
17 Lumbago is a vague term for low back pain.
18 Strains often affect muscles in the neck, lower back, arm, wrist, leg and ankle.
19 Spasms or loss of muscle control sometimes affect sphincter muscles controlling the pylorus (stomach outlet), gallbladder, urethra or anus.
20 Vaginismus is spasm of the vaginal opening (see p 173).
21 Irritable bowel syndrome is caused by spasms disturbing muscular bowel activity, due to nervous stress or enteritis.
22 Cramp is muscular spasm often associated with the calf muscles.

Rheumatism
This is a general term often used for aches, pains, stiffness or limited movement affecting muscles, tendons or connective tissues binding others together. Many doctors prefer the term nonarticular rheumatism for soft-tissue disorders so as to avoid confusion with arthritis, which affects the muscle of the joints. Nonarticular rheumatism includes tendon problems and fibrositis (here covered separately), also scores of other so-called rheumatic diseases, some ill-understood and for which there is no effective remedy. Lack of widespread specialist advice leads many sufferers to try scientifically unproven cures.

Tendon troubles
Tendons are tough and seldom injured. But rising suddenly on the toes in racket sports may rupture the Achilles tendon of the heel, producing intense pain and swelling. Weeks in plaster follow surgical repair. Sometimes strain or rheumatic ailments inflame tendons or their lubricating sheaths, producing conditions respectively called tendinitis and tenosynovitis, with local pain or tenderness. Much walking in new or unsuitable shoes can strain the Achilles tendon. Treatment includes resting the affected joints; physiotherapy; administering drugs or local anesthetic; or surgery.

Fibrositis
This is a vague term describing irritative disorders affecting muscles, tendons and ligaments. People with fibrositis tend to feel tenderness and stiffness in a place that is not in fact the actual site of trouble. Neck injury can thus cause elbow pain. If you are unused to them, strenuous sports or other physical activities may trigger fibrositis. The direct cause is often injury producing neck or back strain. An influenza-type infection or extensive arthritis can also cause fibrositis. Patients may need painkilling drugs, local anesthetics, and local heat. Massage and skilled manipulation of affected areas are also often beneficial.

Cramp
Cramp is pain produced when a voluntary muscle suffers spasm (abnormal contraction). This often occurs in muscle fatigue when oxygen supply to a muscle cannot keep up with demand. Lack of sodium in the body can also trigger cramp by affecting the electrical charge on a muscle. This kind of cramp can happen after heavy sweating, or in bed at night. To relieve cramp, try gradually stretching the affected muscle. Cramp caused by sodium deficiency may be cured by ½ teaspoonful of salt in water. Taking salt tablets and avoiding large meals before events help athletes to avoid cramp. If you get cramp often, see a doctor.

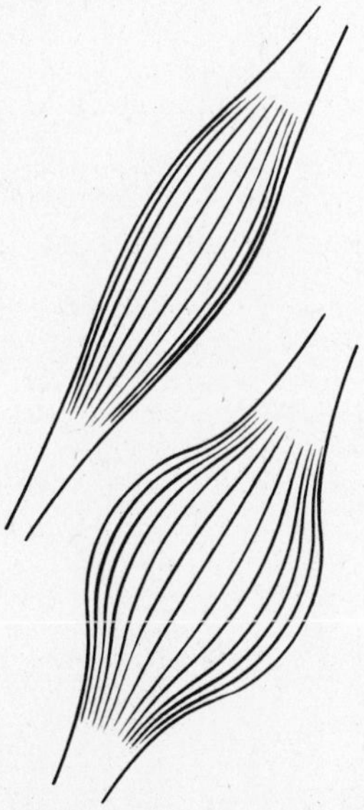

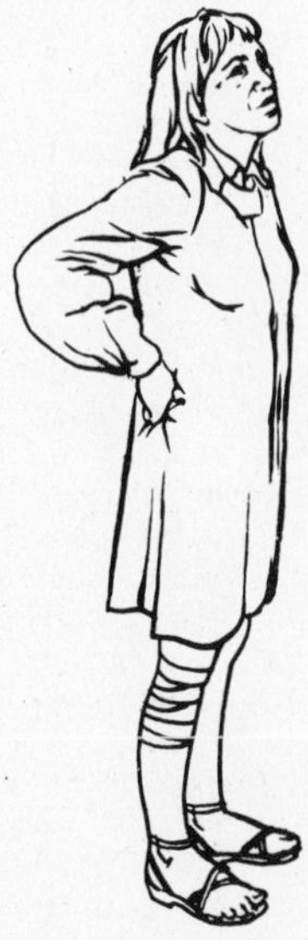

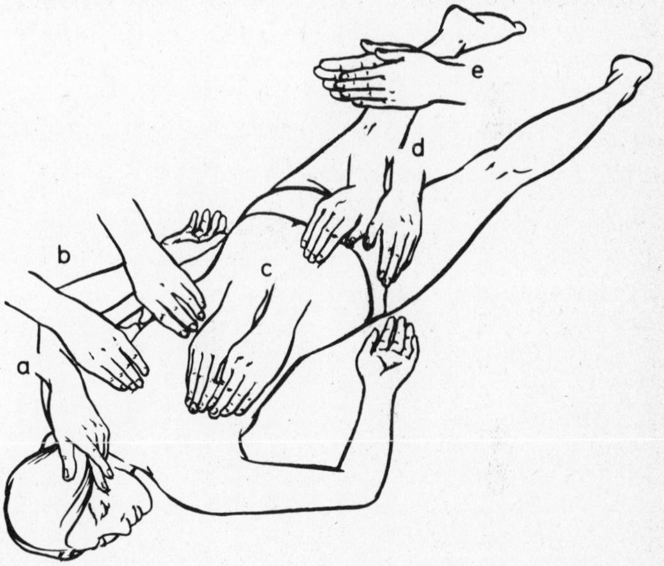

Muscle spasms
These are severe and sudden uncontrolled contractions of voluntary or involuntary muscle. They may occur in various parts of the body in several ways. Steady contraction is called tonic spasm; alternating contraction and relaxation is called clonic spasm. Muscle spasm can have physical or emotional causes. For example, tetany, featuring spasms of the wrists and feet, may be due to parathyroid deficiency (treated by calcium given under medical supervision). Vaginismus (tightening of muscles at the vaginal opening upon attempted intercourse) may be emotional in origin (see p. 173).

Muscle strains
Strains are injuries stretching muscles or tendons without tearing their fibers. A strain is liable to happen if you suddenly twist your arm, slip, or take a wrong step. Any of these acts may overstretch a muscle, causing sudden, sharp pain and local tenderness, but without bruising or swelling. You find you cannot use the muscle as well as usual but it is easier to use and less painful than if it had been sprained. Resting the muscle for 24 hours helps quick recovery. If the muscle is in an arm or leg, support it with an elastic bandage. Daily massage with mild liniment is also useful while the strained muscle remains tender.

Massage
Kneading a person's bare skin can help to alleviate fibrositis and some other muscle troubles. Massage tends to stretch and so relax muscle fibers, reducing knots of hard, tense tissue, and stimulating blood flow. Skilled massage of various areas of the body can relieve muscle tension caused by stress, overwork, and physical strain. Spreading oil or talc on the skin before massage reduces the friction of the hands against the skin. The diagrams *above* show some of the various massage methods. In most of the techniques the masseur fits his hands to the person's muscle contours and works with unbroken strokes of even pressure, starting lightly and then using more body weight to increase the pressure. Many people find massage more effective if the strokes move toward the heart.
a Massage with the fingertips.
b Massage with the thumbs.
c Massage with the fingers.
d Massage with the flat of the hand.
e Massage with the edges of the hands.
Pressure massage involves applying pressure with the fingertips, thumbs, elbows and palms of the hands to specific pressure points in the body; the pressure may last from five to ten seconds, depending on the part of the body being massaged.

Muscles 2

Exercises to build muscular strength and endurance help make the body healthy, firm, strong and well-proportioned. Few of us want massive muscles (women are unlikely to develop them anyway), so exercise repetition is preferable to strenuousness. Inexperienced and older people may suffer strains and sprains, so build your training program slowly, starting with few repetitions, light weights, and long rests between exercises. Wait an hour after eating before you start. Limber up with simple exercises before weightlifting. Exercising for 15 minutes every other day is enough. After exercise take a warm shower and do not eat for 30 minutes. Besides exercising as described here, also try jogging, cycling, and swimming.

Agonists and antagonists
Pairs of muscles working in opposite directions are known as agonists (or prime movers) and antagonists. The biceps and triceps muscles in an arm form one such pair. When a biceps muscle contracts (**a**) to bend an arm, a triceps muscle (**b**) relaxes, so that the biceps acts as agonist and the triceps as antagonist. When a triceps muscle contracts (**c**) to straighten an arm, a biceps muscle relaxes (**d**), so that the triceps becomes the agonist and the biceps the antagonist. Other types of muscle help to make such movements possible. For instance, fixation muscles steady the shoulder blade to make a base for moving the arm.

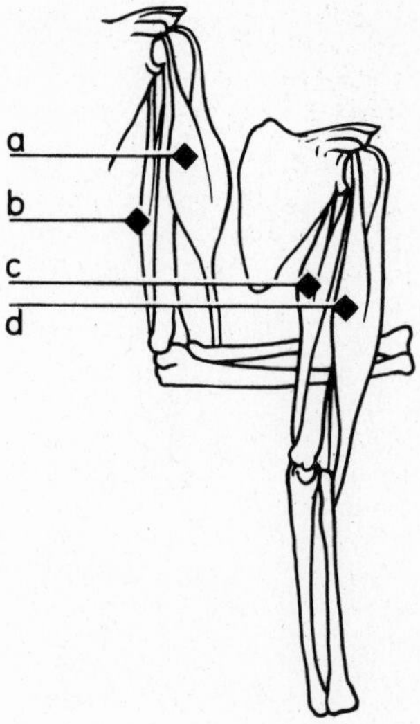

Isometric exercises
Since these use all potential muscle strength instead of the 20–30% customarily exerted, they have significant effects on muscles. To avoid strains or other trouble limit each exercise to 6 seconds and perform it only once a day. Here are some exercises for the upper body.
1 Interlock the fingers of both hands behind your head. Push your hands forward and head back. Repeat with interlocked fingers pressed back against your forehead as you try to force your head forward.
2 Sit at a table or flat-topped desk and press your hands down upon its surface, with your fingers spread wide apart. You can repeat this while standing.
3 Sitting on a chair without arms, grip the sides of the seat and try to pull it upward.
4 Stand near a wall, facing it with your arms straight down and the palms of your hands toward the wall. Press your hands against the wall as hard as possible.
5 Stand facing a doorjamb and place the palms of both hands on opposite sides of the jamb at waist height. Press your hands hard toward each other. Relax and repeat, first at chest level, then at eye level.
6 Stand in a doorway and raise your arms to press the palms of your hands hard against the top of the door frame. You may need to stand on a box.

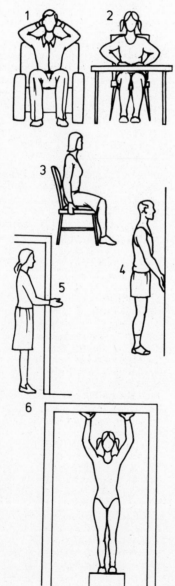

Isometric exercises
Six-second isometric exercises for legs, waist and sides:
7 Sitting on a chair, grip the sides of the seat, stretch both legs in front of you and raise them with the right ankle crossed over the left. Press the inside of your right foot and the outside of your left foot against each other as hard as you can. Then vice versa.
8 Standing with your left side close to a wall, rest the left hand and left foot on the wall. Then push your foot hard against it. Standing with your right side close to the wall, repeat, but now using your right foot.
9 Stand with feet apart while your left heel holds down one end of a towel and your left hand grips the other end of it. Place the right hand on the right hip and pull hard at the towel with your left hand. Keep your head, shoulder, arm and foot in a vertical line. Repeat, using the right hand and foot.
10 Lie on your back with your knees raised, and grip a book in both hands held behind your neck. Now try sitting up by bending but not arching your back. Pull up as far as possible.
11 Lie on your back with your legs straight and feet together, folding both arms behind your head. Try pulling in your abdomen as far as possible.
12 Lying face down, with your hands at your sides, raise one leg and press the foot up under a table. Repeat with the other foot.

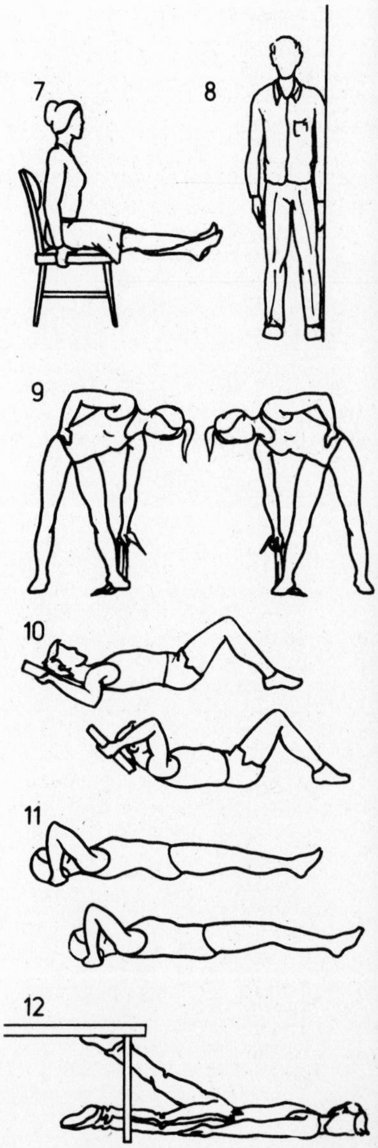

Isometrics
These are static exercises in which one group of muscles exerts pressure on another group or on an immovable object, with no change in muscle length or joint movement (hence the name isometric, meaning "same length"). Isometric exercises are aimed at building muscle strength and tone. They take up little time – just 6 seconds exerting maximum muscle force for one exercise and 90 seconds for 15 exercises covering the whole body. Moreover they require no special equipment. But they leave the heart-lung system unexercised and strain the heart in anyone with heart trouble or high blood pressure.

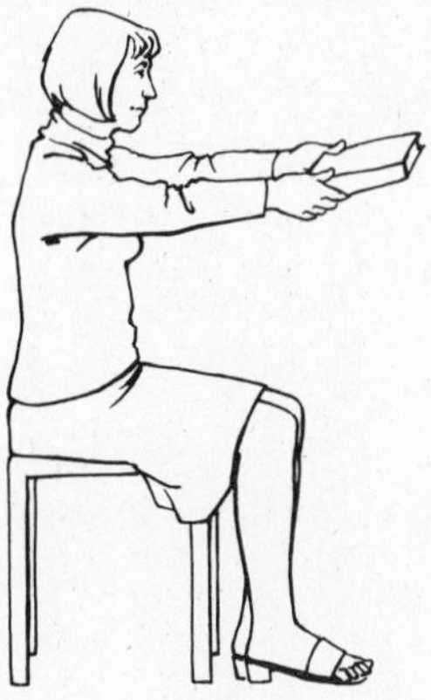

Isotonics
Isotonic exercises involve shifting a resistance through the range of movement possible for a particular joint or joints. This helps to build isotonic strength or endurance. Isotonic strength is best built by means of high-resistance, low repetition exercises. Isotonic endurance is best built by lower resistance, high-repetition exercises. You can measure isotonic strength by the weight of the resistance that you move, and isotonic endurance by the number of limb-muscle contractions achieved against a measured resistance. Weightlifting and other bodybuilding activities are the main isotonic exercises.

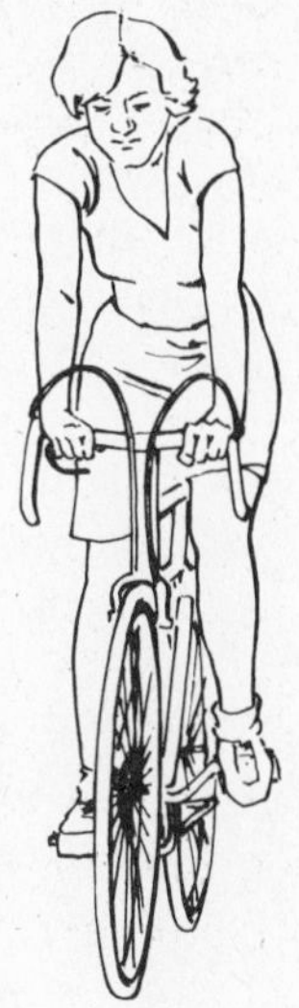

Isotonics for strength
These exercises strengthen various parts of the body. Develop them gradually.
13 Crouch with a dumbbell in each hand, knuckles uppermost, keeping your back straight. Then stand up, bending your arms and lifting the dumbbells to shoulder height. Next, thrust the dumbbells to arm's length above the head. Such exercises help strengthen arm and shoulder muscles.
14 With both hands grip an expander in front of you at arm's length and shoulder level. Keeping both arms straight, pull them out and back until the expander touches your chest. This helps to strengthen chest and upper abdominal muscles.
15 Using weighted boots or foot weights, stand with your hands on your hips and stretch your right leg to the side as far as you can. Then bring the leg across the body as far as you can. Repeat with the other leg.
16 Stand with your feet about 15in apart under a barbell. Bend your knees and grasp the bar with both hands, knuckles uppermost; your hands should be just farther apart than your shoulders. Keeping your chest and head up and your back flat, breathe in and rise to a standing position, pulling the bar up to touch your upper chest under your chin. Turn your hands to bring the palms up, and breathe out. This strengthens the whole body.

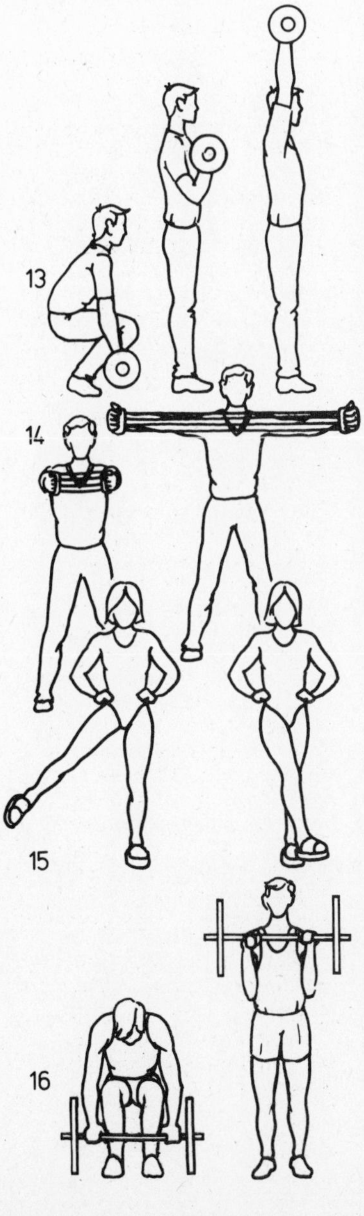

Isotonics for endurance
Shown here are some of the exercises that can be used to build up muscle endurance rather than muscle strength.
17 Push-ups (p.36) are classic exercises for increasing the endurance of the muscles in the arms and shoulders in particular.
18 Squat thrusts (p.41) improve the endurance of shoulder and leg muscles; as you become more competent, increase the demands on your body by standing upright in between each squat thrust.
19 Sit-ups (p.40) are good for exercising the abdominal muscles; as your muscles improve you will be able to perform them without anchoring your feet.
20 To improve the endurance of your shoulder muscles, lie on your back with your hands behind your head as for sit-ups, but only lift your head and shoulders without bending at the waist; repeat this as many times as possible.
21 Sit-ups on a sloping bench will increase your muscle endurance even more than the ordinary version of the exercise.
22 Lie face down on the floor with your arms out to the sides; lift your arms and legs simultaneously as high as possible. Lower, and repeat as many times as you can; the endurance of the muscles of the shoulders, arms, abdomen, hips, thighs and calves will be improved.

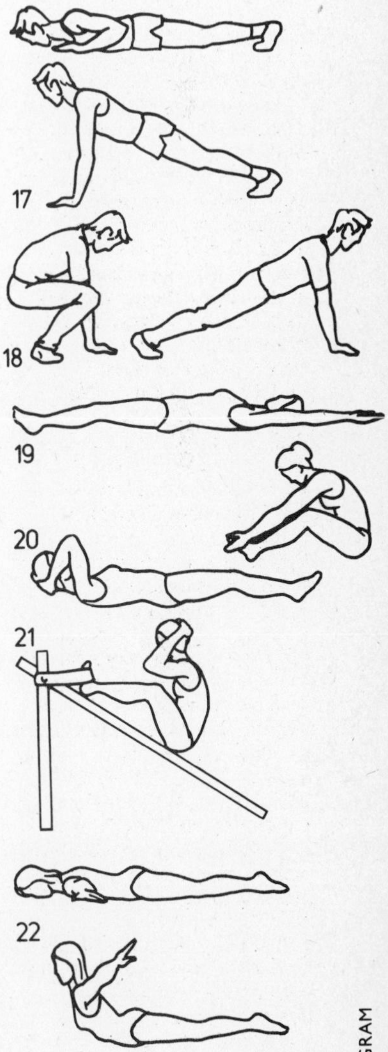

Skin 1

Skin is one of the body's largest, most important organs. It provides a waterproof barrier that keeps germs, dirt and other harmful substances outside the body. Its sweat glands and blood vessels help to control the body's temperature. Sebaceous glands release an oily substance that helps to waterproof the skin and keep the hair shiny. Nerve endings sense heat, cold, pain and pressure. Infections, irritations, faulty glands, cuts and burns, are common causes of skin problems. Good general health helps to ensure a healthy skin, and skin care also involves protecting the skin from intense heat, cold, sunlight, and certain chemicals. On these pages we look at some of the many common skin problems.

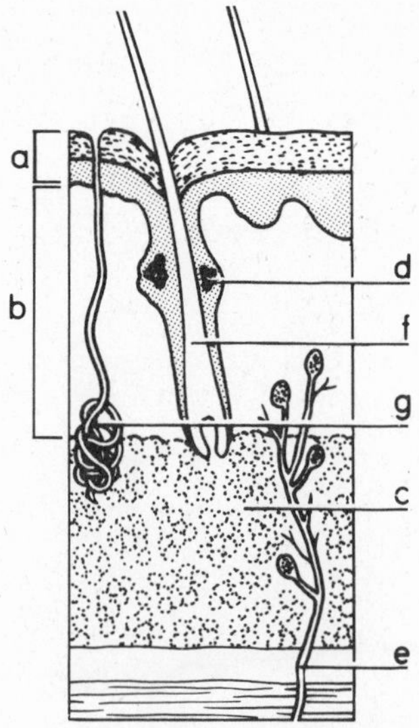

Skin structure
Skin is tissue comprising two main layers. The thin top layer or epidermis consists of flat, dead cells forming a flexible, tough, waterproof surface. Dead cells that rub off are replaced by others. Below this layer is a thicker one: the dermis. This layer contains sweat glands, sebaceous glands, hair follicles (cavities), nerve endings, blood vessels and other units. Below dermis and epidermis is a fatty layer.
a Epidermis
b Dermis
c Subcutaneous tissue
d Sebaceous gland
e Nerve
f Hair follicle
g Sweat gland

Sites of common skin problems
1 Acne, blackheads and sebaceous cysts all tend to be triggered by overproductive sebaceous glands, a condition that often occurs for hormonal reasons in adolescence (see p.78). The areas mostly affected are the face, neck, shoulders and back.
2 Bedsores, or pressure sores, may develop on the elbows, hips, buttocks, ankles and heels of bedridden people. Areas of skin become red and ulcerate. Shifting the patient's position hourly helps to prevent pressure sores.
3 Birthmarks can occur on any part of the body (see p.78).
4 Boils generally occur on the face, neck, back, armpits and buttocks; they are highly infectious (see p.78).
5 Corns and calluses are hardened patches of skin that occur on the toes, heels or balls of the feet as a result of pressure from ill-fitting footwear (see pp. 122–123).
6 Contact dermatitis is a skin inflammation and rash occurring on areas of skin in contact with irritants. Some people react allergically to cosmetics, dyes or other substances that leave most of us unaffected; the skin burns, stings and itches, and it may ooze clear fluid. The areas most affected are the face (from cosmetics or soaps), the neck (from jewelry) and the hands. Steroids taken orally relieve itching, but patients should avoid contact with the irritant.
7 Diaper rash affects babies' skin in contact with urine-soaked diapers (see p.103). A similar rash may appear in older people if they become incontinent.
8 Eczema, or atopic dermatitis, produces red, raised patches on the face or the knee and elbow creases. It is a constitutional disorder that usually appears in infancy; it may clear up at ages 2–3, but recur later in life. Eczema may be subdued by taking oral antihistamines, and keeping irritants away from the skin; using coal-tar ointment may also help.
9 Fungus infections occur in various forms. One form is ringworm, which produces expanding scaly rings on the trunk and elsewhere; this condition can be intensely itchy. All forms of ringworm respond well to griseofulvin taken orally. Another common fungus infection is athlete's foot, which produces painful splits and sores between the toes. Athlete's foot is often spread in baths and locker rooms; drying the feet thoroughly after communal bathing may help to prevent it (see pp.122–123).
10 Herpes is a virus that occurs in two main forms. Cold sores cause painful, irritating patches on the lips and nearby areas; the causative virus remains dormant until triggered into activity by such things as febrile illness, minor injury or strong sunlight. The condition is usually only mildly troublesome and clears up without treatment, but the virus sometimes invades the eyes, bloodstream or brain. Temporary relief may be obtained by treating the cold sores twice daily with camphor spirits, a moist styptic pencil, petroleum jelly or alcohol. Genital herpes affects the genital region and is generally transmitted sexually (see p.177).
11 Hives, urticaria or nettle rash is a skin inflammation causing itchy weals that suddenly appear on any part of the body and come and go for a week or more. Hives is often caused by allergic reaction to certain drugs, foods, infections, or even sunlight; it may also occur from nervous causes. An attack of hives may cause tiredness, nausea and feverishness; a few people suffer a swollen throat that threatens breathing. A short course of steroids may be needed to control severe attacks.
12 Impetigo is an infectious disease that begins with small blisters; within hours these burst and produce a discharge which forms a golden crust on the skin. Impetigo occurs mainly on the face.
13 Molluscum contagiosum is a harmless virus infection that produces painless pink or yellowish pimples in the genital area or sometimes on the face and shoulders. Each pimple is about the size of a pinhead and has a central depression plugged with a whitish cheesy material. If they remain untreated the pimples may persist for months, but doctors can remove them with a caustic substance. Molluscum contagiosum tends to be caught by means of sexual contact, though people can also become infected at public baths. First signs of the disease show up as much as 6 months after infection occurred (see p.177).
14 Prickly heat, or heat rash, occurs on damp parts of the body that are usually covered by clothing, particularly the groin and armpits. The rash produces a prickling irritation. Prickly heat occurs mainly in hot, moist climates.

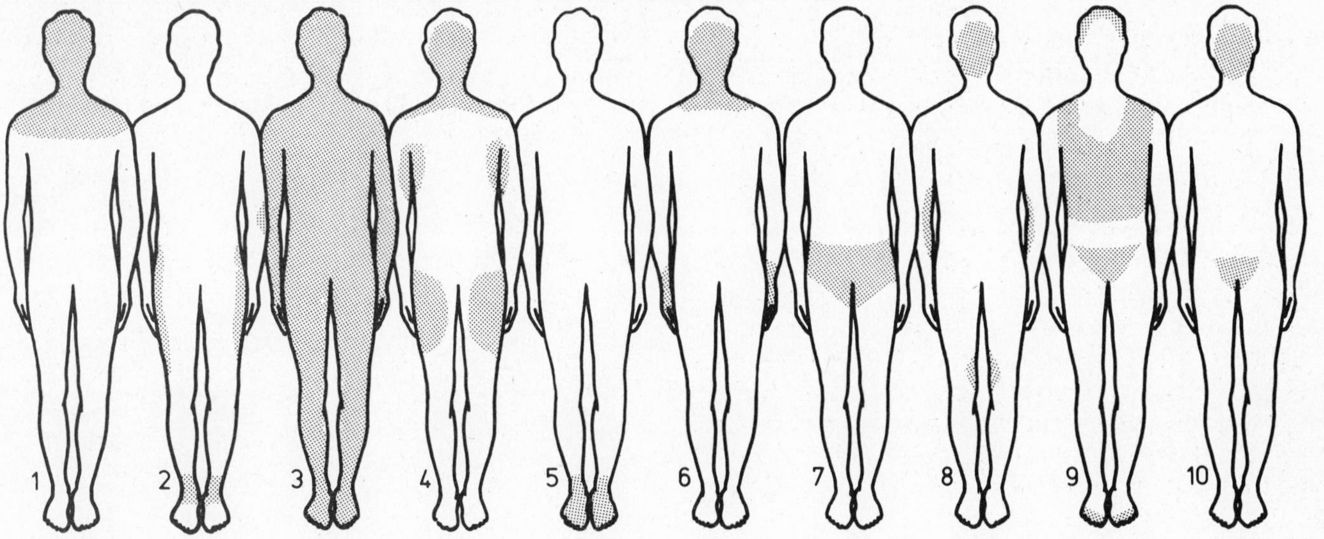

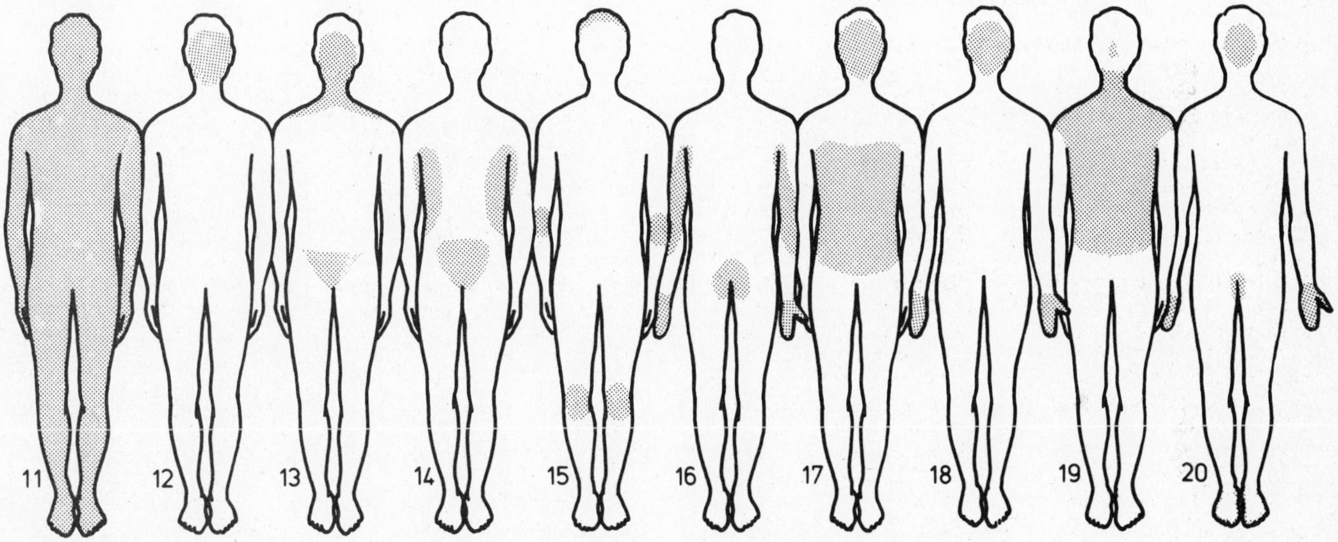

15 Psoriasis features bright red patches covered with loose silvery scales, particularly on the scalp, elbows, knees and lower back. The condition is sometimes disfiguring and itchy, but is noncontagious. Psoriasis may start at any age, and lasts a lifetime with periodic remissions; it affects about 2% of the population. No treatment can completely cure the condition, but controlled exposure to sunlight in a warm climate or else to ultraviolet light brings some improvement. Bathing the lesions daily and scrubbing with a surgical brush may help; in severe cases doctors may prescribe drugs to slow down epidermal cell growth.

16 Scabies, also aptly called the itch, features intense itching, especially at night. The cause is infestation by an almost invisibly tiny species of mite, which is spread by close bodily contact. Females tunnel through the skin to lay eggs, favoring the hands, elbows, underarms, buttocks and genitals. The burrows leave tiny tracks, often hidden by the patient's scratching. Taking a long, hot bath and scrubbing the affected areas makes the mites vulnerable to attack by gamma benzene hexachloride or benzyl benzoate, which should be applied on all the skin from feet to chin. All the family and other close contacts should be treated.

17 Shingles, or herpes zoster, is a virus disease that produces blisters along the line of a nerve on the face or trunk. Pain in the affected area may be quite severe before the blisters erupt; the blisters then burst and dry into crusts. Herpes zoster may cause quite deep scarring, and can be a debilitating disease.

18 Skin cancers may occur on many parts of the body, but the most usual sites are the face and the backs of the hands (see p.78).

19 Sunburn chiefly injures skin on the nose, neck, shoulders, chest and back (see p.79).

20 Warts may appear anywhere on the body, but are particularly common on the face, hands, anal-genital area and the soles of the feet (see pp.78 and 122).

Skin 2

Warts
These are benign skin tumors. Different types may appear on hands, soles of feet, face and in the anal-genital region, but all are probably due to one kind of virus. Warts arrive and disappear surprisingly quickly, but they may remain for months or years. Anyone can get warts, but young skin, being thin, is especially prone. Surprisingly, folklore recipes for charming away warts often seem to work, but coincidence or psychology may play a part in this. Doctors can attack stubborn warts with freezing or cautery. Most warts can be ignored, but painful or cosmetically unacceptable ones can be removed.

Rashes
These come in many forms with many causes. Most clear up upon treatment of their causes, but a few persist. Skin contact with poison ivy, urine or other irritants or allergens causes a skin rash. Swallowing food or drugs to which you are allergic is another cause. Chickenpox, measles and German measles are infectious diseases with a rash as one of their distinctive signs. Psoriasis features an intractable rash probably hereditary in origin. Some rashes respond to various powders, creams or oils, but griseofulvin taken orally is best for ringworm rashes. There is no universal rash remedy.

Birthmarks and scars
Many people have disfiguring naevi (birthmarks) or scars. Naevi result from enlarged blood vessels in skin or an area of dark pigmentation. Moles are brown; strawberry naevi dark red; portwine stains pink to purple. Such marks are most disfiguring when on the face. Strawberry naevi and the paler birthmarks tend to fade in early childhood. But portwine stains, moles and of course scars persist. Fortunately scars and birthmarks can be concealed by special cosmetics that match skin color and can only be removed by cold cream. Tattooing and dermabrasion (abrading skin away) are other ways of treating birthmarks.

Skin cancer
Skin cancers occur mainly in white-skinned people long exposed to strong sunlight, or in anyone who has suffered from considerable exposure to X-rays or substances that include tars and arsenic. Different signs include: scaly, crusted wartlike lesions on freckled skin in solar keratosis (a precancerous condition); an ulcer on the face (rodent ulcer); a fast-growing lump that may break down and bleed (epithelioma); and changes in a mole, such as itching, darkening, inflammation or ulceration (melanoma). Many skin cancers have rolled edges. Most types of skin cancer are treatable, but malignant melanomas are usually fatal.

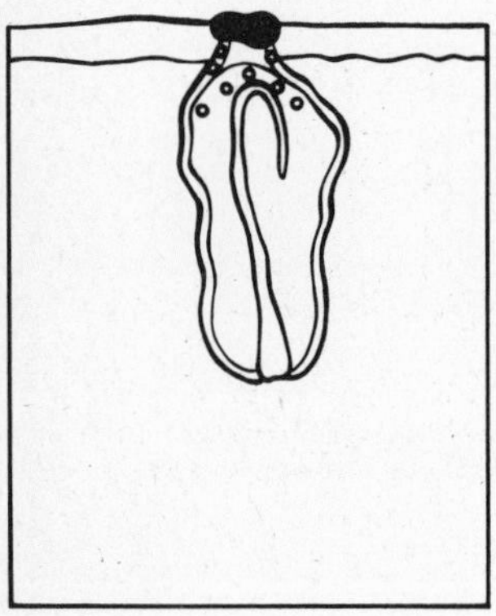

Blackheads
A blackhead (shown *above* in cross section) forms when a hard waxy plug of sebum derived from a sebaceous gland in the skin blocks the gland opening. The plug may blacken in contact with air, producing a blackhead. (If the plug is not in contact with air it is known as a whitehead.) To remove unsightly blackheads, try soaking the skin in warm water. This helps to open pores in the skin and so tends to loosen any sebum plugs present. You can then gently squeeze or wipe out the blackheads. This is most effective when the plugs are recently formed.

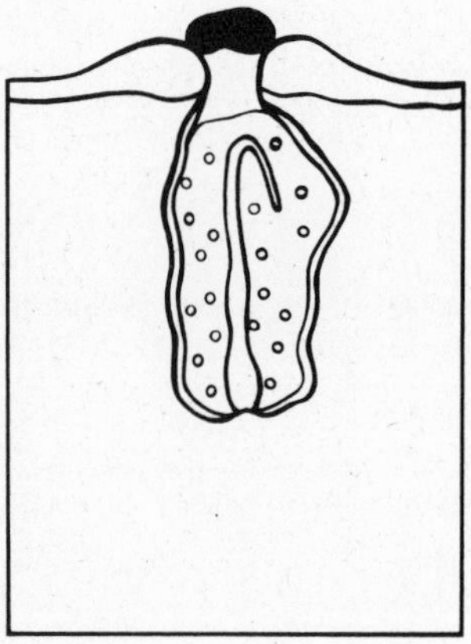

Acne
This involves small, inflamed swellings that develop into pustules, as shown *above*. Acne tends to occur in skin where blackheads have blocked sebaceous glands and these have become infected. Acne mostly affects face, neck, back and shoulders (see p.55). Trouble occurs mainly in adolescence and before menstruation – times during which hormone activity narrows the necks of sebaceous glands. Minimize acne by washing the skin twice a day with antiseptic soap and exposing it to sunlight. Oxytetracycline may help, but has to be taken for two months at least.

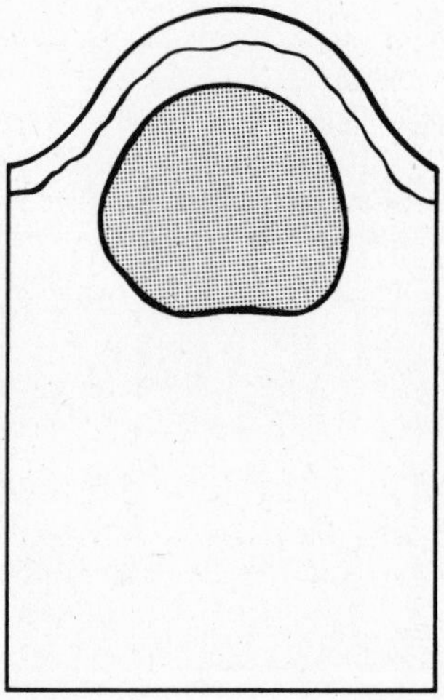

Cysts
Unlike tumors, cysts are sacs containing liquid or semisolid matter *(above)*. Sebaceous cysts, which develop when sebaceous glands become blocked, are a type often found in the skin, especially on the back, head and scrotum. They are firm, round, movable lumps that grow slowly but can get as large as a walnut. Unless they are obvious and unsightly they may need no treatment. But a sebaceous cyst may get infected and inflamed. Applying hot packs several times daily may help to open the blocked duct so that a doctor can drain the contents of the cyst and treat the area with antibiotic ointment. Large or disfiguring sebaceous cysts can be removed.

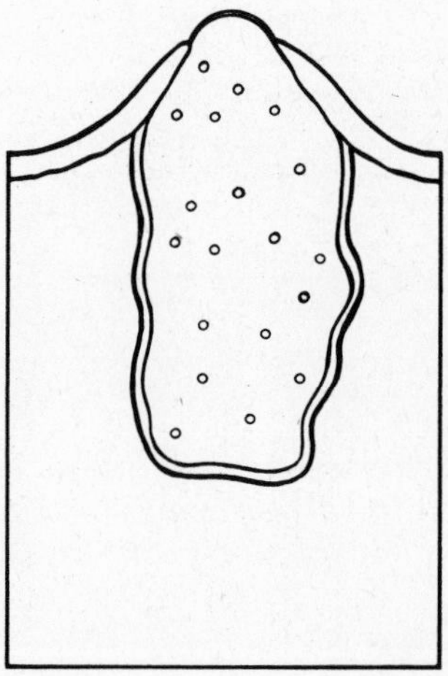

Boils
These painful, pus-filled lumps may develop if staphylococcal bacteria deeply invade a hair follicle and nearby tissue. Early on, a boil is round and red and nearby skin is swollen and tender. Later, as shown *above*, it produces a conical pus-filled head (carbuncles are multiheaded boils). Repeated soaking in warm water speeds up this process and the boil then usually bursts. You can absorb the pus on a piece of gauze, wash the area, dab dry with gauze, add an antibiotic cream, and cover with a sterile gauze pad. If healing takes more than a few days see a doctor. Never squeeze or pinch a boil.

Wrinkles
As we age our skin begins to lose natural oils and moisture. Bundles of collagen protein deep in the dermis begin breaking up (a process hastened by long exposure to sunlight). This makes skin inelastic and wrinkled. Shrinking of body bulk accentuates creases: loose bags hang beneath the eyes; corrugations seam the forehead; crows' feet crinkle the corners of the eyes; and wrinkles ridge the backs of the hands. Externally applied cosmetics cannot rejuvenate old skin, but moisturizing creams and lotions may temporarily help it to look younger. The illustrations show average wrinkling at ages 25 (**a**), 50 (**b**) and 75 (**c**).

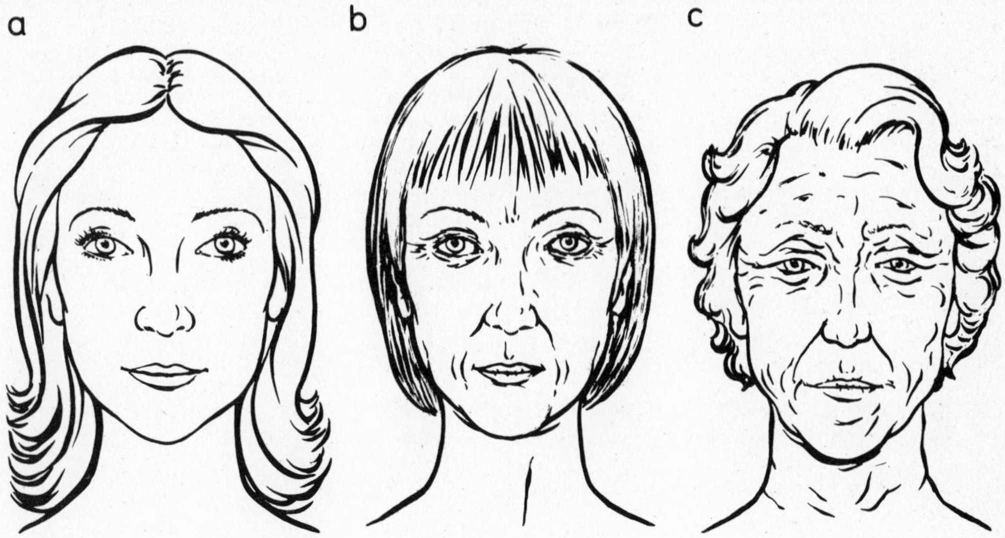

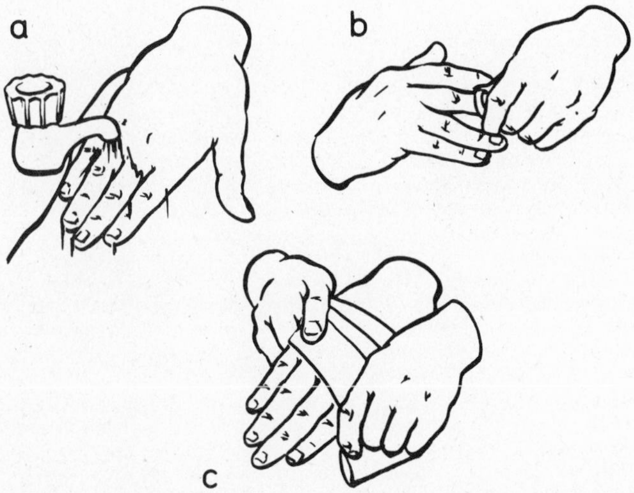

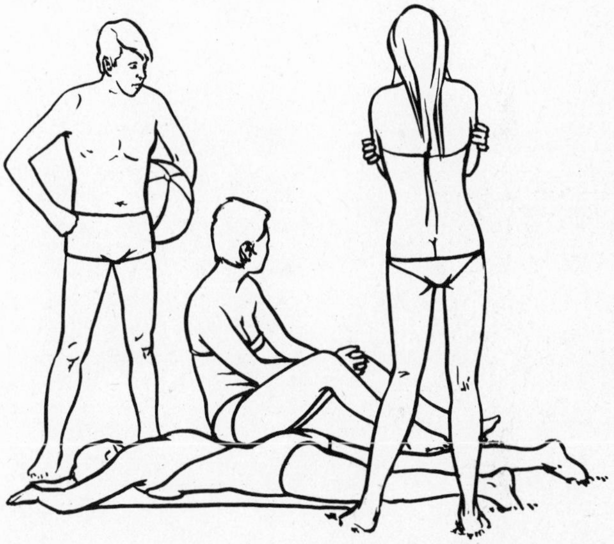

Burns and scalds
Skin may be burned by dry or moist heat; friction; electric current; or strong alkalis or acids. The effects of all are similar. Superficial burns leave the skin intact, but reddened or blistered; deep burns involve any or all of the deeper tissues. Victims often suffer shock and turn pale, with cold, clammy hands and feet. If someone's clothes catch fire wrap him in a blanket, coat, rug or cloth and lay him flat. If he is electrocuted, switch off the current or insulate yourself before removing him.
Do not try treating serious burns yourself; cover them with a clean dressing to prevent contamination and get medical help urgently. Do not try to remove any clothing from the burn. Hospital treatment may include antibiotic therapy and skin grafts if the damage to the skin is extensive.
Minor burns are easy to manage and prompt treatment can often minimize pain and damage.
a Plunge the burned skin under cold running water and keep it there as long as possible.
b Remove any rings or other items that may constrict the tissues if the burned part swells.
c Cover the burned area with a clean (preferably sterile) dressing.

Sun and sunburn
Sunshine on the skin has good and bad effects. It helps our bodies to make vitamin D, and benefits acne sufferers; yet prolonged exposure to it ages skin and may cause cancer. But the problem that concerns most of us is sunburn. Sudden exposure to strong sunshine by people with pale skins is liable to produce first-degree burns showing as red, tender areas of skin that subsequently peel. Nose, neck, shoulders, chest and back are often danger areas. Severe sunburn so inflames the skin that it stops helping to keep the body cool and victims grow dangerously overheated and may even die. Called sunstroke, this is a form of heatstroke if it involves malfunction of the temperature control center at the base of the brain. Keeping the neck covered during long exposure to strong sunlight helps to protect the brain from heat damage. This is especially important in young children. Pale sunworshipers avoid sunburn if at first they start by exposing skin to strong sunshine for only 10 minutes a day and guard the skin with protective oil or cream. Day by day the skin will thicken and brown as granules of the dark pigment melanin rise from deep inside the skin. This thickening and darkening helps protect the skin from harmful rays. After a week, sunbathing for moderately long spells is safe.

Heart

The heart is a hollow muscle lying within the rib cage, well protected against damage by the surrounding bones. The mass of the heart lies centrally in the chest, but the apex, where the beat is most easily felt, tapers toward the left. The heart begins to pump less than a month after conception, and by adulthood is pumping roughly 3000 gallons of blood per day, at an average rate of 70 beats a minute. The heart is responsible for circulating the blood to all parts of the body and therefore for the distribution of oxygen and nutrients. An efficiently functioning heart is one of the prime requisites of a healthy body, and we suggest some of the things that you can do to look after your heart and maximize its efficiency.

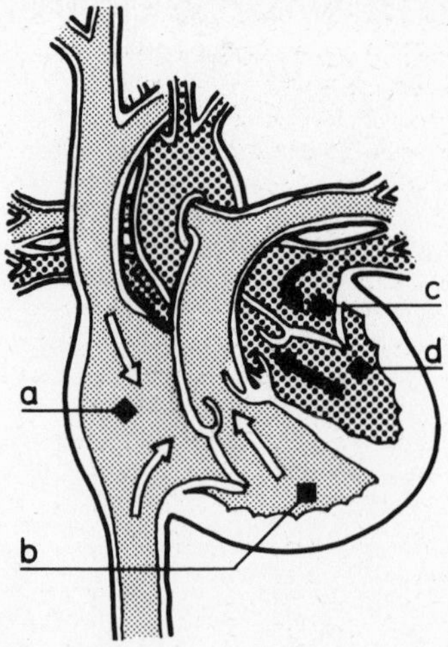

Blood flow through the heart
The illustration shows the path that the blood takes through the heart. Deoxygenated blood enters the upper chamber (atrium) of the right side of the heart (**a**); it is then pumped by the lower chamber or right ventricle (**b**) to the lungs for oxygenation. The reoxygenated blood returns to the left atrium (**c**) and is pumped to the body by the larger left ventricle (**d**). There is a system of valves to control the blood flow and ensure that it occurs in the correct direction.

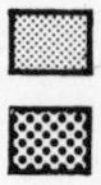

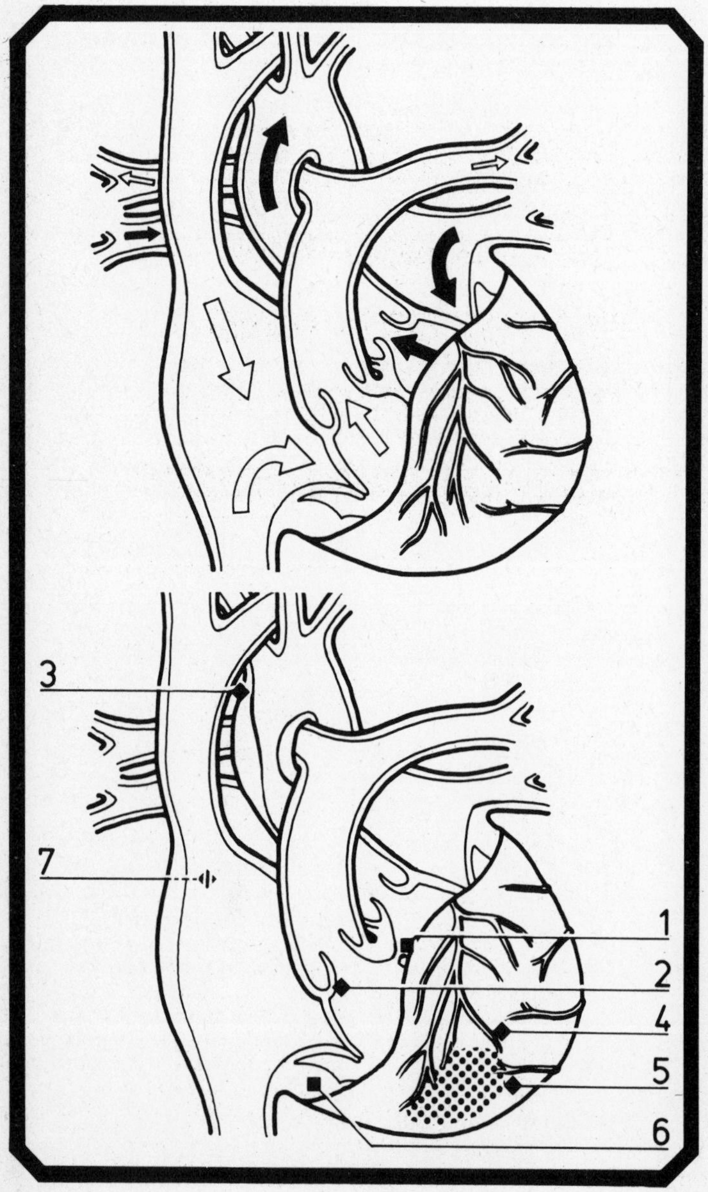

Heart problems
The top illustration shows a cutaway drawing of the heart; the arrows demonstrate the direction of the blood flow. The lower illustration shows some of the problems that can affect the heart.

1 Congenital malformations. Babies can be born with heart problems, sometimes involving a hole in the wall between the chambers of the heart.

2 Diseases of the valves. These can either be congenital, or the result of disease or infection. Valve disease causes blood flow problems, which may weaken the heart and cause it to enlarge.

3 Diseases of the blood vessels. Deposits of fat can be laid down within the walls of the vessels; this is often associated with a raised cholesterol and fat level in the blood. The vessels principally involved are the larger arteries; the problems caused depend on the site of the deposits.

4 Coronary artery problems. The heart gains its blood supply by a system of vessels called the coronary artery circulation. Like the other arteries, this may have fatty deposits in the walls; if the deposits completely block the vessel then a heart attack results. The area of the heart muscle supplied by that vessel is starved of oxygen and dies. If this process happens to vessels that supply the brain with blood, then a stroke is the result. There are various factors that make heart attacks more likely. The most important ones to be avoided are cigarette smoking, raised blood pressure, overweight, lack of exercise, and stress. Certain personality types may be particularly prone.

5 Scar from old heart attack. If a heart attack occurs the scar is permanent, but by avoiding the aggravating situations listed in **4**, the resultant damage can be minimized.

6 Problems with the heart muscle. The heart is a muscular pump; if the blood pressure is raised,which may happen for a variety of reasons (such as kidney disease), the heart enlarges and the valves may work inefficiently. The increase in pressure within the blood vessels may cause damage to the anatomy of the vessel walls and cause a rupture. The most frequent site for this is within the skull, and a stroke is the result.

7 Problems with the heart pacemaker. The heart beats in response to small electrical impulses arising in a bundle of nerve fibers in the center of the heart, controlled by the brain and chemicals in the blood. If this pacemaker is not functioning correctly, disturbances of the rhythm of the heart result.

Efficiency of the heart
This is the ability of the heart to perform its function properly and with the minimum of effort. There are many factors that affect the heart's efficiency, and a surprising number of these, such as diet, weight, exercise and life-style, are under the owner's control. The recent major advances in heart surgery, such as coronary bypass operations, pacemakers and heart transplants, have certainly revolutionized the treatment of previously untreatable cases, but a greater awareness of cardiac health could make many of these operations unnecessary.

Exercise and the heart
The heart is the strongest muscle in the body, and can stand up well to vigorous use, but the hearts of most people, especially if they follow sedentary occupations, are unfit and out of condition – just as their other muscles may be. Regular, sensible exercise will help convert the heart into the efficient organ that it is meant to be, increasing the strength of the heart's muscular walls and also increasing its capability. A heart that is more efficient will have a greater output through increased stroke volume and rate.

Diet and the heart
One of the functions of the blood is to take nutrients from the digestive tract via the intestinal linings and distribute them around the body, and so it is not surprising that the food we eat can have a direct effect on the wellbeing of the circulatory system and the heart in particular. A high intake of fats, especially the saturated animal fats, can greatly increase the fatty acids in the blood and aggravate many forms of heart disease. A diet high in calories can cause obesity, which places extra strain on the heart. The reverse is also true; a low-calorie diet controls body weight and the health of the heart is greatly improved.

Stress and the heart
People who live under a constant strain place an unnecessary and often dangerous burden on their hearts. The stress may arise from overwork, from constant problems in a home situation – such as a failing marriage or difficult children – or from a predisposition in the person concerned to worry and fret excessively. The resulting high levels of cholesterol and adrenalin in the blood have a continuous effect on the heart rate and the heart's health, and high blood pressure or hypertension is another common complication of stress.

The pulse
Your pulse is the measure of your heartbeat – its speed, strength and regularity. The best place to feel the pulse is at the wrist, and you should learn to take your pulse there as a ready assessment of your fitness and also as a check against exercising too strenuously. The method of taking your pulse is described *below right*. The step test shown *below* is an excellent way of checking your fitness program; do the test every two weeks, and plot the results on a graph. The method is as follows.

1a Step up with one foot onto a bench or low chair about 16in high.
1b Bring the other foot up onto the top of the bench.
1c Step down again with one foot.
1d Bring the other foot down to the floor.
Repeat 24 times a minute for 2 minutes.
2 Sit down for 2 minutes, then take your pulse and record the result.
The diagram shows a selection of maximum recommended pulse rates for various ages. **A** shows the typical pulse range for people at rest; **B** shows pulse ratings by age for people unused to exercise, and **C** shows the maximum levels to which you should raise your pulse when you are fitter.

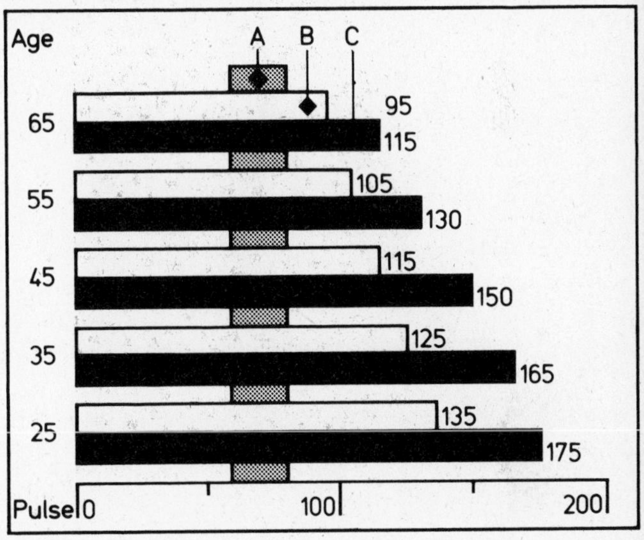

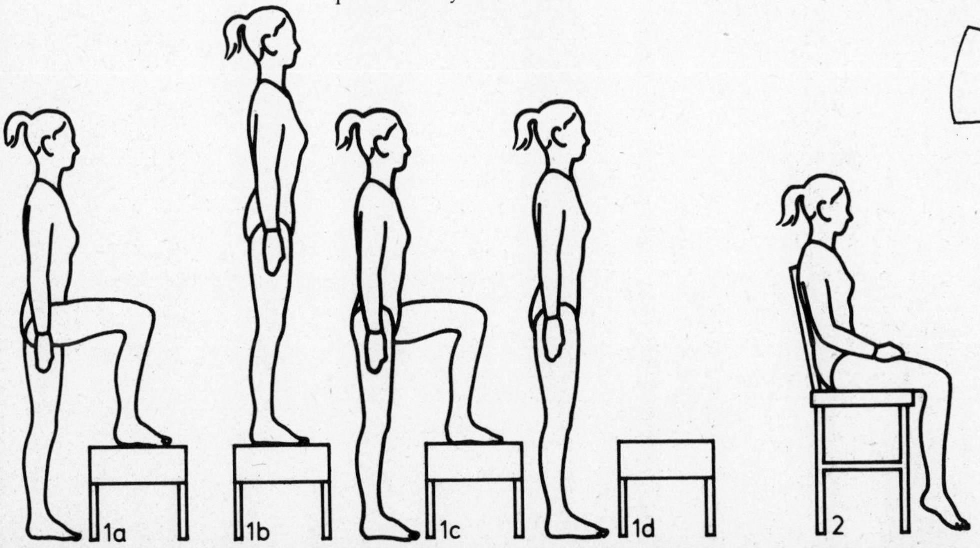

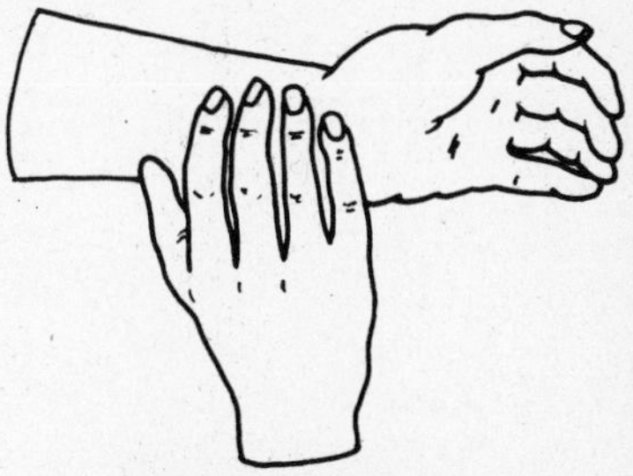

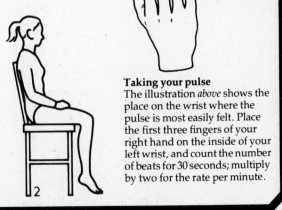

Taking your pulse
The illustration *above* shows the place on the wrist where the pulse is most easily felt. Place the first three fingers of your right hand on the inside of your left wrist, and count the number of beats for 30 seconds; multiply by two for the rate per minute.

Heart and stress

Just as the condition of the body and circulation can affect the heart, so the condition of the mind is reflected in the state of the heart. Stress is one of the major contributing factors to heart disease, partly because it alters the body's systems (such as the blood cholesterol level) in such a way that the heart can be damaged, and partly because those who live under stress are apt to develop conditions that strain the heart, such as high blood pressure from overwork, respiratory problems from smoking too much, poor circulation from lack of exercise and so on. Conscious removal of both the causes and effects of stress recondition the heart and alter the outlook so that heart disease is far less likely to occur, and here we look at some common stress patterns and ways to avoid them.

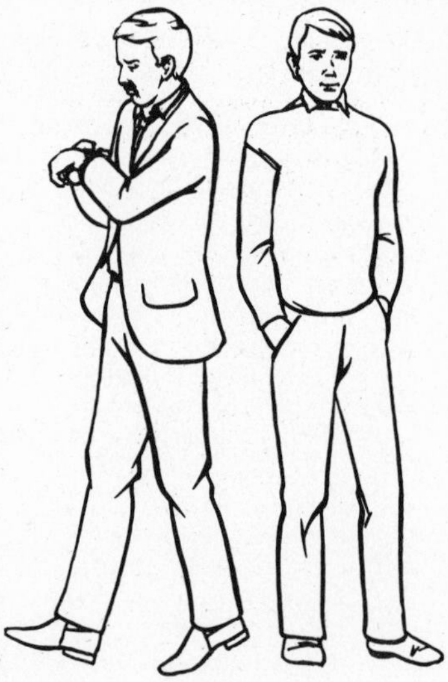

Type A and type B
Personality type is now considered to be a definite risk factor in heart disease, although the direct link is uncertain. Type A, the type most likely to develop heart disease, is the person who drives himself or herself relentlessly, is tense, is often under stress of various kinds, has few or no philosophical or religious beliefs, and has few relaxing hobbies. Type B is more relaxed and easy-going, and takes life at a gentler pace. It is unclear as yet whether type A's likely heart problems come from his genetic makeup or his lifestyle.

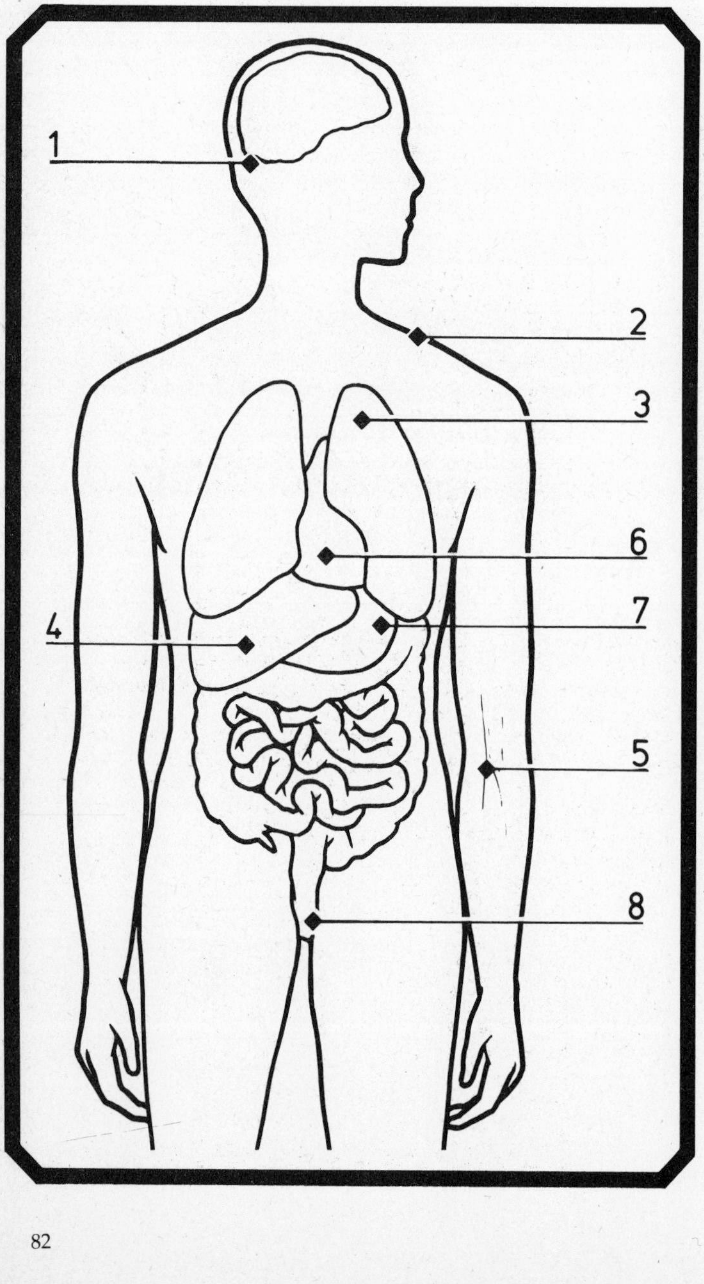

Stress and the circulation
The illustration shows some of the parts of the body that may be affected by the action of stress on the heart and circulation.

1 Pituitary gland; this releases adrenocorticotrophin hormone (ACTH) into the bloodstream, which stimulates the release of adrenaline and other hormones.

2 Skin; pallor may occur as blood is diverted away from the skin to the muscles.

3 Lungs; the rate of breathing speeds up and increases the oxygenation of the blood.

4 Liver; this releases extra sugar into the blood, in order to provide the body with extra energy if required.

5 Blood; the serum cholesterol level of the blood tends to be higher in people under stress because some factor, not yet identified, triggers the mobilization of fat and cholesterol from body deposits. The levels of fibrinogen, platelets and lymphocytes in the blood are all increased; these are defense mechanisms, intended to prepare the blood to clot against excess bleeding if the body is injured, and to help repair any damaged tissues.

6 Heart; the heart rate speeds up dramatically, in order to transport oxygen and nutrients to the muscles more rapidly.

7 Spleen; this releases more red cells into the blood to assist in carrying the extra oxygen from the lungs.

8 Genitals; stress can often cause impotence. Although the origins may be psychological, excessive tiredness and lack of relaxation experienced by a man under stress can be precipitating factors.

Stress and the family
The person who is constantly under stress will find that he or she is missing out on many enriching aspects of family life. If you find that you spend little time playing with your children or talking with your spouse, and if you tend to hurry them along constantly in what they are saying or doing, then stress is affecting your family life adversely. You should make a conscious effort to set aside a sizeable amount of time, both in the evenings and on weekends, to relax with your family and share in their lives; try to leave your day's work behind you when you come home.

Stress and work
The person under prolonged stress tends to be a man or woman who has made vocational success the all-important goal in life. The more successful a person becomes, the greater the number of stressful situations that present themselves. He or she can never relax, but is always "on duty" and worrying about the next task on the agenda. In order to alleviate this situation, the person under stress can learn to delegate as many tasks as possible to trustworthy employees so that the personal load of stress is lessened.

Stress and recreation
Both the quality and the quantity of relaxation and recreation are important to the stressful person. Sports should not be seen as another opportunity for displaying supremacy, but should be an occasion for enjoyment and sociability. Exercise should not be used as a tool to push the body to further extremes of activity, but should be a means of keeping the body healthy and fit as a contrast to the pressures of work. Social events should be attended for the enjoyment they provide, rather than because they present opportunities for furthering a career.

Stress and diet
The stressful person is usually keeping to a busy schedule and consequently frequently skips meals, has a few drinks instead of eating, or eats snacks or takeout foods to stave off hunger pangs. These types of eating habit affect the body adversely and often provide it with inadequate nutrition, and this state of poor digestive health is commonly aggravated in stressful people by the appearance of an ulcer. The stomach tends to become more acid when the body is under stress, and combined with irregular eating habits the stomach and intestine linings may be damaged.

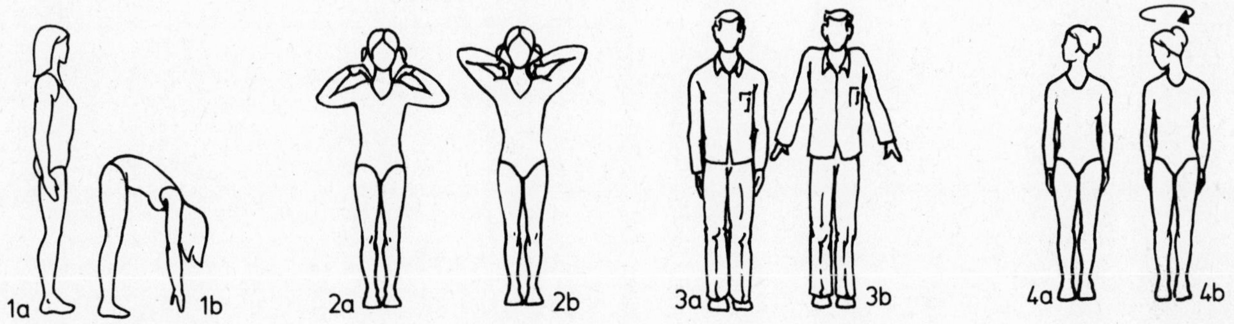

Exercises to relieve tension
These exercises perform two functions for the stressful person. First, they make him or her take the time off to relax, and therefore relieve some of the mental tension, and secondly they relieve some of the physical tension caused by stress. They should be done regularly, concentrating only on the exercise and not on work, time, speed or anything else.
1a Stand upright, with your arms loosely by your sides.
1b Allow your body to flop loosely forward from the waist, and remain in this relaxed position for a few seconds. Repeat several times.

2a Stand upright with your arms out to your sides and your elbows bent so that your fingertips touch your shoulders lightly.
2b Raise your elbows so that your back muscles are stretched, and hold this position for a few seconds. Then relax your arms to the previous position and repeat several times.
This exercise is especially good for relaxing knotted back muscles; other helpful exercises for the same problem include swinging your arms loosely around your body, and alternately humping and hollowing your back.

3a Stand upright with your arms loosely down at your sides and your shoulders relaxed.
3b Lift your shoulders into a shrugging position and hold them there stiffly for several seconds. Then relax them totally so that you are in the starting position. Repeat this exercise several times.
This exercise relaxes the shoulder muscles, which tend to become very tense in stressful people. Another exercise that helps do this involves swinging the arms out to the side and then backward, so that your hands touch behind your back.

4a Stand upright with your head turned to one side.
4b Slowly stretch your neck to the side, then to the back, and then to the other side so that the top of your head moves in a circle in the air. Then repeat this exercise with your head facing the other side.
This exercise stretches the neck muscles and helps prevent the stressful person from developing round shoulders and a hunched stance from constant bending over desks etc.

Heart and diet

It has been increasingly shown over the last decade that an analysis of diet plays a very important role in the understanding of heart disease. Doctors originally realized that a high intake of cholesterol, found particularly in saturated animal fats, was associated directly with atherosclerosis, and patients were put on low-cholesterol diets. However, the serum cholesterol in their blood tended still to remain high, and further research revealed that if the body is low in cholesterol, the liver manufactures it from other fats in the diet. So it became evident that blood cholesterol could only be kept low on a diet low in fats of all kinds, and this has become the almost unanimous recommendation from health sources for a diet toward a healthier heart.

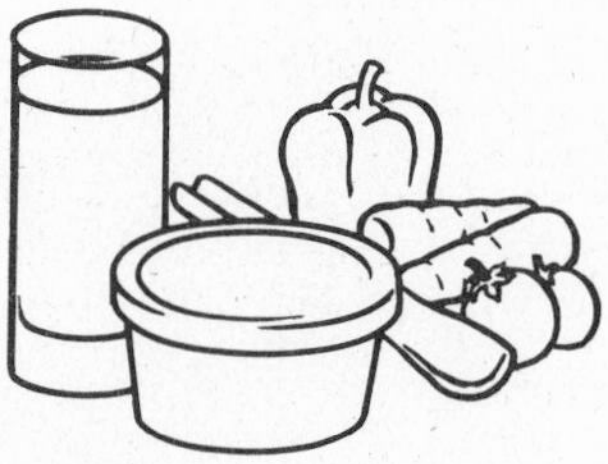

Low-fat snacks
Plenty of nutritious low-fat snacks can be eaten in large quantities without significant fat intake. Fruit juice, fresh fruit and raw vegetables such as carrots, celery, lettuce, cucumber, tomato, pepper, cauliflower, cabbage and spring onion can all be eaten freely. Cottage cheese is extremely low in fat.

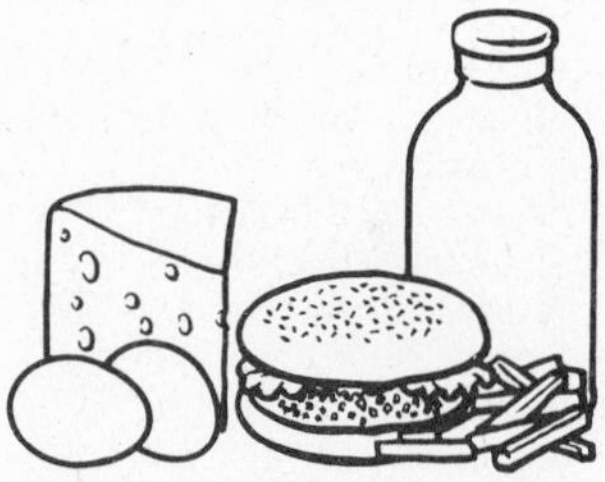

High-fat snacks
If you take a packed lunch to work or have a snack meal in the evening, avoid some of the traditional nutritious foods that can be very high in fat. Cheese and milk, although high in protein and low in sugar, are also high in fat. Potato chips, hamburgers, cold meats and hard-cooked eggs should also be avoided.

In this panel we give some dietary guidelines for people with a heart condition or who are anxious to avoid one.

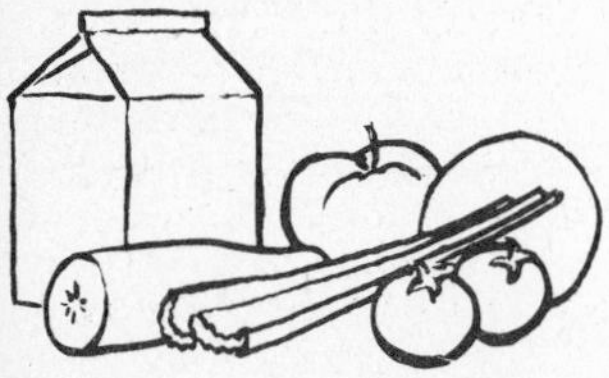

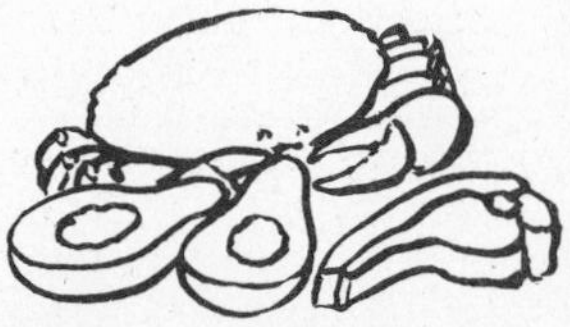

Do

- Seek specialist dietary advice if you or other members of your family have high blood pressure or a history of heart disease.
- Reduce your overall intake of fats as well as reducing cholesterol in the diet if you want to reduce your risk of heart disease.
- Remember that some foods that are low in fat (eg crab) are high in cholesterol and so should be eaten only very occasionally.
- Eat smaller portions of meat – no more than 6oz (170g) a day, and preferably less than this.
- Increase your intake of fresh vegetables and fruits (except avocados and olives, which are comparatively high in fat and so are best avoided).
- Eat breads, cereals and flour products that do not contain large amounts of fat or sugar.
- Substitute skim milk for whole milk, and eat low-fat yoghurt.

Don't

- Let fats account for more than 30–35% of your daily food consumption (compared with 40% in the diet of most Americans).
- Eat more than 300mg of cholesterol per day (compared with a typical US daily consumption of 600–700mg).
- Eat more than three egg yolks per week, including those used in baking.
- Use saturated fats (animal fats) for cooking when unsaturated fats (vegetable oils) can be used instead.
- Eat meat that is obviously fatty; even lean meat has a high fat content.
- Eat nuts, which have a high fat content.
- Eat whole-milk dairy products (including milk, cream, butter, hard cheeses and ice cream).
- Just substitute margarine for butter; a low-fat spread should be used in its place.

Reducing fat in the diet
Although the relationship between diet and heart disease is still not fully understood, current research suggests that persons can reduce their propensity to heart disease by reducing the amount of fat in their diet. When special diets for persons at risk from heart disease were first prepared, the main emphasis was on reducing the intake of cholesterol. This still remains an important feature of this type of diet, but following the discovery that a person's liver manufactures cholesterol from other fats when the cholesterol content of the diet is very low, it is now more usual to recommend that all fats in the diet should be significantly reduced.
On these pages we compare the cholesterol and fat contents of some different types of food. To allow a scientific comparison of one food with another we have in each case given the cholesterol or fat content per 100 grams of food. When planning your diet, however, it is important to bear in mind the weight of a typical portion. It would, for example, be physically impossible to eat 100 grams (roughly 3½ ounces) of vegetable oil at one sitting, but there would be nothing greedy about eating the same weight of meat.

Cholesterol content of foods
Included in the list *below* are some of the foods to watch when trying to reduce cholesterol intake. Figures given are milligrams per 100g of food. Also note that whole milk has 14mg of cholesterol per 100g whereas skim milk has only 2mg.

Very high: over 500mg
Brains (2000mg)
Egg yolk (1480mg)
Kidney
Liver (chicken, turkey)
Very high: 200–500mg
Liver (beef, lamb, pork)
Fish roe
Butter (250mg)
Sponge cake
Egg, scrambled
High: 100–200mg
Shrimp
Crab
Whipping cream
Mayonnaise
Cream cheese
High: 80–100mg
Beef
Pork
Lamb
Chicken
Cheese (most types)
Doughnut
Mackerel
Lobster
Medium: 50–80mg
Clams
Cod
Tuna
Margarine (0–50mg depending on brand)
No cholesterol
Egg white
Vegetable oils

Preparing meat
The high fat content of many meats can be reduced by careful preparation and cooking. Cut all visible fat from meat before cooking. Never fry meat, or baste it during cooking. Grill bacon, sausages, chops etc on a rack so the fat drips away. Meat soups and stews should be prepared as follows. First simmer the meat so the fat melts and floats to the top. Then refrigerate the liquor until the fat solidifies. Finally remove the solidified fat and finish cooking the meat. To cook fish, wrap it in foil so the moisture is retained and there is no need to brush with oil or fat.

Low-fat baking
The first rule in low-fat baking is to use no shortening of any sort; if some fat is necessary to the recipe, then use unsaturated oil instead. Eggs are very high in cholesterol and so should be avoided; many recipes can be made leaving out the eggs, and if this does not work use low-cholesterol dried egg. Do not use any butter, but replace it with unsaturated margarine; instead of cream use skim milk. Use non-stick baking pans so that you do not need to grease them. Use cocoa, chocolate, nuts and coconut only sparingly in your baking as they are all high in fat.

Snacks and party food
Fast food such as hamburgers, tacos, fish and french fries, with all the dressings and sauces that go with them, are usually loaded with fat, so it is much better to make your own snack food. Delicious low-fat sandwiches can be made with such combinations as: cottage cheese with pineapple or celery; salmon and cucumber; chicken and tomato; green salad etc. Of course all potato and corn snacks are fried and therefore very high in fat. At parties avoid cheese snacks, olives, coleslaw and dips unless you know their exact contents; if you are giving a party yourself provide dips made from cottage cheese with fingers of raw vegetables.

Dressings and sauces
These need not be foregone altogether by those seeking to eat a low-fat diet, but should be prepared carefully so that they avoid high-fat pitfalls. Salad dressings, if based on oil, should use an unsaturated one, but ideally you should experiment with non-fat dressings based on vinegar or lemon juice; also, some stores stock non-fat dressings. Do not use any prepared mixes, and do not add any cheese except cottage cheese. Cream or milk sauces can be made using skim milk. Mayonnaise is very high in fat, and ketchups, mustards and seafood sauces also generally contain a fair amount of fat.

Fat content of meat and fish
Meat is a major enemy of people on a low-fat diet. Fish is generally much lower in fat, although the cholesterol content is relatively high. Figures *below* are grams of fat per 100g of food.

g
53 Bacon, fried, crisp
42 Pork sausage, cooked
40 Beef, rib, lean and fat, roast
39 Salami, dry type
28 Pork, lean and fat, roast
27 Lamb, shoulder, lean and fat, roast
25 Luncheon meat, canned
22 Ham, lean and fat, roast
20 Hamburger, broiled
15 Pork, lean only, roast
14 Beef, rib, lean only, roast
11 Mackerel, fried
11 Veal cutlet, cooked
10 Liver, beef, fried
9 Lamb, shoulder, lean only, roast
8 Haddock, fried
7 Chicken, breast, flesh and skin, fried
6 Salmon, canned
5 Cod, fried
3 Chicken, flesh, broiled
2 Crabmeat, canned
1 Clams, canned

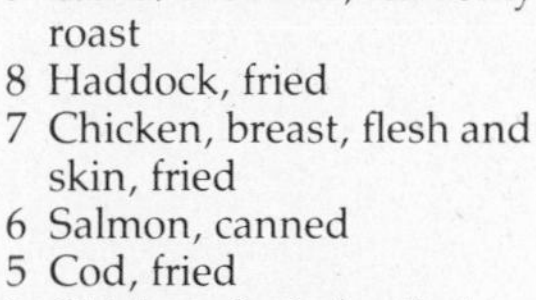

Fat content of baked products and snacks
Virtually all store-bought cakes, pastries, cookies and crackers are high in fat, although most breads are low. Chocolate, peanuts and potato chips are all very high in fat. Figures *below* show grams of fat for each 100g of food.

g
43 Peanuts, chocolate-coated
40 Potato chips
36 Chocolate, semi-sweet
33 Piecrust, baked shell
30 Cookies, chocolate-chip
24 Danish pastry, plain
23 Pecan pie, one-crust
19 Doughnut, cake type
15 Fruitcake, rich
14 Fudge, plain
12 Cupcake, no icing
11 Apple pie, two-crust
11 Crackers, Graham
11 Caramels, plain
9 Waffles
8 Pizza, cheese
7 Pancakes, wheat flour
7 Gingerbread
4 Fondant, uncoated
3 Bread, most types
>1 Jello
>1 Meringue

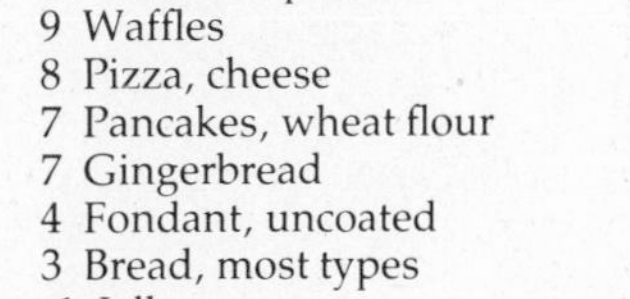

Fat content of dairy products and eggs
Listed *below* are the fat contents (grams of fat per 100g of food) of selected dairy products, dairy product substitutes and eggs. Note that regular margarines have almost the same fat content as butter; use low-fat spreads, which are also low in cholesterol. People on a low-fat diet are recommended to avoid all cheeses except cottage cheese.

g
82 Butter
81 Margarine, regular
41 Low-fat spread
38 Cheese, cream
38 Cream, whipping
35 Non-milk creamer, powder
32 Cheese, blue
32 Cheese, Cheddar
24 Cheese, Camembert
18 Egg, yolk only
16 Ice cream, rich
11 Ice cream, regular
9 Condensed milk, sweetened
8 Evaporated milk, unsweetened
4 Milk, whole
1 Yoghurt, low-fat
>1 Cheese, cottage, uncreamed
>1 Milk, non-fat, skim
>1 Egg, white only

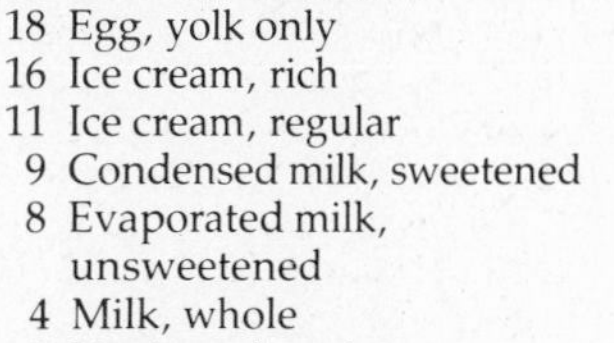

Fat content of vegetables, fruit and nuts
Almost all vegetables and fruits are very low in fats (less than 1g per 100g of food). Avocados and olives are notable exceptions, and nuts are very high in fats. Cooking methods obviously affect the amount of fat consumed. Figures *below* show grams of fat per 100g of food.

g
62 Dried coconut
61 Brazil nuts
49 Peanuts
33 Onions, fried
22 Mushrooms, fried
12 Potatoes, french fried
11 Olives, black
10 Avocado, average
4 Potatoes, mashed with milk and butter

Fat in salad dressings
Salad vegetables with their minimal fat content are ideal for persons on a low-fat diet, but the fat content of many salad dressings must be taken into account. Figures *below* show grams of fat per 100g of food.

g
100 Salad oils
79 Mayonnaise, home-made
53 Blue cheese
50 Thousand Island
40 Commercial, mayonnaise-type, regular
12 Commercial, mayonnaise-type, dietary
1 Yoghurt, low-fat
1 Cottage cheese
>1 Vinegar
0 Lemon juice

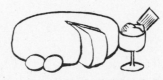

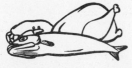

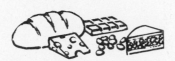

Heart and exercise

Regular, sensible exercise is one of the greatest tonics that you can give your heart. As the muscle walls of the heart strengthen, they pump the blood more efficiently and the circulation improves. This enables the body's other muscles to work harder, as more oxygen is reaching them and the heat and waste substances that they produce are being dispersed more rapidly; the person feels fitter and more capable of exertion. Of course a heart unused to exertion should not be subjected to sudden or strenuous exercise as this can be dangerous; the level and intensity of exercise should be increased only gradually over several weeks.

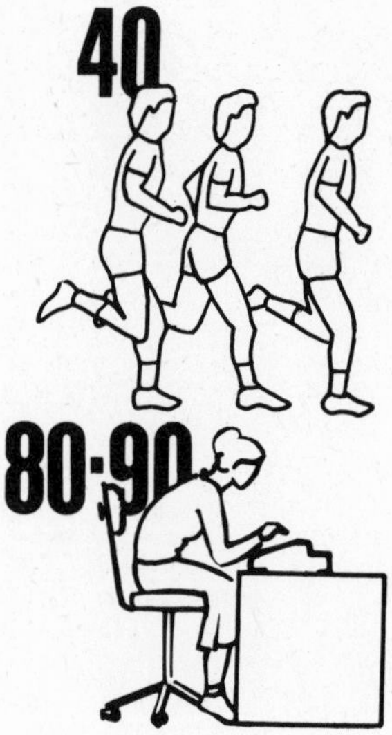

The fit and unfit heart
The fit heart is an efficient heart, and only has to pump the blood slowly as it is pumping a large volume at one time, and also pumping it strongly. The normal pulse of a trained endurance runner may be as low as 40 beats per minute. The unfit heart, on the other hand, is an inefficient heart. It has to pump the blood rapidly as its volume of pumped blood is small and its pumping action is poor; the pulse rate of a sedentary worker can be as high as 80–90 beats per minute.

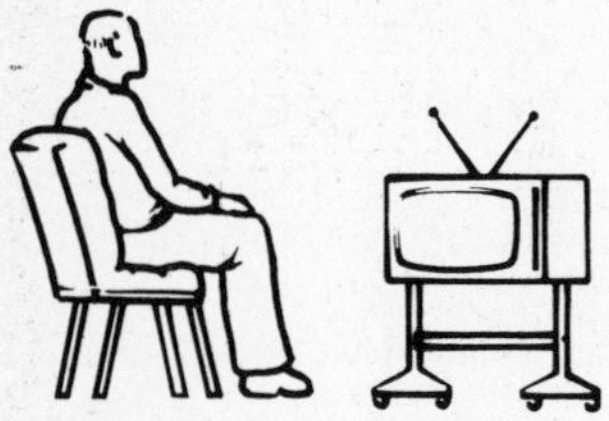

Good and bad lifestyles
The age of convenience has removed many of the natural exercise activities from our lives. Cars, trains, buses and airplanes have taken the time and effort out of travel, and electric tools and gadgets have reduced the amount of time spent in manual labor. Television has brought an enormous increase in sports spectatorship rather than participation, and the pollution and overcrowding of more urban environments has made walking a far less appealing exercise than it used to be. Despite the recent crazes for jogging, health farms etc the population in general has become more and more sedentary.

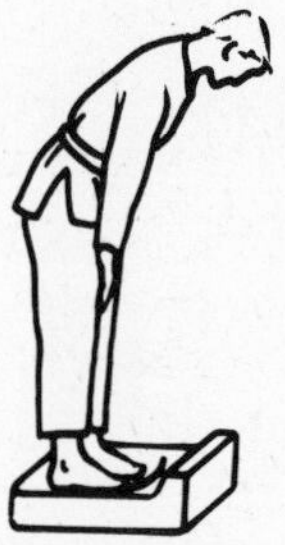

Medical advice and self-care
If you are middle-aged or elderly, or if you have been unused to exercise for several years or longer, then it is strongly advisable to consult a doctor before embarking on exercise of any sort. He will confirm that you are in a suitable condition, and will advise you on how quickly or slowly to increase your level of exercise. You should look after yourself by making sure that you do not exercise too strenuously if you are overweight, by losing the excess pounds, and also by checking your pulse regularly and not exceeding the recommended maximum for your age and fitness level.

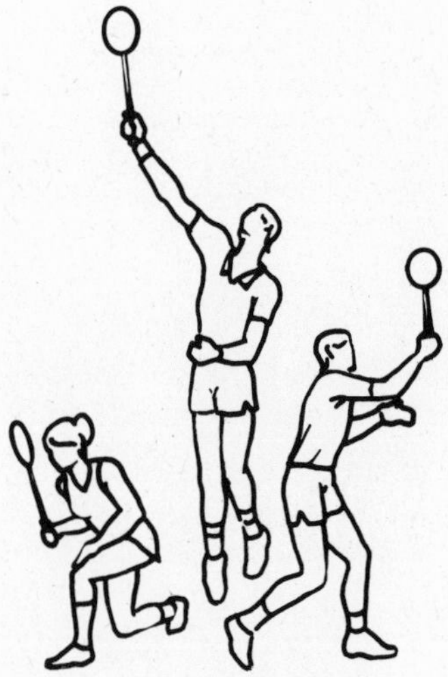

Exercise in daily activities
Your daily routine can be altered to provide many opportunities for exercise. Instead of taking the car to work, try walking or cycling; if you take a bus or train, get off a couple of stops early and walk the rest of the way. Use stairs rather than the elevator. Use your lunch hours for walking rather than just eating, drinking and sitting around. Join a sports club with members of your family or friends, and encourage one another to play regularly; if you drink or smoke heavily, cut down drastically so that the good you are doing your body by exercise is not counteracted.

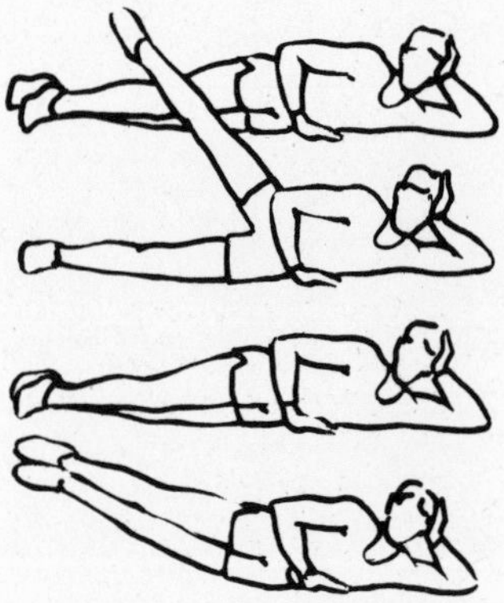

How to tackle exercise
Set aside regular times to exercise, otherwise the activity will be squeezed out of your routine. Take regular rests during your exercise period, especially in the early weeks, and check your pulse; if you are near your maximum rating (see p. 81) stop for a while until your pulse slows, and then continue. Always precede and follow a bout of exercise with gentle calisthenic, or mobility, exercises; these allow the blood flow to speed up and slow down gradually. It is unwise to drink very cold drinks or take a cold shower immediately after exercising as the shock to the body can strain the heart.

Exercises

Before and after every bout of scheduled exercise, gentle exercises such as these should be done in order to speed up and slow down the blood flow gradually. This protects the heart from strain, and stops the blood from "pooling" in the legs when exercise has stopped but the heart is still pumping strongly. The exercises also allow the body to warm up and cool down gradually so that there is no temperature shock, as might be experienced for instance after vigorous exercise on a very cold morning. Any bending and stretching or loosening exercises will serve the purpose; we illustrate two.

1a Stand straight with your left hand on your hip and your right arm curved above your head.

1b Bend over to the left with small "bouncing" movements. Then change arms and bend to the other side. Do this exercise several times on each side.

2a Stand straight with your legs together and your arms by your sides.

2b Jump into the air, raising your arms and kicking your legs apart; land in the original position. Repeat several times.

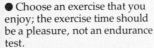

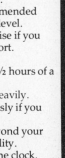

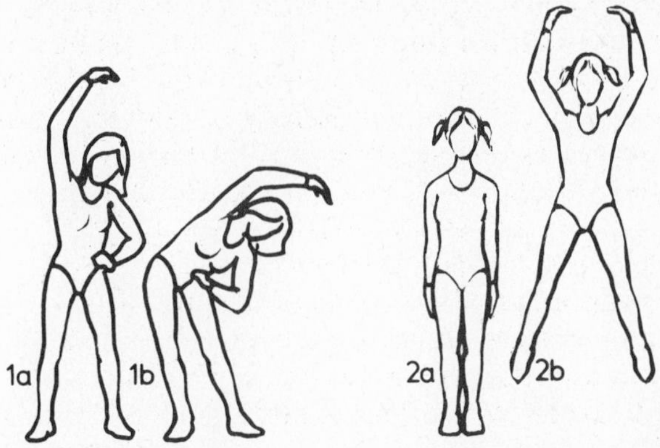

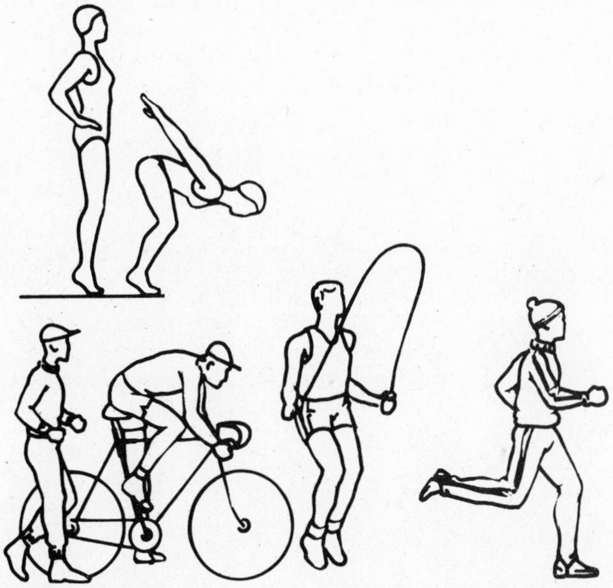

Exercise activities

Aerobic exercises, those that take extra air into the lungs, are excellent for strengthening the heart and providing the blood with plenty of oxygen. Activities such as brisk walking, swimming, cycling, jumping or skipping with a rope, and jogging are recommended for those starting out on a regular course of exercise for the first time in several years. As your fitness increases you can enter into other, more strenuous aerobic activities such as racket sports, sprinting, competitive swimming and canoeing, cross-country skiing and running etc. In any case remember that all exercise activities should be built up very slowly; exercise for only a very few minutes each time for the first week or so, then gradually increase as you feel yourself getting fitter and more capable. Never exercise to the point of exhaustion. Stop at once if you feel faint, dizzy or sick, if you become pallid or get spots before your eyes, if you become very short of breath, or if you feel a pain in your chest or head. If these symptoms recur each time you try to exercise, take them as warning signs and see a doctor. Rather than exercising against the clock, or increasing your targets in set times, make relaxation and enjoyment the key elements of your exercise times.

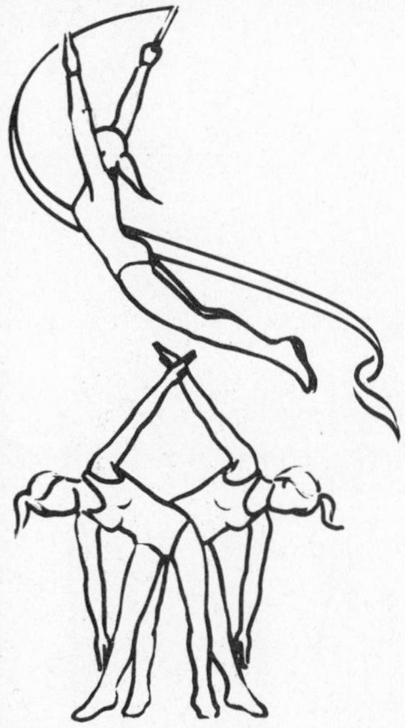

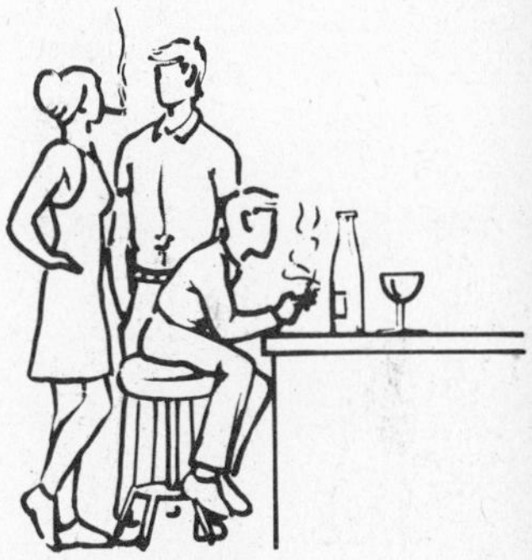

Do

- Choose an exercise that you enjoy; the exercise time should be a pleasure, not an endurance test.
- Check up with a doctor if you have not exercised regularly for a long time or if you have any other health doubts.
- Choose an exercise within your capabilities.
- Lose any excess weight.
- Warm up and cool down with appropriate exercises each time.
- Walk instead of using other transport whenever possible.
- Keep a close check on your pulse rate, both during and after exercise.
- Vary your exercise activity if you get bored.

Don't

- Exercise strenuously without medical supervision.
- Exceed the recommended pulse limit for your level.
- Continue to exercise if you feel pain or discomfort.
- Eat large meals.
- Exercise within 1½ hours of a meal.
- Smoke or drink heavily.
- Exercise strenuously if you are overweight.
- Push yourself beyond your achievement capability.
- Exercise against the clock.
- Force yourself to do an exercise activity you dislike.
- Have a cold drink or take a cold shower immediately after exercise.

Circulation

Much as a pump drives hot water through the pipes of a central heating system, the heart drives blood around the body through a closed system of tubes called blood vessels. The blood that flows through these tubes nourishes all body tissues. Its main ingredients are the straw-colored fluid called plasma (protein cells in water); red blood cells, which supply oxygen obtained from the lungs; and white blood cells that scavenge dead tissue and help to defend the body against invading germs. It also contains platelets (used in the clotting process), salts, electrolytes, vitamins and minerals; all of these elements have to be present within fine quantity limits to maintain a healthy body.

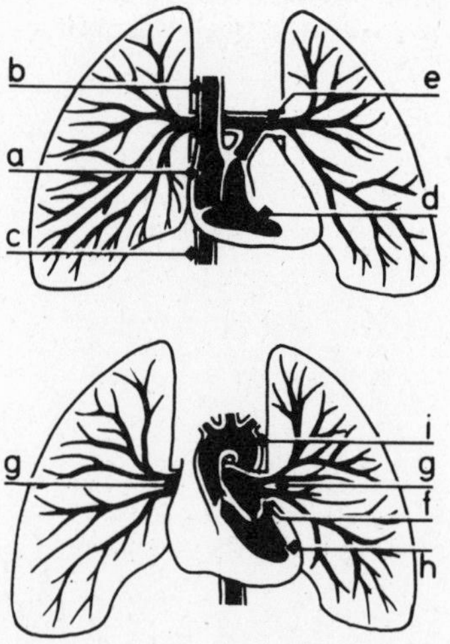

Oxygenation of the blood
The heart pumps two kinds of blood: deoxygenated and oxygenated. The diagrams show these two aspects of the circulation. In the top diagram, deoxygenated blood enters the right atrium (**a**) via the superior (**b**) and inferior (**c**) vena cavae, and is pumped by the right ventricle (**d**) to the lungs via the pulmonary artery (**e**). In the bottom diagram, oxygenated blood from the lungs enters the left atrium (**f**) via the pulmonary veins (**g**), and the left ventricle (**h**) pumps it out via the aorta (**i**). Veins are blood vessels that carry blood toward the heart, arteries carry blood away from it.

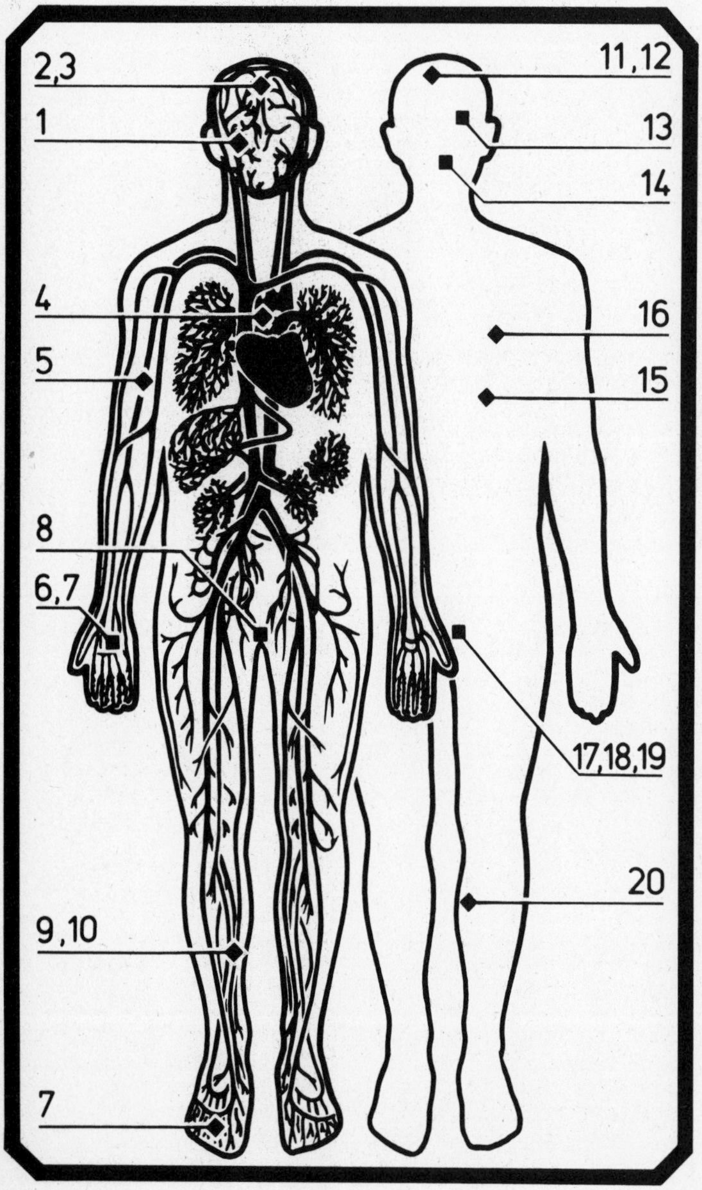

Locations of problems
The left half of this illustration shows sites of major and minor circulation disorders.
1 Anemia, any of several red blood cell defects affecting the whole body.
2 Fainting, caused by a briefly reduced blood flow to the brain.
3 Stroke, caused by a blocked or burst artery affecting the brain.
4 Atherosclerosis, a thickening and narrowing of the arteries caused by deposits of cholesterol and other debris (see p.80).
5 High blood pressure; the causes of this are often unknown, but some cases are caused by kidney disease.
6 Raynaud's disease causes spasm of the digital arteries.
7 Chilblains, painful or itchy swellings that may occur on cold hands, feet or ears because of poor circulation.
8 Piles, swollen veins in the rectum.
9 Varicose veins, swollen veins occurring in the legs if the venous valves are defective.
10 Thrombophlebitis, a blood clot and inflammation that affects deep or surface leg veins. This condition often occurs in the bedridden, but exercising the legs helps to prevent it. Deep-vein thrombosis requires medical treatment.

Danger signs
The right half of the diagram shows the locations of circulation disorders, and other problems that may be indicated by circulation abnormalities.
11 A combination of light-headedness, lethargy, morning headache, flushed face, and ringing in the ears may indicate high blood pressure.
12 Confusion, dizziness, slurred speech or paralysis of limbs may mean that a stroke has occurred.
13 The insides of the eyelids are usually pale if the person is anemic.
14 Blood in sputum may indicate an injury or disease in the lungs.
15 Blood in vomit may be caused by injury or disease in the digestive tract. If any blood is lost in this way, seek medical help immediately.
16 Fatigue, combined with breathlessness after exertion, may indicate anemia, although many other illnesses may also produce these symptoms.
17 Vaginal bleeding between periods or after the menopause should always be investigated.
18 Blood in urine is usually caused by a minor infection but should be investigated.
19 Blood in stools may be caused by piles, or may indicate an ulcer or other serious complaint. Any bleeding that persists should be medically investigated.
20 Cramping pain and swelling in the calf may suggest deep-vein thrombosis and should be treated medically.

Blood pressure
This is the force with which the blood presses on the walls of the arteries. It is measured with a sphygmomanometer, consisting of a gauge and an inflatable cuff (*right*), and a stethoscope. Two readings are taken, as the heart contracts and then relaxes, which show the systolic and diastolic pressures respectively. If these are too high your doctor will prescribe drugs and probably advise you to restrict your salt intake and avoid obesity, as untreated high blood pressure, or hypertension, can be fatal.

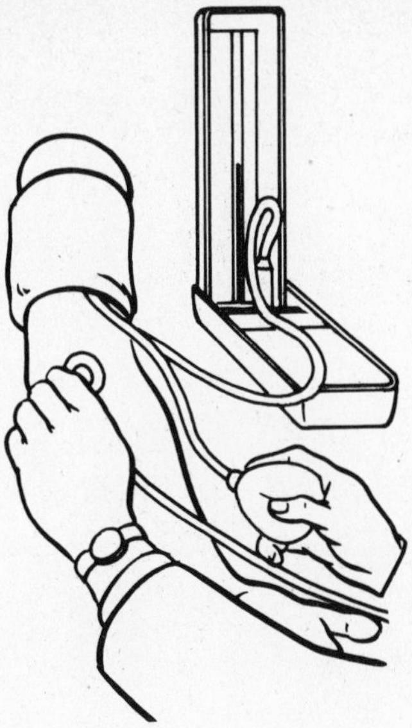

People at risk
Some types seem more prone than others to major circulatory problems. Below age 40 coronary disease is almost entirely a male disease. Muscular and overweight men are most often the victims of early heart attacks and these types of attack tend to run in families. Otherwise groups at risk from major circulatory problems include the obese, heavy smokers, the inactive and those under stress. The chart *right* shows the percentage of US male (**A**) and female (**B**) deaths from cardiovascular diseases that occur in various age groups.

A	B	Age
0·4%	0·3%	0-24
3%	1%	25-44
8%	4%	45-54
18%	10%	55-64
71%	85%	65+

Fainting
This happens when the brain is briefly starved of oxygen. It can occur through shock, or fear, on jumping up after kneeling, after a long soaking in a hot bath, or in early pregnancy. Warning signs are turning pale, a cold sweat on the face, dizziness and nausea. If you feel dizzy and about to faint, sit with your head between your knees as shown *right*. This improves blood flow to the brain and should prevent actual blackout. If a person does faint, lie him or her down with the feet raised and loosen tight clothing around the neck, chest and waist. Recovery takes no more than a minute or two.

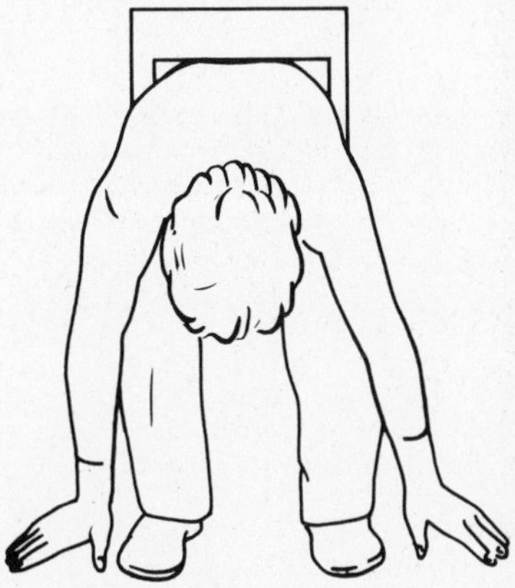

Bleeding
Clotting factors in the blood soon tend to seal a small cut. It may help if you press a clean cloth pad (such as a folded handkerchief) against the wound. If bleeding persists add more layers of cloth, increasing the pressure and keeping the injured part still. To stop copious bleeding press together the wound edges with a clean cloth or even your fingers, and raise the cut limb; prevent shock by lying the patient down with feet above head level. If possible clean a small wound with antiseptic, and sterile gauze swabs. Then cover with clean gauze kept in place by a bandage or adhesive tape, and seek medical aid.

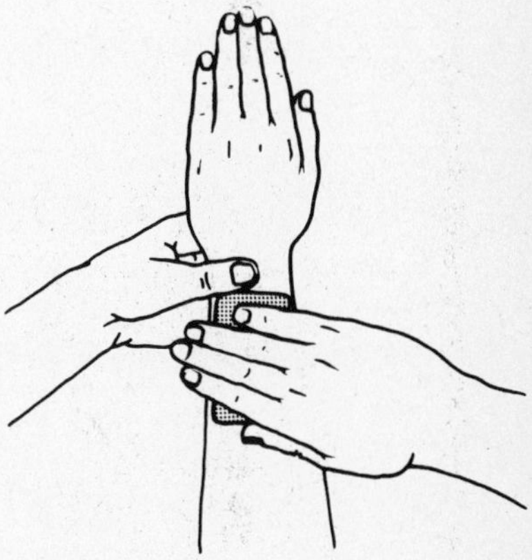

Anemia
This describes several defects of red blood cells, all of which make the victims feel weak, tired and even breathless. One cause common in underdeveloped countries is lack of iron intake in the diet, but this is rare in the Western world except among pregnant women and premature infants. Loss of blood caused by a bleeding ulcer or cancerous lesion, or by persistently heavy menstrual periods, can also lead to anemia, as can various malabsorption diseases or a poor metabolism. Sickle cell anemia, aplastic anemia and thalassemia are congenital or acquired blood disorders.

Varicose veins
Superficial leg veins sometimes become swollen and tortuous, causing aching or discomfort. This happens when defects occur in valves controlling the flow of blood up the veins to the heart. Blood pools in the superficial veins making them bulge (surrounding muscle prevents this happening to the deep veins). About 10% of people are born with faulty valves that may cause varicose veins if their work involves unrelieved standing so that the calf muscles cannot pump the blood "uphill." Pregnant women and obese people are more at risk than others. For treatment see pp.120–121.

Hemorrhoids
Hemorrhoids (piles) are varicose veins that occur in the rectum and anus when faulty valves let blood flow the wrong way and pool; the surrounding vein swells and may grow inflamed. Internal hemorrhoids occur high in the anal canal. External hemorrhoids protrude from the rectum. Hemorrhoids may be itchy or painful, with bleeding, infection or ulceration. But symptoms may also be mild and disappear for long periods. In fact, hemorrhoids tend to give trouble only when their effects are accentuated by such conditions as pregnancy, chronic coughing and chronic constipation.

Clotting
Blood clots may form in blood vessels if these are roughened by deposits or are injured by accident, surgery or childbirth. Cellular blobs called platelets pile up in the damaged vessel, triggering production of a mesh of fibrin fibers. These trap blood cells and platelets, to form a clot that hampers or blocks blood flow through the vessel. A thrombus is a clot that stays where it was formed. Often new blood vessels grow around a vessel blocked by a thrombus. An embolus is a thrombus that breaks away and flows through the bloodstream until it lodges somewhere else. Doctors may use anticoagulants to disperse dangerous clots.

Respiratory system 1

This system's task consists of supplying the blood with oxygen (vital for the body's life processes) and ridding it of carbon dioxide waste. Entering the system through the nose, air is filtered, warmed and moistened and then flows on down through the pharynx, larynx, and windpipe (or trachea). This tube divides into two bronchi which feed air to the two big, spongy masses of tissue called the lungs. Inside each lung, bronchi divide and subdivide like tree roots, ending in tiny hollow cups called alveoli. Tiny blood vessels connected to these alveoli absorb oxygen and lose carbon dioxide gases; breathing in draws oxygen into the lungs; breathing out expels carbon dioxide.

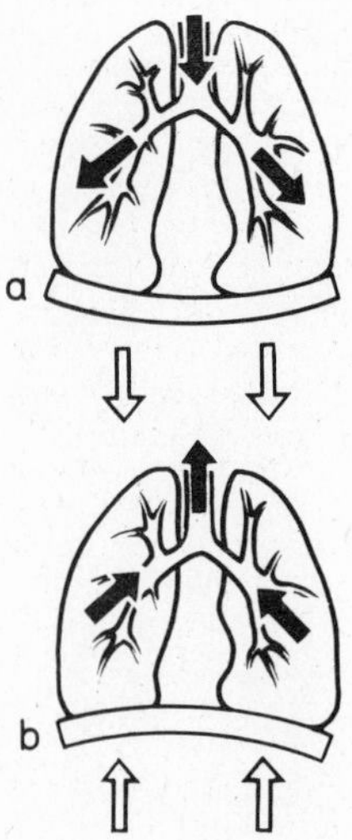

How the lungs work
Lungs let air in and out by expanding and contracting passively. They are operated by the muscles of the ribs that curve around them, and by the diaphragm – a sheet of muscle lying just below them. Breathing in (**a**) occurs when the diaphragm moves down and the ribs move out. This enlarges the chest cavity containing the ribs, and so creates a partial vacuum. To fill that vacuum, air flows into the lungs and these expand because their tissue is elastic. Breathing out (**b**) occurs when the diaphragm moves up and the ribs move in. This reduces the chest cavity so that air is forced out of the lungs.

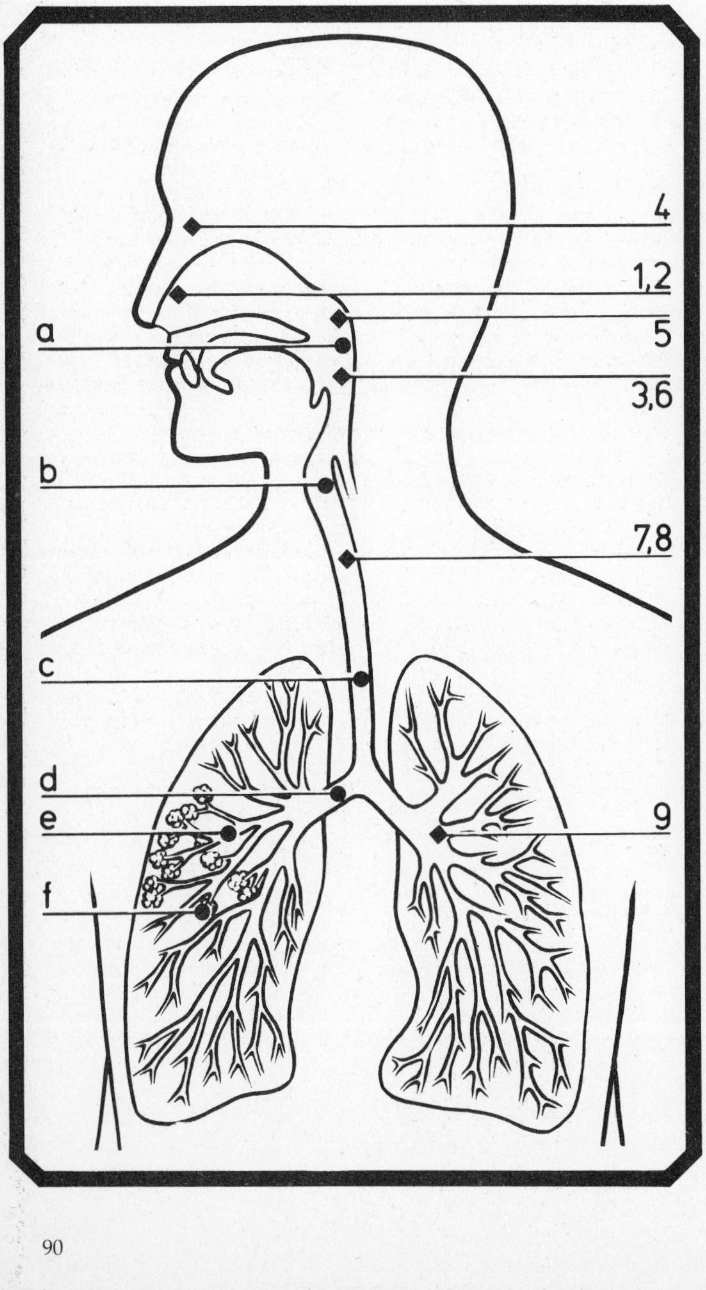

Parts of the respiratory system
a Pharynx.
b Larynx.
c Trachea.
d Bronchus.
e Bronchiole.
f Alveoli.

Minor problems
The illustration shows the sites of some of the relatively minor problems that can affect the respiratory system. Most of the problems that affect the trachea or above are minor, and will clear up of their own accord or with simple treatment. Some troubles that occur in the lungs are more stubborn as these parts of the respiratory system are less easily accessible.
1 Nasal polyps are soft growths hanging from the mucous membranes lining the inside of the nose; they may occur singly or in groups. If they block the nasal airway, they should be removed surgically.
2 A nose blocked by mucus can usually be cleared by blowing the nose. If you use nose drops, make sure that they are a brand approved by your doctor, as frequent use of some nose drops can damage the linings of the nose and the sinuses.
3 The common cold virus causes sneezing, watery eyes, a watery nasal discharge, and often a sore throat. The condition usually lasts only 2–3 days, but secondary infections may set in.
4 Discharges from the nose with simultaneous headaches are usually caused by sinusitis, an infection of some of the cavities in the front of the skull. Long-term antibiotic treatment or sinus clearing surgery may be required.
5 Adenoids, the glands at the back of the nose, become chronically enlarged in some children and cause mouth-breathing by day and snoring by night. The adenoids usually shrink back to a normal size eventually.
6 A sore throat is usually caused by a viral infection, and is best treated by sucking candies that lubricate the throat with saliva. Gargling and sucking antiseptic throat lozenges may ease the condition or may make the throat feel even sorer. A recurrent sore throat linked with tonsillitis (inflammation of the glands at the back of the throat) may require removal of the tonsils.
7 Coughing may be caused by inhaling a particle of food or debris, inhaling saliva, or developing an infection of the nose, throat or lungs.
8 Hiccups, caused by spasms of the diaphragm, are often cured by holding the breath briefly or applying gentle pressure to the chest.
9 Overbreathing is a nervous condition usually caused by anxiety.

Coughs
Coughs are caused by irritation of the respiratory tract, for instance by infection or by inhaled food or smoke particles. If your cough is merely tickling and irritating, suppress it with a cough mixture, but if you have a rattling cough that produces sputum, an expectorant will help clearance. Coughs that cause pain just below the breastbone or lower in the chest suggest tracheitis or pleurisy, and call for medical advice. So, too, does a child's cough that ends with a "whoop" or gasp (see p. 93). Any cough or hoarseness that persists without apparent cause should be investigated.

Overbreathing
Overbreathing, or hyperventilation, occurs when anxiety causes apparent air hunger; the person concerned feels that he or she is not receiving enough air, and takes deep gulping breaths. In fact the opposite is true; the person is overbreathing and receiving too little carbon dioxide, which can cause dizziness, tingling in the skin, cramp in the hands, and feelings of panic. Relief can be obtained by holding a paper bag over the person's mouth for a few breaths so that carbon dioxide is reinhaled; this will correct the imbalance. If a bag is not available, you can cup your hands over the person's mouth.

Hay fever
This is a common allergy where the body reacts abnormally to breathed-in pollen by producing an antibody that combines with the pollen, so stimulating the release of histamine. This in turn swells blood vessels and produces a runny, itchy, blocked nose; sneezing; bloodshot eyes; and a sore burning sensation in the mouth. Hay fever occurs in spring or summer when pollen is plentiful. House dust, animal scurf and other allergens have a similar but continuous effect on some people. Victims should try to avoid the allergens, and antihistamines, steroid drugs, and specific desensitization may help.

Posture and breathing
Slouching as you sit, stand or walk (and wearing restrictive clothes) hinders efficient breathing and may contribute to impaired lung function. Practice sitting with a straight back in a chair that supports the head and back. Alternatively stand with your head up, neck straight, shoulders down and back, stomach and buttocks in, but hold yourself naturally, not stiffly. You might also try standing with arms down by your sides, then inhaling deeply as you raise your arms outstretched to shoulder level. Breathe out fully as you lower your arms.

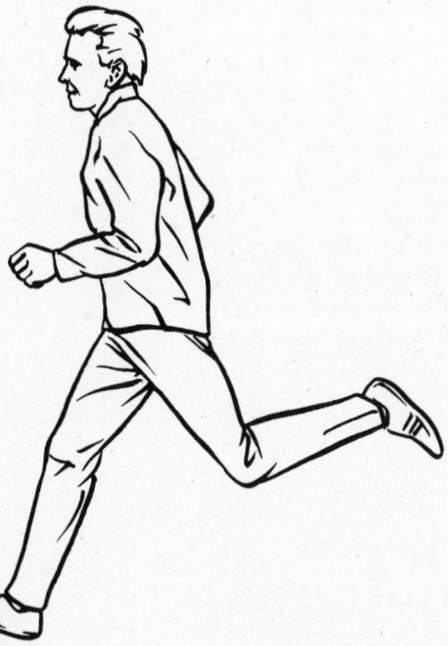

Exercise and the lungs
Because the lungs are simply passive, spongy bags, they themselves are not improved by exercise. But by exercising the muscles that work the lungs you help these to achieve their maximum efficiency. Keeping up such exercise throughout life not only helps you feel fit but may help to slow down the rate at which the lungs lose efficiency with age. Anyone taking exercise that is vigorous enough to make him pant should not need other breathing exercises. There are various aerobic exercises – those designed to increase the body's needs for oxygen and so to make the whole circulatory-respiratory system work harder. Healthy people can try walking quickly, jogging, cycling, swimming, jumping rope or any combination of these. In running, inhale air deeply through the mouth, breathing from the abdomen so that the stomach expands on breathing in and flattens on exhaling. Rhythmic breathing, not gasping, is the aim. Rhythmic breathing and striding are helped by "running tall" and swinging the arms at the sides rather than across the body. For further advice on aerobic exercises, see also pp. 38–39.

Do
- Have nasal polyps removed if they obstruct nasal breathing.
- Keep the nasal airways open during a cold or other nasal infection – preferably by gently blowing the nose into a handkerchief.
- Seek medical help for chronic nasal and sinus infection.
- Use soothing medicine or suck candies for a sore throat caused by a virus infection.
- Seek medical help if you lose your voice or it stays hoarse for more than a few days.
- Hold your breath to cure hiccups.
- Place a paper bag over the mouth to stop overbreathing.
- Seek medical help for coughs that give pain, end in a whoop, or last for more than a few days without obvious cause.
- Try medically approved drugs or desensitization if suffering an allergy such as hayfever.
- Cultivate good sitting, standing and walking posture.
- Exercise the lungs to help keep them effective.

Don't
- Bother you doctor if you just have a cold – he can't cure it either.
- Suppress a cough that helps to produce sputum.
- Ignore a blocked nose and breathe through your mouth; this will get you into bad breathing habits and will not help to cure the source of the problem.
- Blow your nose so violently as to cause a nosebleed.
- Use nasal sprays or ephedrine or isoprenaline drops without medical approval.
- Ignore chronic discharge of mucus into nose and throat; it could be a symptom of more serious problems.
- Ignore a persistent or painful cough, or a persistently lost or hoarse voice.
- Gargle or suck antiseptic throat lozenges without medical approval.
- Have adenoids and tonsils removed unless tonsils have proved persistently troublesome.
- Slouch, so that your lungs cannot fully expand or contract.

Respiratory system 2

Most major respiratory diseases are those that affect the lungs, sometimes starting as milder conditions higher up in the respiratory tract. The main causes are certain infections, inhaled particles of proteins and dust that affect the lungs, accidentally inhaled objects like pins and pieces of food, and cancer. Some lung troubles soon clear up but others progress or leave damage likely to be extended by later attacks. In certain conditions the lungs become so ineffective that untreated patients die of oxygen lack. Fortunately, antibiotics, surgery and self-help can prevent or minimize effects of some lung diseases that used to be fatal in the majority of cases.

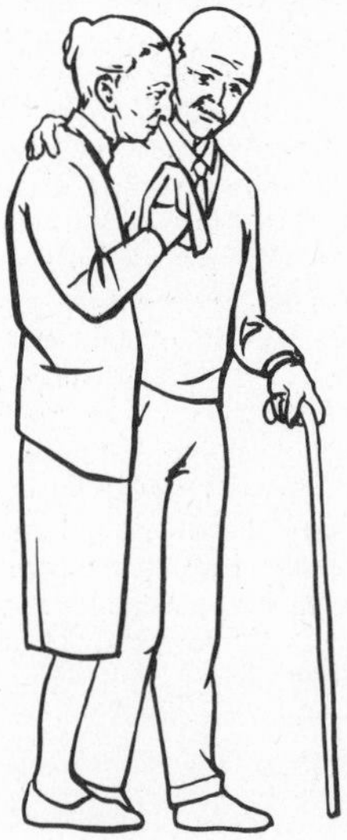

People at risk
The very young and very old are especially liable to serious respiratory troubles. Mothers who smoke may give birth to babies with respiratory diseases or susceptibility to chest infections and sudden unexplained death. Children who catch whooping cough or measles or accidentally inhale such things as peanuts may suffer permanent lung damage, and untreated sinus or tonsil troubles may lead to chronic bronchitis. Anyone who is overweight or smokes is at risk, and among old people even a mild influenza attack may cause potentially serious lung complications.

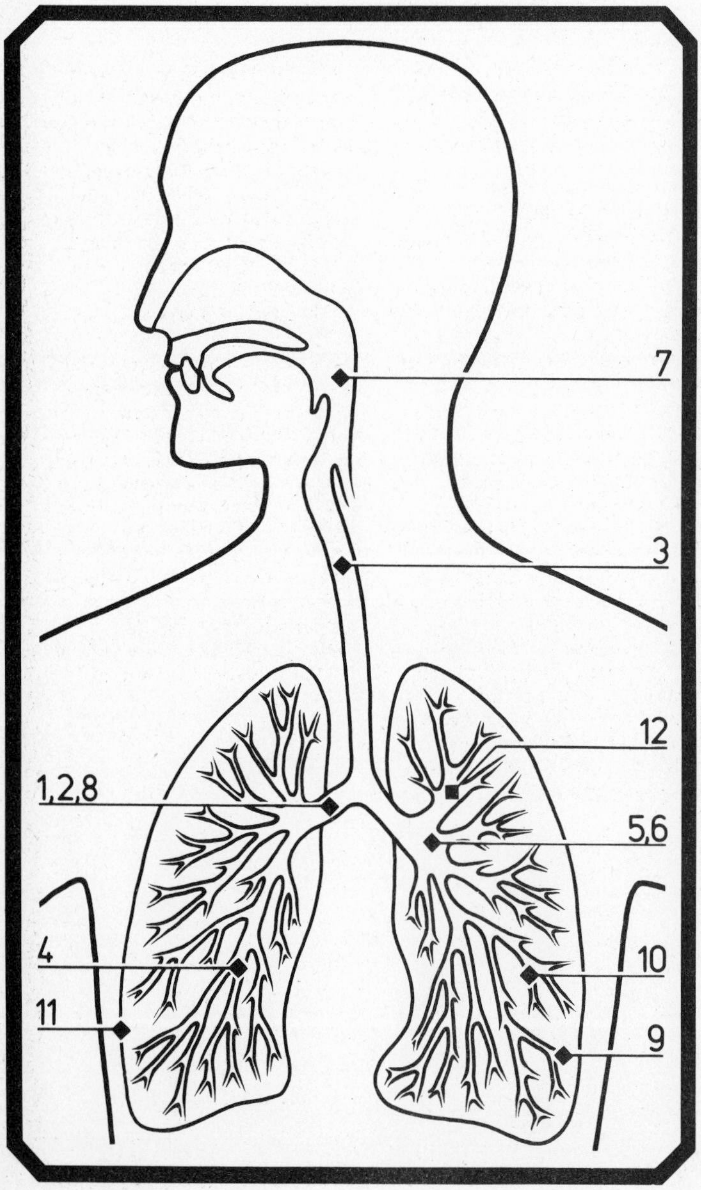

Serious respiratory problems
These are problems that can have more serious consequences than those listed on page 90, but early treatment may help to minimize their effects.

1 Asthma narrows the airways of the respiratory system and produces extra mucus, making it difficult to exhale.
2 Whooping cough occurs when the germ Bordetella pertussis attacks the bronchi, inflaming lung tissue and producing thick fluid that hampers breathing. Treat with bed rest, fresh air and prescribed antibiotics.
3 Choking is often caused by inhaling a foreign body. Many a life has been saved by striking the victim sharply several times between the shoulders, or by using the Heimlich maneuver (see p. 96).
4 A lung abscess involves damage, infection and loss of use of a small part of the lung, often due to inhaling a peanut or broken tooth.
5 Pneumoconiosis describes a group of dust diseases caused by inhaling particles of coal, silica, asbestos, or cotton (see p. 93).
6 Tuberculosis is a germ-borne disease that can form cavities in the lung with fatal results. However, it can be treated very effectively by the use of antibiotics such as streptomycin.
7 Influenza occurs when a virus invades the respiratory system, producing a running nose, sore throat, cough, generalized aching and other symptoms. Bed rest, painkillers, and plenty of fluid to drink are usually treatment enough. Only old patients and those with heart trouble or bronchitis need contact their doctor.
8 Bronchitis is inflammation of the bronchi, causing the coughing up of yellow sputum. Acute bronchitis may cause painful breathing.
9 Bronchiectasis involves permanent dilatation of the smaller bronchi. Antibiotics, postural drainage and surgery may be helpful.
10 Pneumonia is inflammation of the lung due to infection; parts of the lung fill with fluid and become airless. Lobar pneumonia affects one or more lobes of the lung; so called bronchopneumonia affects both lungs in a patchy way.
11 Pleurisy is inflammation of the pleura – the membrane that covers each lung and the chest wall. It may accompany pneumonia, carcinoma (cancer) and pulmonary infarction (caused by obstruction of local circulation). There may be pain in the side of the chest, or shortness of breath.
12 Lung cancer causes pressure on the surrounding structures and often the development of secondary cancerous deposits in the brain, bone, liver, adrenals and skin. The disease is usually fatal.

Asthma
The narrowed airways and breathing difficulty produced by asthma attacks tend to be caused by an allergy, usually to house dust. Infection, sudden activity or excitement may provoke an attack. Ways of preventing attacks include desensitization (which works best in the young), and trying to avoid the conditions listed above. Removing pets may be necessary if animal fur acts as an allergen. Doctors prescribe dilator drugs as aerosol sprays, tablets, powders or injections to dilate airways and curb the output of mucus. Some treatments prevent attacks; others relieve symptoms already present.

Air pollution and illness
Atmospheric pollution and smoking are the prime causes of chronic bronchitis, a major cause of illness and death in industrialized countries. Reductions in air pollution produce a decrease in chronic bronchitis, but an increase in the incidence of smoking causes an increase in the incidence of chronic bronchitis. People working with asbestos, silica, and other dangerous dusts may avoid potentially fatal lung diseases if they wear protective clothing and masks. If you think you are at risk, consult your doctor.

Immunizations
You can now have yourself or your children immunized against several respiratory diseases that were once major killers. Vaccination against whooping cough and diphtheria is given with other vaccinations during the first year of life. Whooping cough vaccine rarely causes serious side effects, but the disease may cause bronchiectasis or other serious complications, so have your child vaccinated unless your doctor advises against it. Vaccination against tuberculosis can be given, if wished, at 10–13 years. There are influenza vaccines, but to be effective they must match the prevalent strain of virus.

Lung cancer
Cells in the bronchi start to grow in an uncontrolled way and invade other tissues with usually fatal results. Lung cancer is caused by the deposition of carcinogenic material in the airways, from smoking, polluted urban air, or the inhalation of asbestos dust or certain other dusts produced by mines or factories. By far the biggest culprit is smoking. Lung cancer kills many thousands each year, yet could be almost entirely prevented if people stopped smoking and lived and worked in clean air. Warning signs include coughing and spitting blood-stained sputum, weight loss, malaise and lassitude (see p. 166).

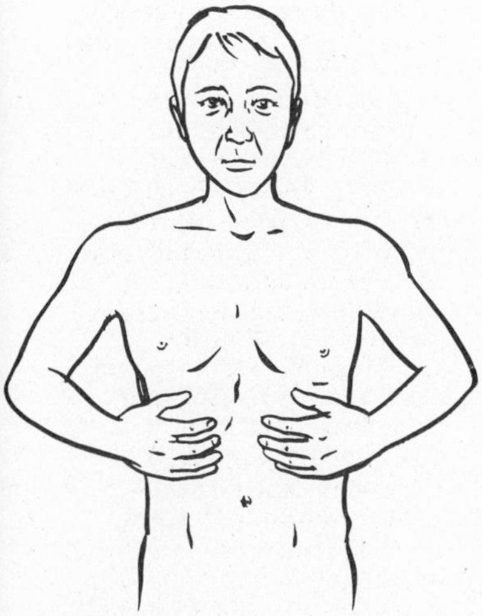

Treating bronchitis
In an acute attack stay in bed in a room with warm but not dry air until your temperature is normal. Antibiotics and a soothing inhalant help; use a cough suppressant only if you have an irritating, unproductive cough. Treat aches with analgesics that do not irritate the stomach. Chronic bronchitics should practice breathing out, sitting relaxed with fingernails on the lower rib cage. As you gently breathe out you feel your rib cage sink below your fingertips. As you gently breathe in you feel the rib cage rise. Practice controlled breathing for several minutes twice daily.

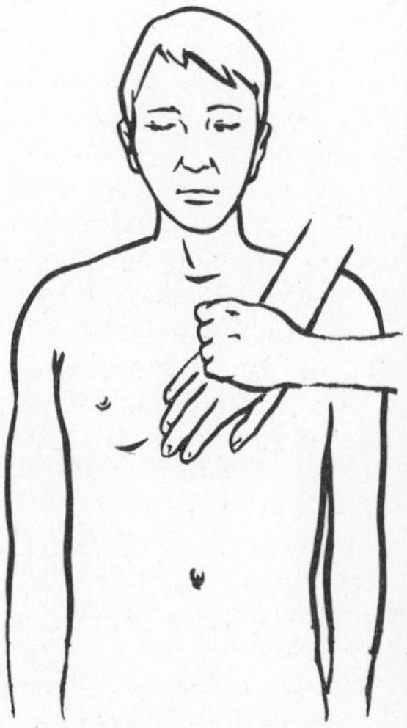

Treating pneumonia
Severe pneumonia needs hospital care; antibiotics help in treating bronchopneumonia and lobar pneumonia. The patient sits up in bed in a well-ventilated warm room, at first taking only milk, orange juice or similar fluids, with some solid food after a day or two. Postural drainage (lying tilted with the affected part of the lung uppermost) may assist coughing up sputum, and so may placing a hand on that part of the patient's chest and punching the hand with a clenched fist. Similar treatment aids lung abscesses, bronchiectasis and cystic fibrosis.

Do
- Take bed rest for any infections involving high temperatures.
- Take care not to inhale any particles of food.
- Store peanuts out of the reach of small children.
- Call a doctor for all but slight chest infections.
- Cough up infected sputum.
- Try postural drainage to help clear infection.
- Try to live and work in clean air.
- Use the lungs fully; breathing exercises may help.
- Keep your weight down.
- Maintain an adequate, balanced diet.
- Expose your skin to sunshine at least occasionally.
- If asthmatic, avoid stress, sudden activity and, if possible, known allergens.
- Have your children immunized against whooping cough, diphtheria and tuberculosis, unless advised otherwise by your doctor.
- Use a smog mask if exposed to bad air pollution.

Don't
- Allow small children to eat peanuts, or to play with beads, dried seeds, or any other items small enough to be inhaled.
- Allow yourself to become alcoholically intoxicated; this can lead to the aspiration of food or vomit, which can be fatal or which may lead to aspiration pneumonia.
- Become overweight.
- Smoke.
- Work in dusty air – especially if the type of dust present is known to harm the lungs.
- Call the doctor for influenza unless the patient is old or has a heart or chronic chest ailment.
- Enter stuffy rooms if you are subject to chest troubles.
- Breathe cold, damp air if you are subject to chest troubles.
- Slouch.
- Underuse your lungs.
- Ignore signs that may indicate lung cancer or other serious diseases.

Digestive system 1

The digestive system is basically a tube designed to break down food particles for use inside the body. The tube starts at the mouth and ends at the anus. Between the two, different parts of the digestive system play specific roles as food dismantlers. As the food passes through the system, it gets chewed, moistened, churned and then digested until its particles are molecules small enough to filter through the tube wall into the bloodstream, where they circulate around the body to provide essential nutrients. Meanwhile the residue continues through the digestive system and exits from the anus.

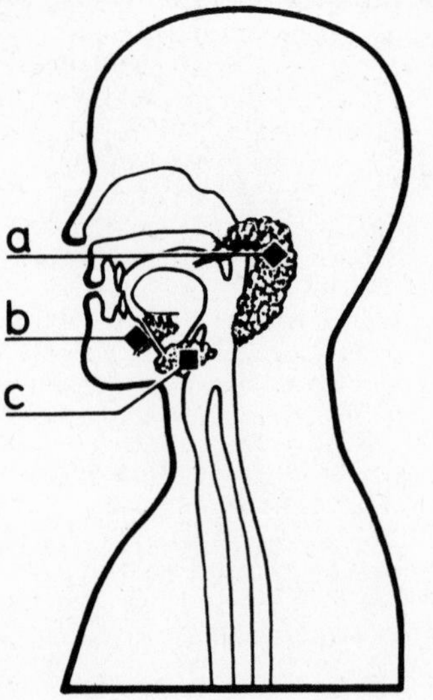

Salivary glands
As food is chewed it is moistened by and mixed with saliva from the salivary glands. There are three pairs of these glands; their positions are shown in this diagram of the left side of the head.
a Parotid gland.
b Sublingual gland.
c Submandibular gland.
Saliva contains the enzyme ptyalin; this breaks down starches into simple sugars, and initiates the process of digestion.

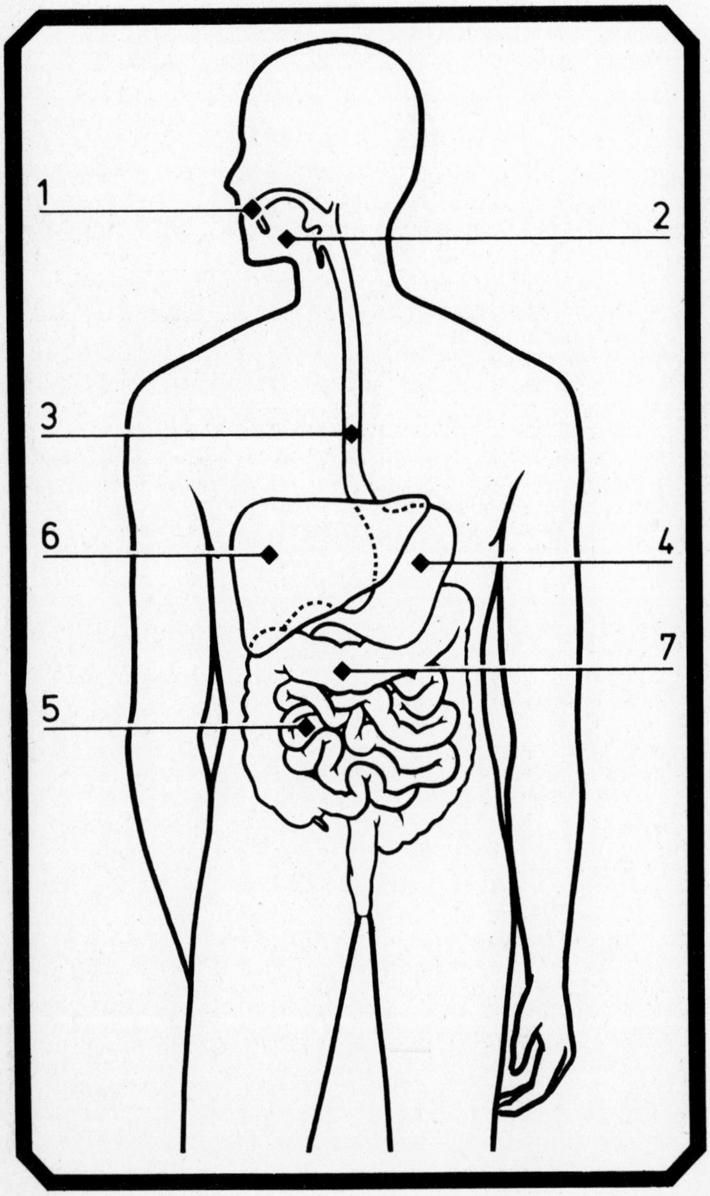

Digestive system
The illustration shows the various parts of the digestive system; here we list problems that commonly arise in these areas.
1 Teeth; these chop up food into small particles so that it is easy to digest. Aching teeth and painful gums are usually caused by poor dental hygiene (see pp. 64–67).
2 Salivary glands; these make the digestive juice saliva, which begins converting starch to sugar. Painful swelling of these glands occurs in mumps.
3 Esophagus (gullet); this pushes food down to the stomach by means of waves of muscular contraction. Burning chest pain may indicate heartburn or other forms of esophagitis.
4 Stomach; this mixes the food with digestive gastric juice containing the enzyme pepsin, which digests meat, and hydrochloric acid. Stomach problems include indigestion and gastritis; many stomach complaints produce symptoms that include nausea.
5 Small intestine; digestion of fats, proteins and starches is completed in this tube, which is over 20ft long. The active agents are digestive juices from the liver, gallbladder and pancreas. Digested foods pass through the wall of the small intestine into the bloodstream. The duodenum, or upper part of the small intestine, is the site where duodenal ulcers occur.
6 Liver, pancreas and gallbladder; these all produce digestive juices – for further information see pp. 106–107.
7 Large intestine; this portion of the digestive tract receives and stores undigested ("waste") foods from the small intestine. It also absorbs some water and minerals, and breeds bacteria; the waste and bacteria combine to form the feces, which are expelled from the rectum via the anus. Problems of the large intestine include constipation and diarrhea, which can both have various causes, and appendicitis, which is inflammation of a short cul-de-sac of intestine.

Food
Foods contain chemicals that we need for building and repairing body tissues, providing energy, and regulating how the body works. Organic (carbon-based) nutrients include proteins (essential for body building and repair) and carbohydrates and fats (providing energy) as well as vitamins (which help the body to work effectively). We also need inorganic nutrients such as minerals and water. Fats and proteins largely come from animals and seeds, and plants provide most carbohydrate foods. A balanced diet will build and maintain a healthy body (see pp. 22–25).

Digestive process
This process breaks down the big, complex molecules of food. Proteins are progressively split up into amino acid molecules by juices in the stomach and the small intestine. Fats turn into glycerol and fatty acids through the action of enzymes from the pancreas and small intestine, helped by bile from the liver and gallbladder. Starch and complex sugars become simple sugars under the attack of saliva, pancreatic juice and small intestine juice. The products of digestion form units small enough to pass into and through the cells that line the small intestine.

Metabolic problems
Some people have inborn defects of metabolism making them unable to use certain nutrients. People with celiac disease cannot digest the gluten in wheat; they lose weight, develop anemia and a swollen abdomen, and yield fatty stools. Infants with galactosemia cannot cope with lactose (milk sugar) or galactose (a sugar produced by digesting lactose). They fail to gain weight and suffer from liver trouble; in time there may be cataracts and brain damage. Phenylketonuria victims cannot use one constituent of proteins. Such conditions proved untreatable until special diets were devised for them.

Diets for special needs
If certain foods have marked effects on the body, special diets may be needed. Pregnant women need at least some foods rich in iron and calcium. Young children benefit from food rich in iron, calcium and vitamin D. Some special diets ease particular conditions. Celiac sufferers thrive on a gluten-free diet. Infants with galactosemia need lactose-free milk preparations. Those with phenylketonuria receive a protein digest without the problem ingredient. People with high blood pressure and some kidney disorders often need to reduce sodium intake, especially in the form of salt.

Appetite problems
Loss of appetite is a common symptom in children and adults, and frequently its cause is not serious. It may occur as a result of anxiety, depression, excitement, stress, or even early pregnancy. Children who lose their appetite may be overtired, anxious or incubating an infection, or they may have been eating snacks between meals. People obsessed with slimming may suffer anorexia nervosa, a psychiatric state where they deliberately starve themselves (see pp. 28–29). Most cases of loss of appetite disappear when the underlying physical or emotional problem is dealt with. Overeating may be overindulgence in food and drink on one particular occasion; this may lead to indigestion or even nausea and vomiting. In this case a bland diet will be needed to quiet the stomach. Alternatively, overeating may be psychological in origin, either a temporary reaction to stress of some kind or a lifelong compulsion leading to obesity. Obese people are breathless, tired, and liable to respiratory diseases, diabetes, varicose veins, diseases of the heart and kidneys, and atherosclerosis. Compulsive eaters eat when they feel bored, depressed, guilty, frustrated or lonely; they will probably need psychiatric help to change their eating habits.

Bad breath
Unpleasant-smelling breath has several possible causes. An infection such as sinusitis, pyorrhea or gingivitis may give rise to an unpleasant odor, and so may a failure to clean your teeth properly. A recent meal containing strong-smelling ingredients such as garlic, onions or curry may cause the breath to smell, and so may smoking or drinking alcohol. If your stomach is empty of food, or if you have not drunk anything for several hours, your breath may begin to smell, or if you persistently breathe through your mouth rather than your nose. If you suspect that your bad breath arises from an infection, see your doctor or dentist so that he can work on curing the condition; make sure that you clean your teeth regularly, and also that you have something to eat or drink every few hours, even if it is only a glass of water. For temporary bad breath caused by strong food or drink, try an antiseptic mouthwash, or suck chlorophyll tablets or strong mint-flavored candy.

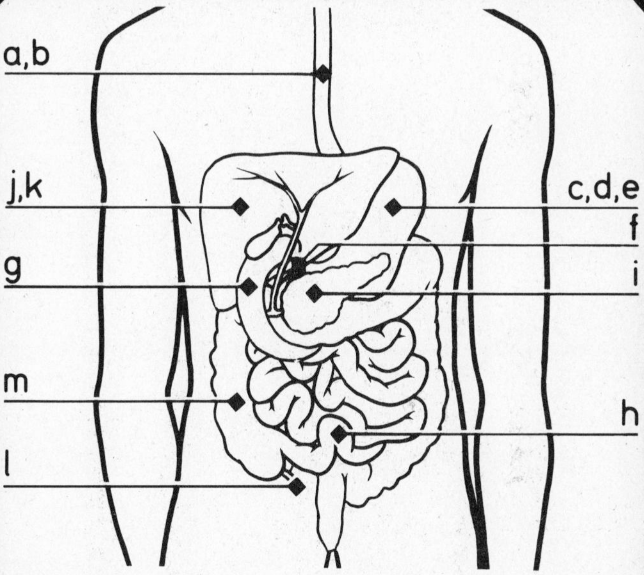

Vomiting
Physical causes of vomiting include the following.
a Intolerance of a particular food.
b Narrowed esophagus.
c Gastritis: inflammation of the stomach lining.
d Gastroenteritis: inflammation of the stomach and intestine linings because of food poisoning or other irritation.
e Stomach ulcer.
f Pyloric stenosis: narrowing of the muscular ring between the stomach and the small intestine.
g Duodenal ulcer.
h Ileitis: inflammation of the ileum, or lower part of the small intestine.
i Pancreatitis: inflammation of the pancreas.
j Hepatitis: inflammation of the liver.
k Cirrhosis of the liver.
l Appendicitis.
m Diverticulitis: inflammation of a pouch in the colon.
Cancer of various parts of the digestive tract may also cause vomiting. Treatment for simple vomiting attacks is bedrest, with no food or drink until the vomiting stops. Continuous vomiting calls for urgent hospital treatment.

Digestive system 2

For varying reasons most people experience a few minor digestive upsets at some stage in life. Infants suffer colic, flatulence and other troubles; children (and adults too) may suffer choking fits when food gets lodged in the throat. For some people, every journey is marred by motion sickness, and vacationers in foreign countries are notoriously prone to attacks of food poisoning, especially when the local water supply is suspect. A few unfortunate individuals swallow poisonous substances that may prove fatal unless remedies are swiftly applied. Many people are frequent sufferers from indigestion with no apparent cause. Many of the common digestive problems, such as indigestion, are linked with poor eating habits.

Man's digestive system is designed to function optimally on several small or medium-sized meals per day, but many people abuse their digestive system by eating too much, too little, too irregularly, or too quickly. They may fail to eat a balanced diet, or they may poison their systems with more alcohol or carbohydrate than their bodies can readily cope with. Smoking, stress and constipation (itself usually a product of poor eating habits) compound the problem. Happily there is much that can be done in the realm of personal health care to overcome many of the common problems that affect the digestive system.

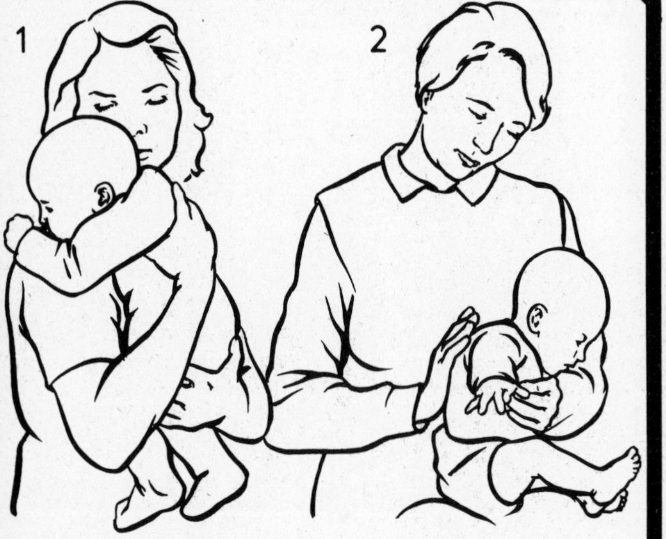

Babies' digestive problems
During feeding, a baby swallows air that forms a bubble in his stomach. Burping the baby at least once during each feeding and again afterward helps to prevent discomfort. There are several ways of doing this: two of them are pictured here.

1 The mother holds the baby against her shoulder while she gently rubs his back.

2 The mother holds the baby sitting upright in her lap as she gently rubs his back. Vigorous back-slapping is usually a waste of time. Feeding too quickly or not being fully burped may cause colic in a baby aged between two weeks and three months. The attacks of severe abdominal pain often come on in the evening, and the baby screams, while lying on its back with clenched fists and legs drawn up to the body. Cuddling or tightly wrapping up the child may bring relief. Medical opinion is divided about the true cause of colic. Gentle regurgitation of some milk after feeding is common in young babies, and no cause for concern provided the baby is still gaining weight. True vomiting may be due to an infection or obstruction, and calls for medical advice.

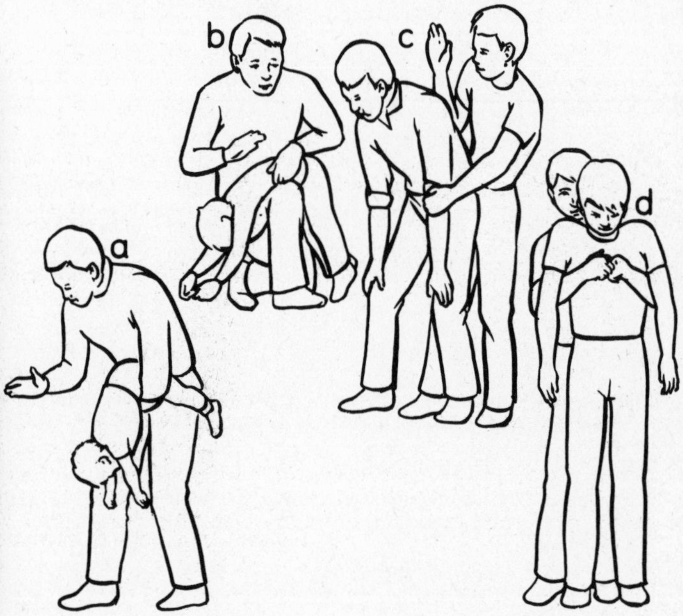

Choking and obstructions
Food, vomit or other objects lodged in the windpipe may cause choking, unconsciousness and death unless prompt action is taken. The illustrations show possible courses of action for attempting to remove an obstruction.

a If the person choking is an infant, grasp him by the legs and hold him upside down; smack him sharply several times between the shoulder blades. If the child is very small, make sure the head is supported as you turn him upside down to avoid injury to the neck.

b Lay an older child across your knee, head hanging down, and do the same.

c For adults, strike several sharp blows between the shoulder blades.

d If the smacking method is not effective with an adult, stand behind the person with your fists clasped against his upper abdomen, then push them up hard toward you. This is the Heimlich technique.

It is best not to try to remove an obstruction with a hooked finger or tweezers, since this almost invariably forces the obstruction farther down the windpipe. If the victim fails to breathe after you have shifted the obstruction, give mouth-to-mouth or mouth-to-nose artificial respiration. Detailed instructions for this can be found in first-aid manuals; ideally everyone should be taught this life-saving routine.

Indigestion
Also called dyspepsia, this condition involves heartburn, mild stomach pain, and possibly a bloated feeling after eating. Eating too quickly or taking too much food in one meal may cause indigestion, and so may the production of too much stomach acid. Chewing food thoroughly, avoiding half-cooked and gas-producing foods, avoiding fatty and rich foods and eating little and often may help to prevent or ease indigestion. Milk will often relieve the symptoms; antacids should be used sparingly. Sleep propped up by pillows at night, and keep a bland drink handy for relief of nighttime indigestion.

Motion sickness
People who get seasick, car sick, train sick or air sick are reacting to kinds of motion that turn the head in several dimensions at the same time. The balancing organ in the inner ear sends confusing signals to the brain's vomiting center, especially if the sufferer is watching the horizon (eye signals reach the brain before those from the inner ear). Shutting the eyes or lying down may minimize the symptoms. Travel sickness pills help by making the balancing organs less sensitive, but must be taken before you start your journey.

Food poisoning
This almost always occurs as a result of poor food hygiene. Symptoms typically comprise vomiting, diarrhea and abdominal pain; they may start up to 24 hours after eating food contaminated with bacteria, but within an hour if the poisoning is caused by bacterial toxins. Take plenty of fluids to replace those lost, and call a doctor if the symptoms persist for more than 24 hours or are severe. Food poisoning is often caused by germs that have been spread via insects (especially flies), unwashed hands, dirty kitchen utensils or polluted water (see p.19).

Poisoning
The first priority if you suspect that someone is poisoned is to seek medical advice immediately. If the person is conscious, find out what they have eaten or drunk; if the person is unconscious, or if the victim is too young to talk, look about for any sign of the poison such as pills, chemical containers etc. Telephone your local poison advice center immediately; the number should always be clearly written by the telephone. Tell the center the symptoms that the victim is showing, and what he or she might have swallowed. If the substance can be positively identified, they will advise you on the next course of action.

Flatulence
Eating foods that produce gas in the digestive system may produce functional indigestion (that is, indigestion that has no organic basis) as well as belching or passing wind. If you suffer from persistent flatulence, you should seek a doctor's advice so that any medical cause, such as gastritis or an ulcer, can be ruled out. If no medical problem exists, then you may find that changes in your eating habits will ease the problem. Gas-producing foods include brussels sprouts, cauliflower, turnips, peas, beans, cucumbers, green peppers, cabbage, radishes, and melons; these foods should be avoided as much as possible. Carbonated drinks are also likely to cause gas problems. You may experience less discomfort if you avoid lying down after a meal; allow plenty of time after your evening meal before going to bed. Eat slowly, chew each mouthful thoroughly, and do not talk while eating; all these measures will help to prevent you from swallowing air as you eat.

Acidity in foods
Many foods that taste acidic produce in the body an alkaline ash, and similarly many foods that lack any acid or sour taste produce an acid ash in the body. A healthy body automatically adjusts any acid/alkali imbalance, but if the functioning of the body is impaired in any way one of the elements may become temporarily or permanently dominant and cause distressing symptoms, as in indigestion, peptic ulcers, acid kidney stones etc. In such cases, the diet may need to be adjusted to neutralize the condition. Foods that produce an acid ash include cereals, cheese, corn, cranberries, eggs, fish, lentils, meats, peanuts, plums, prunes, rhubarb and walnuts. Foods such as butter, lard, vegetable oils, cornstarch, sugar, cream, coffee and tea are neutral, producing neither an acid or an alkaline ash, while almonds, brazil nuts, coconut, most vegetables and fruits other than those previously listed produce alkaline ash.

Do
- Burp babies gently during and after feeding.
- Cuddle a baby suffering from colic.
- Act instantly to give first aid to someone who is choking.
- Try milk before antacids to relieve indigestion symptoms.
- Try closing your eyes, lying down and taking preventive pills to relieve travel sickness.
- Wash hands and kitchen utensils before preparing food.
- Wash raw fruit and vegetables.
- Take plenty of clear fluids if you are suffering diarrhea from food poisoning.
- Store perishable foods such as meat, milk, fish, fats and cooked foods as cold as possible.
- Seek medical advice if you suspect poisoning.
- Allow plenty of time to eat.
- Chew food thoroughly before you swallow it.

Don't
- Irritate the stomach by heavy drinking or smoking.
- Irritate the stomach by prolonged use of aspirin.
- Overuse laxatives.
- Eat gas-producing foods if you are liable to indigestion or flatulence.
- Eat fatty and other rich foods if you are liable to indigestion.
- Eat badly-cooked food.
- Eat food that has been kept lukewarm.
- Worry about acidity in foods unless your doctor tells you that it matters.
- Take fruit juice on an empty stomach if you are liable to indigestion or if you have a peptic ulcer.
- Swallow air excessively as you eat.
- Eat hurriedly.
- Swallow large lumps of food.
- Eat more than you need.
- Swallow food or drink hot enough to scald your throat.
- Eat under stressful conditions.
- Drink tap water or ice made from it when supplies may be polluted.

Digestive system 3

Most of the digestive tract conditions featured on these pages are fairly serious. Some cause prolonged discomfort, some can be debilitating, others are acutely painful. A few can prove fatal if left untreated. However, almost all respond to self-help that can be given in your own home or workplace. For example, by taking care what, when, and how you eat you may be able to heal a peptic ulcer. Drinking plenty of fluids is a commonsense way of restoring body fluids lost through vomiting or diarrhea.
Modifying your daily pattern of activity helps some digestive ailments. People with esophagitis benefit by lying down after eating, while hiatus sufferers are better if they stand. Care with lifting heavy loads may prevent a hernia, and will certainly reduce the risk of worsening a hernia that is already present. Some of the conditions we describe will clear up with very simple treatment; others are chronic and can only be suppressed, so that although the underlying condition remains, you can spare yourself acute attacks of pain or discomfort that might occur otherwise. Of course you cannot cope with all the problems. Appendicitis, strangulated hernia, and chronically bleeding ulcers call for surgery. Then, too, many of the symptoms we describe could fit several ailments. In most instances you need medical help to establish diagnosis and treatment.

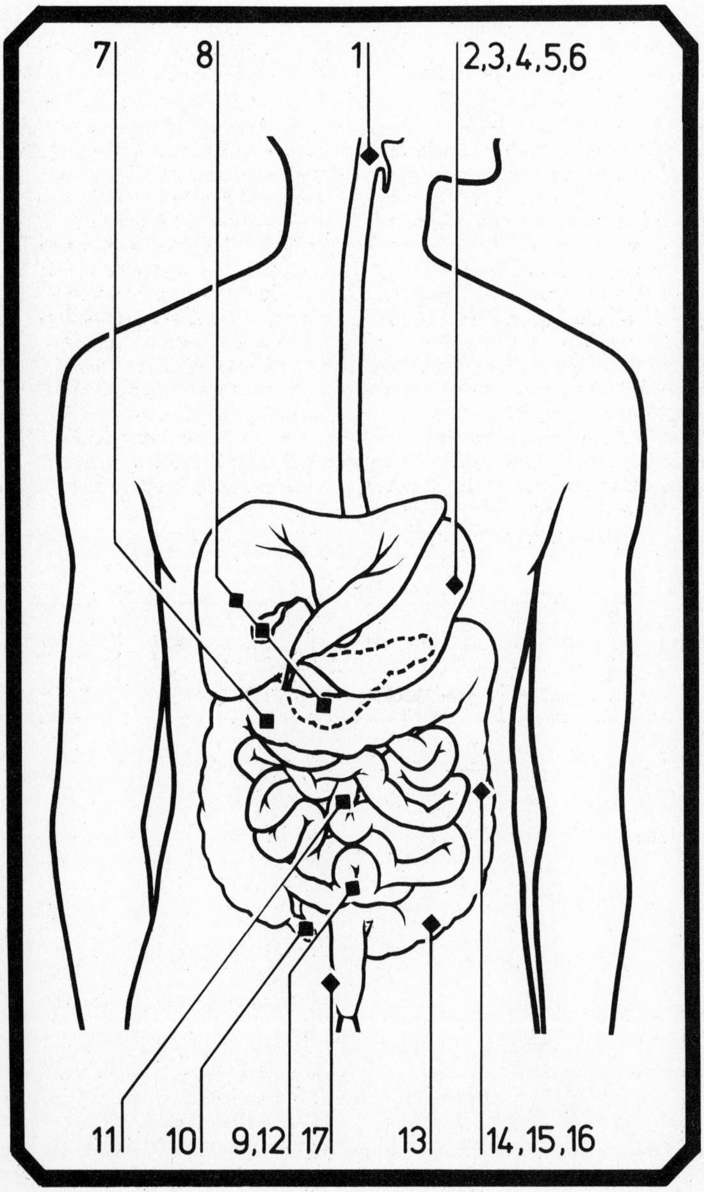

Digestive tract troubles
The diagram shows sites of some tiresome or painful conditions of the digestive system, mostly responding to treatment at home.
1 Esophagitis – inflammation of the gullet (esophagus) – occurs through irritation due to hot or abrasive foods, smoking, infections etc. Swallowing is difficult and there is burning chest pain. Take bland foods, have plenty to drink, and lie down for an hour or two after meals.
2 In hiatus hernia the stomach pushes up into the esophageal area, giving chest pain that is worst after eating or on lying down. Eating small meals often and not swallowing air, gas-producing foods, tea, coffee, or alcohol helps, and so does not lying down after meals.
3 Dyspepsia (especially indigestion) usually results from excess acid secreted in the stomach.
4 Gastric ulcer is an eroded area of stomach lining, which may bleed if it involves a blood vessel.
5 Gastritis is inflammation of the stomach due to irritation.
6 Gastroenteritis is inflammation of the stomach and possibly all the digestive tract.
7 Duodenal ulcer is an ulcer in the duodenum, caused by excess acid.
8 Liver, pancreas and gallbladder problems are described on p.106.
9 Ileitis (Crohn's disease) is inflammation of the lower small intestine producing weight loss, anemia, perhaps diarrhea and other symptoms. Bed rest, bland diet, vitamin-mineral supplements, and plenty of liquids help to treat it, but medical advice should be sought.
10 Appendicitis, inflammation of the appendix, needs surgery.
11 Umbilical hernia is a navel swollen by a protruding piece of intestine. Common in babies, this usually needs no treatment and regresses by age 2.
12 Inguinal hernia of the groin may get pinched, causing acute pain, vomiting, and swelling in the groin; if left untreated, peritonitis may result.
13 Femoral hernia, occurring at the top of the thigh, may also get strangulated.
14 Colitis is inflammation of the colon, due often to mild infection producing diarrhea.
15 Irritable colon can involve alternate constipation and diarrhea, with bloated abdomen and discomfort. A bland, fibrous diet and bed rest help acute attacks.
16 Diverticulitis is the inflammation of pouches that may form in the colon, giving left-sided abdominal pain and fever.
17 Piles (hemorrhoids) are varicose veins of the rectum (see p.100).

Gastritis
This is a general term for inflammation of the stomach due to irritation. It involves abdominal pain, vomiting, diarrhea, loss of appetite and fever if the cause is some kind of infection. Other causes include alcohol, spicy food, stress, aspirin, or concentrated alkali or acid. Often the best treatment is simply resting the stomach by eating nothing and taking plenty to drink (but not alcohol, coffee, tea or colas) and not smoking. You may find that analgesics such as acetaminophen (not aspirin), and antacids and antinauseants help relieve the symptoms. If the vomiting persists, though, you should call a doctor.

Gastroenteritis
This condition is closely related to gastritis but involves more of the digestive system; inflammation occurs in the linings of the stomach and the intestine. Nausea, vomiting, diarrhea and cramping pains in the abdomen occur. Often the victim feels weak and faint, with a fast pulse and clammy, cold skin. Food poisoning, allergy or irritant foods or chemicals may be to blame. Bed rest and a light, liquid diet is the main treatment (it is important to replace liquid lost by diarrhea). Nausea may be alleviated by antacids and antinauseants.

Appendicitis
This is inflammation of the appendix – a tiny dead-end opening off the large intestine. A blocked appendix swells, gets infected and, if not removed, may burst, with potentially fatal results. Symptoms include loss of appetite, and severe pain that comes and goes in the navel area; the pain finally settles in the right lower abdominal region, which grows tender to the touch. There may also be nausea and vomiting. Anyone who has suspected appendicitis should call a doctor and avoid eating, drinking or taking any drugs, especially laxatives.

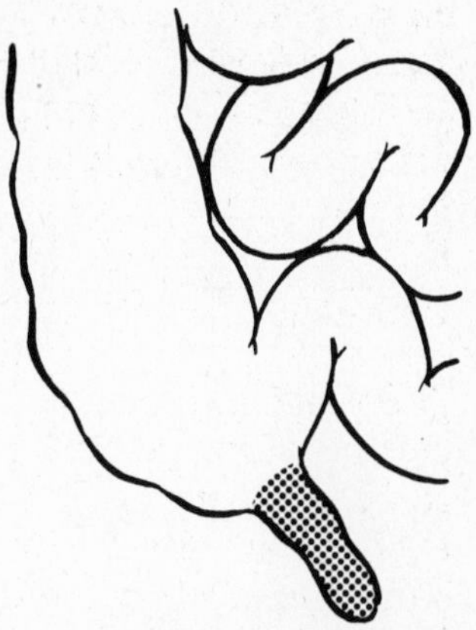

Hernias
Hernias (ruptures) occur where part of the intestine pokes through a weak part of the abdominal wall. Inguinal hernia occurs in males of all ages where thigh meets abdomen. Femoral hernias (commonest in women) occur at the top of the thigh. Umbilical hernias (often seen in infants) protrude from the navel. Some hernias regress naturally, and others can be pushed back into place. But if a hernia gets nipped at its entrance the resulting strangulated hernia causes pain and vomiting and needs urgent medical aid. In hiatus hernia the upper stomach bulges up where the esophagus passes through the diaphragm.

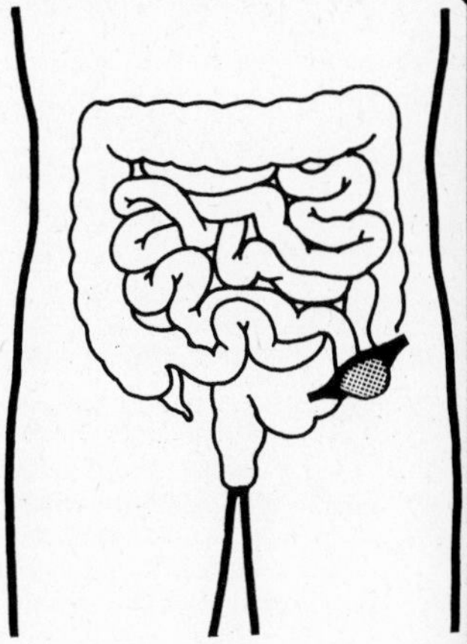

Avoiding hernias
Some hernias occur because channels fail to close properly during pre-birth development, but most hernias develop when muscular exertion forces the abdomen through a weak part of the abdominal wall. To avoid this kind of hernia do not exert unusually sudden muscular force that raises pressure within the abdomen. Do not cough violently or strain the bowels. Raise any heavy weight from a squatting position (**a**) rather than just remaining standing and bending at the waist (**b**); correct lifting posture prevents back strain as well as hernias.

a

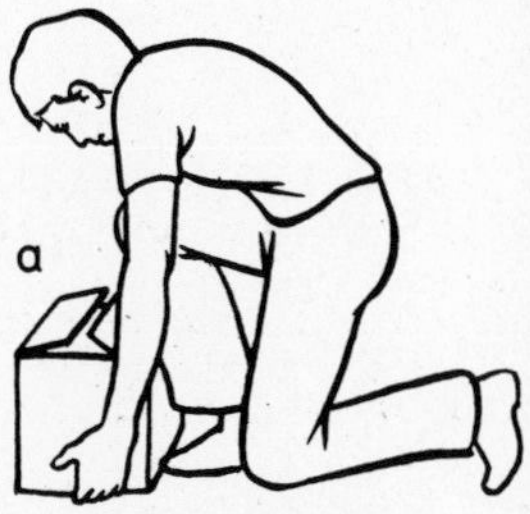

b

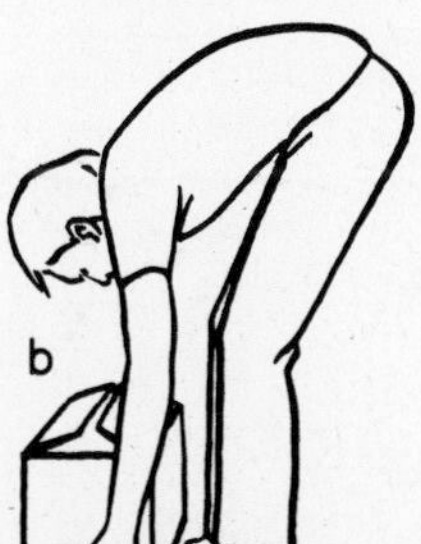

Peptic ulcers
There are two types of peptic ulcer: duodenal and gastric. About 90% of peptic ulcer sufferers are men and most of their ulcers are duodenal. (In women, gastric ulcers outrank duodenal ulcers.) Duodenal ulcers can occur from age 20 onward; gastric ulcers are uncommon in people under 40. Ulcers often occur in people who are very competitive; who are under stress or short of sleep; who drink and smoke heavily or eat rich food; or who suffer frequently from stomach infections and produce excessive stomach acid. Giving up smoking and taking a rest from work heals most duodenal ulcers.

Food for ulcer sufferers
The food lists *below* show a few do's and don'ts for peptic ulcer sufferers. The principles behind these lists of foods are omitting the foods that stimulate the output of digestive juice and foods that chemically or mechanically irritate the inflamed lining of the stomach or the duodenum, but including foods that reduce acidity in the stomach. Modern drugs help to make strict diets unnecessary, and fruits and vegetables (once banned) are now considered harmless. Try to keep to a well-balanced diet, and eat small, light, frequent meals rather than large, heavy ones.

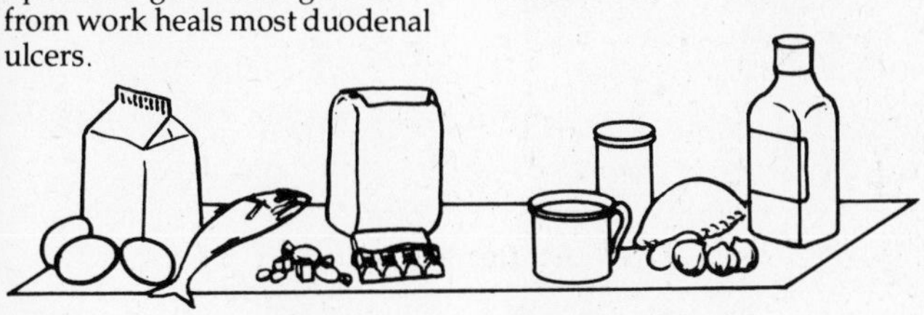

Eat	Limit	Avoid
Milk	Sugar	Rich fatty foods
Eggs	Candies	Fried foods
Fish	Chocolate	Spicy foods
		Pastry
		Strong coffee
		Strong tea
		Cocoa
		Cola drinks
		Alcohol
		Meat extracts (in gravies etc)
		Spices
		Pickles
		Most fruit juices
		Fibrous meats
		Whole grain cereals
		Smoking

Digestive system 4

The area that most people call the bowels is properly named the colon or large bowel (the small bowel being the small intestine). This end part of the digestive system absorbs fluid, and forms and expels feces. Many defects in our modern living styles force our bowels to cope with unnatural habits such as rushed, irregularly-spaced meals and an excess of processed foods; in order for the bowels to work correctly they should be treated correctly, particularly by following good dietary principles. The effort needed to keep the bowels healthy is minimal compared with the trouble that they can otherwise cause – especially as our bodies age. While even healthy bowels are liable to invasion by germs or worms, most common conditions respond to simple treatment.

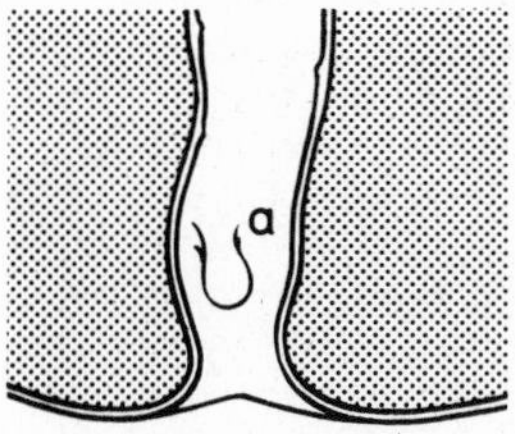

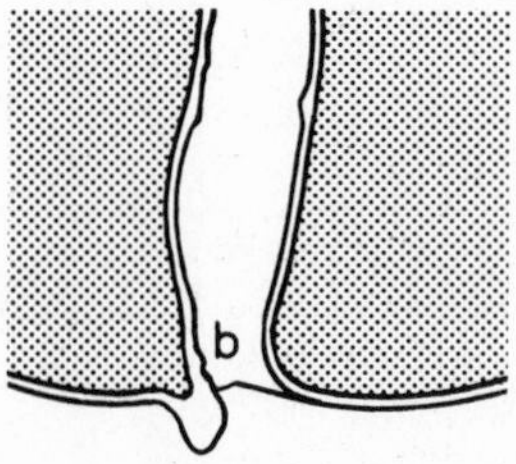

Hemorrhoids (piles)
Internal hemorrhoids (**a**) can occur high in the anal canal; external hemorrhoids (**b**) protrude from the rectum. Eating extra fiber in your diet and not straining at stool may stop symptoms; a greased finger can sometimes push external hemorroids back into place. Itching may be relieved by sitting in warm water for 30 minutes. Various local anesthetic preparations deaden pain and relieve itching. Hemorrhoids that continue to give trouble should be seen by a doctor; if necessary the enlarged veins can be treated by injection or removed by a simple, safe operation.

Diarrhea
This happens when the bowels try to purge themselves of some irritant or poison. The bowels respond to irritation by producing extra mucus and speeding up the rate at which waves of muscular contraction force feces through the bowel. This means there is less time than usual for the intestines to absorb water. This usually results in colicky pain, and an irresistible urge to open the bowels frequently, passing movements that are thin and watery. Acute diarrhea usually lasts only a day or two. If the cause is anxiety, it may clear up unaided. Diarrhea due to food poisoning is treated by avoiding milk drinks and solids but taking clear liquids such as fruit juices and soups in order to replace the salts and water being lost (otherwise you may get dehydrated). Taking an adsorbent such as kaolin may help; adsorbents coat the walls of the digestive tract, and absorb irritating substances. Low doses of paregoric will help to slow down contractions of the bowel and so make fewer bowel movements necessary; codeine may relieve abdominal discomfort. Start a bland diet as the diarrhea improves. Seek medical advice if diarrhea is severe or persistent, or if it alternates with constipation.

Constipation
Opening the bowels infrequently and producing hard stools with difficulty is likely to happen to anyone who eats little food, takes little fluid, has a diet low in fiber, takes no exercise, or persistently ignores the need to open the bowels. Habits such as hurrying to work straight after breakfast, or rising late in the morning, may be to blame. Other possible causes of constipation include depression, some medicines, and certain physical diseases. Some doctors consider that opening the bowels only once every two days or so has no very harmful effect. But constipation can cause piles, and it seems at least possible that major bowel disorders can be triggered by chronic constipation. All basically healthy people can cure constipation by taking exercise, drinking plenty of fluid and including sufficient fiber in their daily food (see p.101). It helps, too, if people cultivate a regular morning bowel movement. There should seldom be a need for artificial laxatives. If constipation persists, see your doctor, for there may be some underlying cause requiring medical treatment.

Worms
Various parasitic worms invade the digestive system.
a Threadworms or pinworms are common in children. Resembling tiny white threads ¼ in long, they live in the colon, emerging at night to lay eggs around the anus. This produces itching that causes scratching, leading to reinfection via the mouth. Meanwhile worms show up in feces. One dose of piperazine will clear an infestation; all the family should be treated.
b Common roundworms look like white earthworms up to 4 in long; they invade the small intestine, and are spread via contaminated food. Treatment is as for threadworms.
c Tapeworms comprise up to 30 ft of flat, white segments, that live in the intestine and break off to leave it via the feces. Tapeworm infestation results from eating underdone pork, beef or fish; treatment is by drugs.
d Hookworms are about 1 in long; they cause anemia by sucking blood when lodged in the intestine. They occur in warm climates; eggs exit via the feces, hatching into larvae that invade the skin of barefooted people. Patients need drugs, iron supplements and a high-protein diet. Wearing shoes or sandals in warm climates, combined with good sanitation and foot hygiene, prevents infestation.

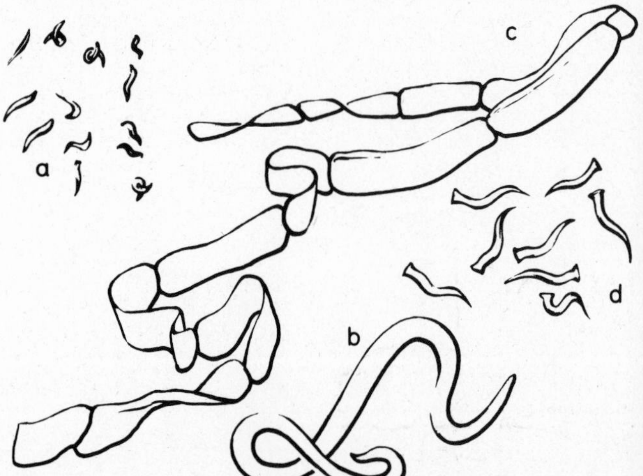

Pregnancy
Constipation, flatulence and piles may occur in pregnancy. If necessary, constipated women can try magnesia or senna as a laxative, but should not take liquid paraffin preparations or strong purgatives. With luck, constipation will clear up if they eat plenty of fibrous fruit, and take some bran, as well as drinking plenty of fruit juice and other liquids. Relieving constipation will help to prevent or relieve piles. Flatulence (excess wind in the intestines) is best prevented by avoiding gas-producing and indigestible food. Severe diarrhea in pregnancy requires medical attention.

Babies
Babies sometimes suffer from constipation and diarrhea. If a very young baby passes hard movements with difficulty add sugar water to its feedings (one level teaspoon of brown sugar to 4 oz water). Constipation that occurs on weaning may call for adding fruit juice to the baby's cereal. Avoid giving laxative medicine except as your doctor may prescribe. If a young baby fed on milk frequently passes loose, green foul-smelling movements give only frequent glucose water drinks (1 level teaspoon of glucose to 2 oz water) and call your doctor. But remember that young healthy babies pass several soft movements every day.

Adults
Short-term constipation and diarrhea, often linked with travel and sudden change of diet, are common problems. Business travelers and vacationers may suffer from gastroenteritis produced by contaminated food. Some individuals seem to respond to stress at work or in the home with bowel conditions including irritable colon. Busy people who save time by relying heavily on processed and convenience foods may lack dietary fiber and so increase the risk of contracting piles, appendicitis, bowel cancer or ulcerative colitis.

Old people
Old people are more liable than younger ones to certain bowel complaints as the large bowel deteriorates and eating habits change. Pouches called diverticula occur where the large bowel bulges through weak parts of the muscular wall. Infected pouches give rise to diverticulitis. As muscles generally lose tone, straining at stool becomes more likely to produce a hernia. If overstraining collapses the rectum wall, a fecal mass may become trapped inside the rectum and keep overflowing; eating enough dietary fiber helps to prevent this situation from developing.

Foods high in fiber
Listed *below* is a selection of commonly available high-fiber foods. Figures refer to the number of grams of fiber for every 100g of food.

g	
44	Wheat bran
27	All bran
15	Puffed wheat
14	Almonds
14	Coconut, fresh
13	Weetabix
12	Peas, frozen, boiled
12	Ryvita
11	Cornflakes
9	Brazil nuts
9	Dates, dried
8	Wholewheat bread
8	Peanuts
7	Beans, haricot, boiled
7	Granola
7	Blackberries
7	Raisins
6	Spinach, boiled
6	Corn, canned
5	Rice, brown, boiled

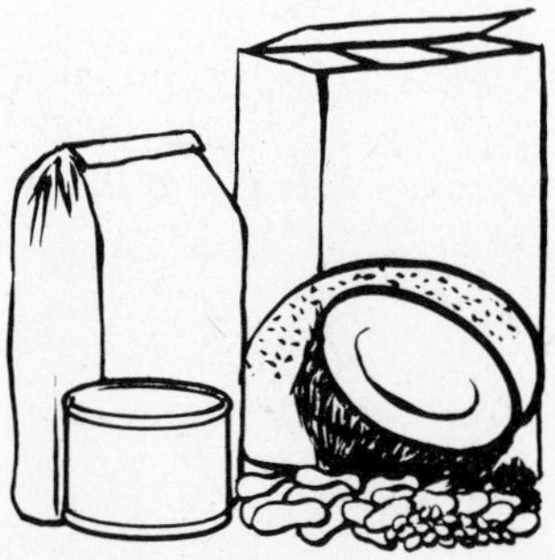

Fiber in the diet
Fiber or roughage plays a vital role in the diet. The human digestive system cannot digest fiber, but uses it to help retain toxic substances that would otherwise pass into the bloodstream. Fiber produces soft, bulky and easily evacuated stools and speeds up their elimination. A fiber-rich diet can alleviate some bowel conditions and help to protect the body against appendicitis, bowel cancer, colitis, diverticulitis, heart disease, hemorrhoids and hernias. Groups of people that eat very high-fiber diets are largely free of many Western ailments.
When we talk of fiber in food we mean indigestible cellulose; this occurs only in cereals, vegetables, and fruits. Cooking tends to break down cellulose cell walls, so most of the food taken for its fiber value should be eaten raw; cereal fiber is best.
Eat wholewheat bread; the fiber content of wholewheat bread is 8.5g per 100g, compared with 5.1g for brown bread and only 2.7g for white bread. Also brown rice has a much higher fiber content than white rice: 5.5g per 100g after cooking compared with 0.8g. For breakfast try bran with other bran cereals, perhaps mixed with chopped apple (2.0g per 100g) or banana (3.4g per 100g).

Do
- Make sure to include enough fiber in your diet by eating some raw cereals, fruits and vegetables rich in roughage. Natural bran is probably best.
- Treat diarrhea by taking clear liquids to make up for fluids lost by the body.
- Prevent constipation by exercising, forming regular bowel habits, and eating some roughage.
- Try to cure constipation by exercising, eating roughage, and drinking plenty of liquids before you turn to artificial laxatives.
- Try treating hemorrhoids and diverticulitis by adding fiber to your diet.
- Treat the entire family if one member has a threadworm infestation; to prevent reinfestation, encourage the affected person to sleep in gloves and pajamas and keep the fingernails cut short.
- Wear shoes if you travel to an area where hookworm occurs.
- Seek medical advice if a young baby passes many loose, greenish, foul smelling movements daily.

Don't
- Strain at stool; this is a habit that is very likely to produce hemorrhoids and hernias.
- Take solid foods or milk if you are suffering from acute diarrhea.
- Eat a diet based heavily on convenience and processed foods.
- Engage in habits that lead to chronic constipation.
- Take laxatives for constipation if you develop any signs that may indicate appendicitis (see p. 99).
- Try curing constipation with strong purgatives or liquid paraffin.
- Worry if a young baby passes half a dozen or more soft motions daily, unless these are loose, green and foul smelling.
- Give a baby laxative medicine unless it has been prescribed by a doctor.
- Ignore a change in bowel habit that persists more than two or three days – see your doctor about continuing diarrhea, constipation or alternation of the two.

Urinary system 1

The urinary system is a purifying mechanism that traps wastes and poisons that accumulate in the blood and then expels them in urine, an amber-colored fluid that is 4% dissolved solids and 96% water. Urine excreted by the kidneys travels through two tubes called ureters into the bladder, a muscular bag capable of storing several pints of urine. However, nerve signals usually make the bladder empty when it holds no more than one half pint. From the bladder, urine leaves the body via a tube called the urethra, shorter in women than in men. Control of urine flow is a landmark in child development, and setbacks in achieving this control are common childhood problems. Studying the urine of a person of any age affords doctors insight into a variety of medical conditions.

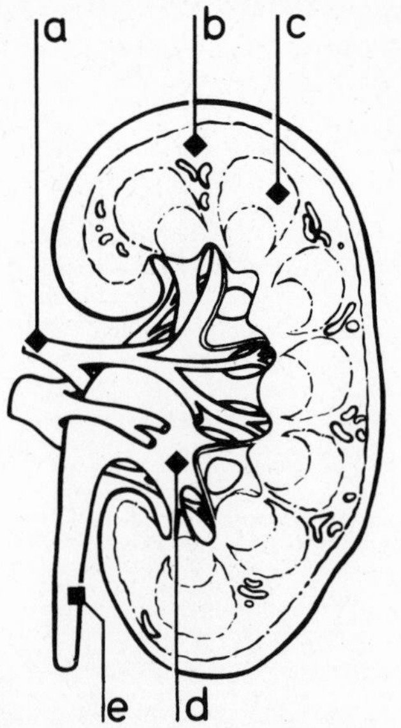

Healthy kidneys
Kidneys are two bean-shaped organs flanking the backbone just above the small of the back. They cleanse blood; maintain the body's salts-and-water balance; and keep its fluids slightly alkaline. Blood enters kidneys via the renal artery (**a**). In the cortex (**b**) or outer part of each kidney a million nephrons (blood-cleaning units) filter out impurities. These collect in the medulla (**c**) or inner part of the kidney. This reabsorbs nutrients and excretes waste products in the urine, which passes through the renal pelvis (**d**) into the ureter (**e**). Healthy kidneys process over 170 quarts of fluid daily, but excrete only about 1½ quarts.

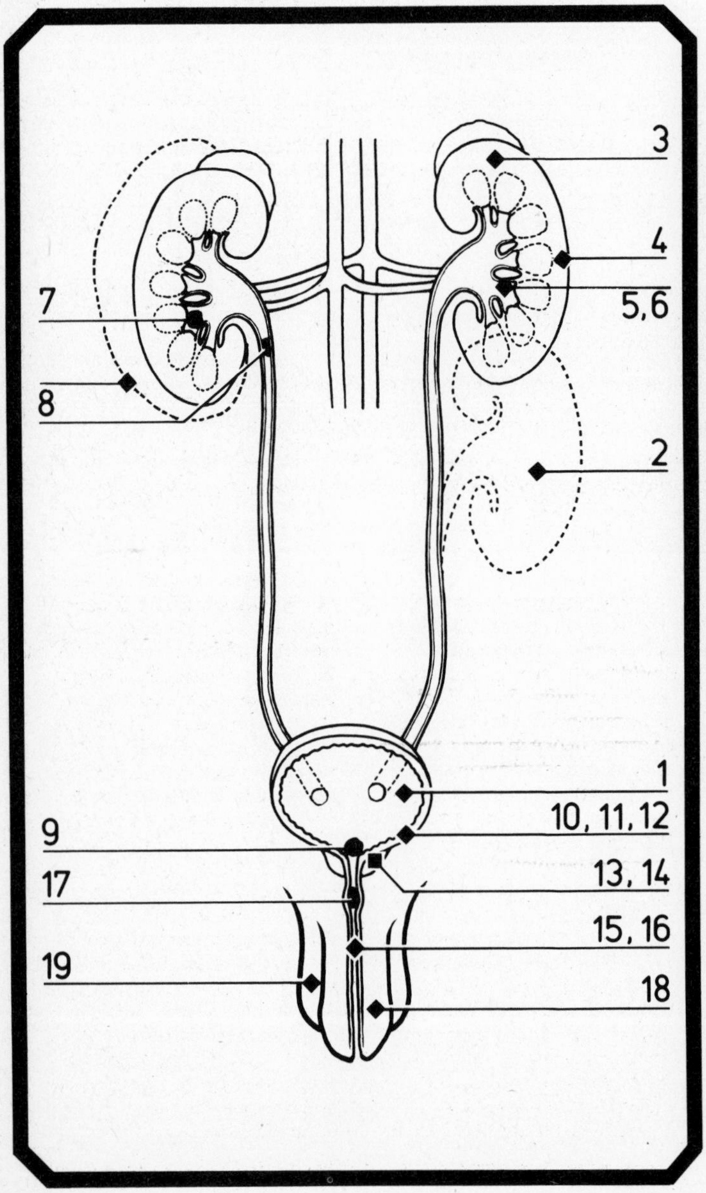

Sites of urinary tract problems
A few of these problems need no attention. Most respond to surgery or lesser treatment. Cancers (not shown) vary in type, site and curability.

1 In diabetes insipidus a faulty hypothalamus stops vasopressin secretion, so kidneys reabsorb too little water. The result is high urine output and intense thirst. Treatment involves replacing vasopressin by injection or nasal spray.
2 Ectopic kidney is a kidney in an abnormal position (such as two kidneys on one side of the body). Ectopic kidneys are liable to kidney stones, infection and blocked urine flow.
3 Single kidney: some people are born with only one kidney, but one can do the work of two.
4 Glomerulonephritis involves inflammation of the glomeruli, filtering capillaries within the kidney's nephrons. Water accumulates in body tissues and there may be kidney damage and heart failure.
5 Pyelonephritis (kidney infection) may produce kidney damage and toxins in the blood.
6 Acute kidney failure can cause loss of kidney function, pulmonary edema, hemorrhage, and uremia (poisoning by toxins accumulating in the body).
7 Kidney stone in the kidney itself. Movement of the stone may damage kidney tissue.
8 Kidney stone in a ureter. If it blocks the ureter urine accumulates above the stone, distending the ureter and enlarging the space inside the kidney. Kidney tissue grows thinner and may be destroyed.
9 Kidney stone in the bladder.
10 Cystitis: inflammation of the bladder (see p.104).
11 Extroverted bladder is a congenitally incomplete bladder causing urine leakage and requiring surgery.
12 Some physical and psychological problems can cause lack of bladder control, giving rise to incontinence.
13 Enlarged prostate gland. If this blocks the bladder mouth, the bladder wall thickens and accumulating urine dilates the ureters and enlarges the space inside the kidneys whose substance grows thinner and may be destroyed.
14 Prostatitis: inflammation of the prostate (see p.105).
15 Urethritis is inflammation of the urethra (see pp.105 and 177).
16 Urethral stricture may be due to infection, especially gonorrhea, or injury.
17 Kidney stone in the urethra.
18 Hypospadias and epispadias are conditions where the male urethral opening is on the top or bottom of the penis shaft rather than in the glans penis.
19 Diaper rash occurs on skin soaked with urine, especially in babies. Incontinent adults may also suffer skin troubles.

Pregnancy testing
Doctors can diagnose pregnancy six weeks after the last period by detecting the presence of human chorionic gonadotrophin (HCG), a hormone appearing in pregnant women's urine. Drops of urine and anti-HCG (which neutralizes HCG) are added to a glass slide, with, a minute later, latex rubber particles coated with HCG. If the urine contains HCG tiny visible particles remain smooth (**a**). If a woman is not pregnant the particles clump together, forming milky "curds" (**b**). Home pregnancy testing kits are now available commercially, which can detect pregnancy even earlier from a sample of urine.

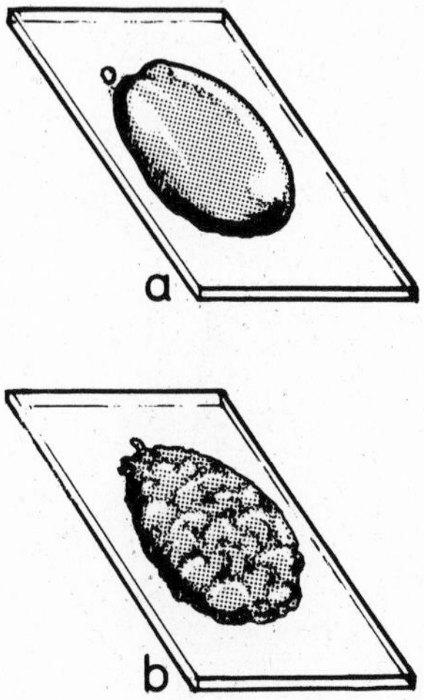

Changes in urinary habits
These may be temporary and of no significance. People tend to urinate less often than usual in hot weather, or if they have drunk less than normal. Drinking more than usual causes them to pass more urine, perhaps more frequently, than normal. Otherwise an increased volume of urine or an urge to pass urine more frequently than usual suggests the onset of one of several diseases, some of them not even originating in the urinary tract. Anyone waking at night tends to want to pass water, but if you wake often with this urge, it is advisable to see a doctor. Excessive urination in the night is termed nocturia.

Changes in urine
Just as with urinary habits, changes in the color or smell of urine may have harmless natural explanations. A deep color may mean urine is simply concentrated (as in someone who has drunk nothing for some hours). Discoloration can be due to eating licorice or beet. If you are taking penicillin your urine will smell rather like burned rubber. Otherwise, unusual color or the presence of froth or cloudiness may indicate infection or some other disease. Special tests sometimes reveal bacteria, sugar, albumen, pus, inorganic crystals or other foreign bodies in the urine if disease is present.

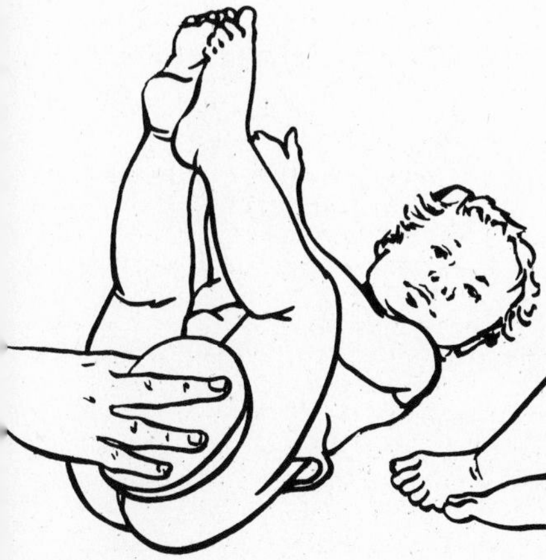

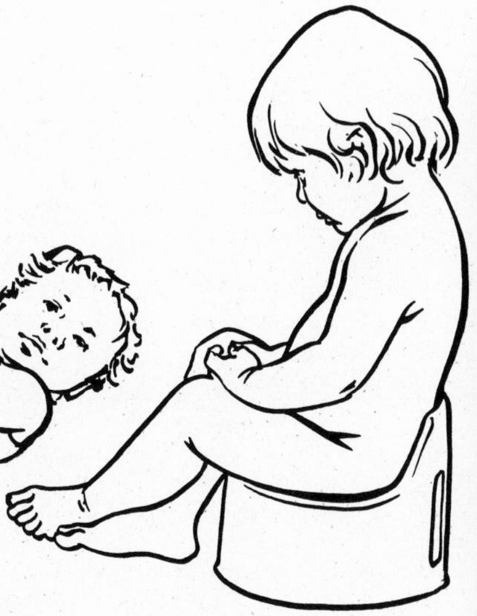

Diaper rash
Until bladder control begins to develop, babies may pass urine so frequently that their diapers are almost constantly soaked. Freshly passed urine rarely irritates the skin, except in cases of extreme sensitivity, but if a urine-soaked diaper remains on the baby then bacteria on the skin may act upon the urine to produce ammonia. It is generally ammonia, produced in this way, that causes diaper rash; the rash is really a mild ammonia burn. Changing the diapers frequently will help to prevent diaper rash, and so may an application of zinc oxide cream at every diaper change.

Toilet training
Some parents put young babies on the potty after feedings, but generally this is futile until bowel and bladder control begin developing. By 15 to 18 months, a child may signal that his diaper is wet or soiled, and should be encouraged to do so. Bit by bit his signals will come early enough for you to put the child on his pot in time. When this happens always show that you are pleased. But don't expect the child to use the pot each time you produce it, and do not scold when he has an accident. Children just old enough to use a flush toilet need assistance and reassurance at first: fitting a special infant seat will often help.

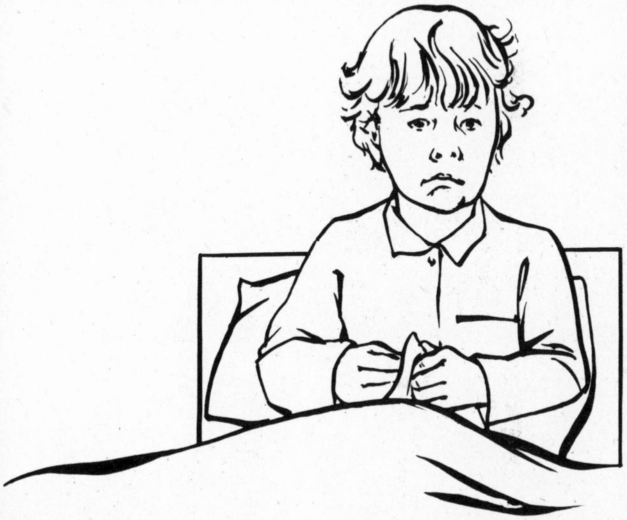

Bedwetting
Most children are dry at night by 3 years old, with just a few accidents until they reach 4. Children who are persistently wet by day after 3 or by night after 4 may be late developers and grow out of it in time. Others who were already dry may suffer a relapse. Bedwetting of this type often happens among those aged 4 to 7. Physical causes of bedwetting among young children include late development of the brain's bladder control center. Another cause may be worry created by a child's overanxious parents who may force toilet training. Later on, physical illness or emotional upset perhaps caused by starting school or birth of a sibling or lack of parental affection can trigger an episode of enuresis (bedwetting). Never punish bedwetting; this only makes it worse. Simply change the wet bedclothes and pajamas, and give the child a goodnight hug. Greet dry nights with praise. Try to avoid the problem by giving nothing to drink at least two hours before bedtime. Make sure he urinates just before going to bed, and wake him and put him on the potty after an hour or so (most bedwetting happens in the first three hours). Older children may respond to a battery-powered device which sounds a bell or buzzer as the first drops of urine reach the undersheet. This wakes the child in time for him to use the toilet. Sometimes a doctor may prescribe drugs or even psychiatric help.

Urinary system 2

Conditions outlined on these pages range from the inconvenience of incontinence and the severe discomfort of cystitis to diseases that could kill if left untreated for a week. Many urinary troubles involve infection established in the urinary tract after sexual contact, injury or operation. Women are particularly liable to urinary tract infections because the short urethra offers less protection to the bladder, ureters and kidneys than a man's much longer urethra provides. Fortunately, common infections respond to sulfonamide drugs or drinking plenty of fluids. More serious is infection linked with urine stagnating behind some blockage in the urinary tract. This condition, and any other liable to cause kidney damage, needs urgent medical help.

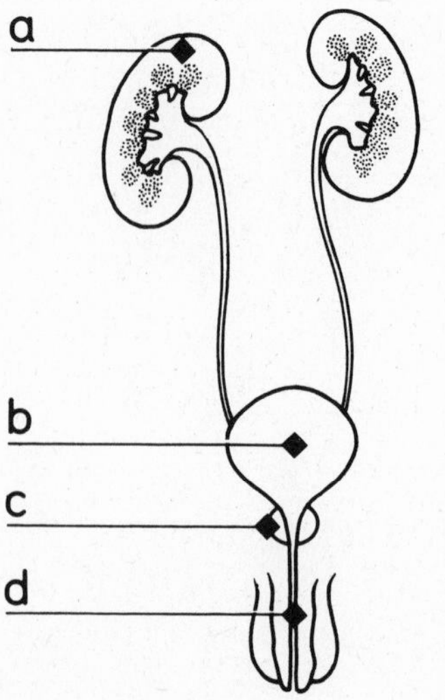

Infections
Each part of the urinary tract is liable to infection.
a Pyelonephritis (kidney infection) occurs if bacteria invade the kidneys from nearby tissues or via the bloodstream, lymph system or bladder. Girls and pregnant women suffer more than other groups.
b Cystitis, or inflammation of the bladder, is often due to bacteria invading via the urethra or sometimes via the kidneys.
c Prostatitis is inflammation of the prostate gland, usually due in younger men to bacterial infection via the urethra.
d Urethritis – inflammation of the urethra – occurs if bacteria invade the urethral opening.

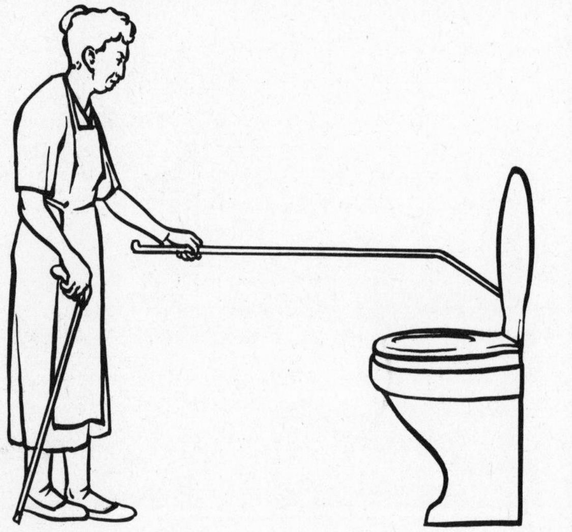

Older people's problems
Infection, local nerve damage, muscle atrophy and mental deterioration may all cause urine incontinence. Old people are more likely to leak urine than most, especially if they become senile and lose awareness of their bladder. In some older women, coughing, laughing or lifting cause so-called stress incontinence; or there may be a sudden, uncontrollable desire to pass water (urge incontinence). Such problems are worst among those too frail to leave their beds. Anyone suffering incontinence should see a doctor. If the trouble stems from an infection he may help to cure it; even if no cure is possible, there is much that can be done. Avoid drinking less, but drink little after about 5pm. If possible, visit the bathroom at two-hourly intervals, even if you do not want to. If you suffer stress incontinence, stop the flow after passing water for a second, then continue: this may rebuild weak internal muscles. A handy bottle or commode may help prevent accidents. So may wearing slacks or panties with loose elastic, or (for men) pants with an easy fastening such as Velcro. A firm handrail and a raised toilet seat may assist getting up and down. Protective pads and underwear, and special urine-collecting bags (worn under clothing), may help people who are always wet.

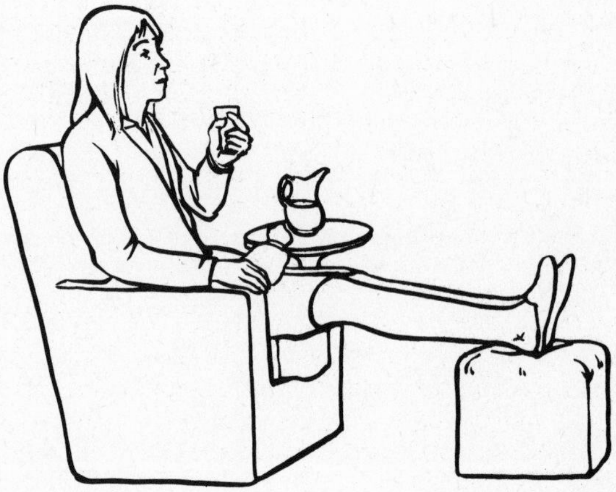

Cystitis
This is inflammation of the bladder, often with urethritis (inflammation of the urethra), and is especially prevalent in women. Acute cystitis gives rise to a frequent urge to pass water although this process produces pain or burning. There may be pain in the lower abdomen, even incontinence, and blood or debris in the urine which smells foul. The cause is often infection by bacteria from the bowel invading via the urethral opening, but sometimes via the kidneys. External infection may be caused by wiping the bottom carelessly, sexual activity, or cross-infection from the vagina. Noninfectious cystitis may be caused by tissue irritation or injury due to riding, frequent intercourse, contact with chemical irritants (such as foam baths or contraceptive creams), prolapsed uterus, surgery, or childbirth. If an attack starts, collect a urine specimen in a clean, closed bottle for your doctor, who will prescribe antibiotics for infectious cystitis. To minimize the effects of an attack, drink plenty of cold water or fruit juice (at least one pint an hour); a mild analgesic and warmth against the back and between the legs will help to make you more comfortable until the attack passes.

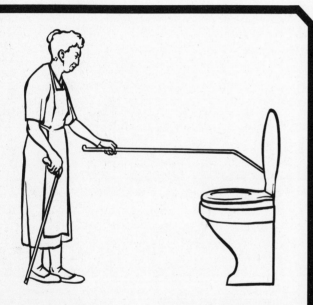

Kidney stones
Stones may form in kidneys from dissolved substances that have precipitated out from urine and grown around bacteria or other tiny nuclei. Why they form is often unclear. But infection, urinary tract obstruction, prolonged bed rest, excessive sweating, gout, and drinking too little fluid are known causes. Small, smooth stones escape in urine. Large stones stuck in the kidney or ureter can cause bleeding, savage pain and – if blocking the urine flow – back pressure and kidney damage; such stones must be removed by surgery. Otherwise doctors may prescribe specific drugs or diets and suggest drinking plenty of water.

Injuries
Surrounding fat guards kidneys against most injuries, but kidney injury is still possible. A severe blow may bruise kidneys so that they bleed, producing bloodstained urine. Crushing injuries may be severe enough to require surgery for repair or removal of a damaged kidney. Severe pelvic injury can cause bladder damage necessitating surgical repair. Injury to the urethra is more common than injury to kidneys or bladder. There may be hemorrhage, and urine leaking into nearby tissues may narrow the urethral tube, with consequential infertility and even impotence. Here, too, treatment has to be by surgery.

Kidney failure
Sudden kidney failure can be due to burns, injury, shock, heart attack, drugs or certain other factors. Once the kidneys stop purifying blood, poisons build up in the body producing coma and death within a week unless the patient receives prompt treatment. This includes bedrest; a diet low in protein, nitrogen and potassium; and drugs or fluids (given intravenously) to prevent shock. But the amount of fluid must be carefully controlled. If the trouble involves infection, doctors will give antibiotics. Severely ill patients may need to use an artificial kidney machine until their own kidneys restart.

Artificial kidneys
People whose kidneys become permanently useless may be kept alive indefinitely by using an artificial kidney several times weekly to purify their blood. A tube that has been inserted in an arm or leg artery passes the blood through layers of semipermeable membranes that filter out waste products – a process called hemodialysis. The purified blood flows back into the patient's body through a tube inserted in a vein. Peritoneal dialysis, in which the peritoneal cavity is filled with the purifying fluid, is used by some people. Dialysis is costly and time consuming, and kidney transplants are to be preferred.

Warning signs and symptoms
Most of the following signs and symptoms could suggest serious disease or be troublesome enough to merit medical aid. Ignoring some of these conditions could be fatal.

1 Pain in the kidney area, fever and shivering may mean an acute kidney infection. Nausea, headache and a general feeling of malaise may accompany a chronic kidney infection.
2 Reduced output of (maybe brownish) urine, painful sides, puffy eyes and face, and mild fever could be caused by acute glomerulonephritis (inflammation of glomeruli).
3 Sudden drop in urine output with drowsiness, dry skin, nausea, and diarrhea may mean acute kidney failure, needing urgent treatment.
4 Mild pain in the kidney area perhaps with blood in urine, anemia and bloated abdomen can indicate kidney stones.
5 Excruciating pain spreading from kidney area into abdomen and genitals with sweating and nausea, probably indicate that a kidney stone has blocked a ureter.
6 Pain or a burning sensation on passing water and an urgent need to urinate often suggest that someone has urethritis or cystitis or both.
7 Tenderness felt in the rectum, with fever, harsh pain, and difficulty passing water suggest prostatitis, requiring antibiotic treatment.
8 Watery or thick greenish-yellow discharge from the penis suggests gonorrhea or nonspecific urethritis (see p.177).
9 Difficulty in starting to pass water or a poor stream can mean infection, tumors somewhere in the urinary tract, or loss of muscle control.
10 Inability to pass urine may indicate blockage of the urinary tract somewhere between the kidneys and urethral opening. The cause could be inflammation, injury, a kidney stone, or a benign or malignant tumor. In older men an enlarged prostate gland may be to blame.
11 Passing water more often than usual could mean urinary tract infection, but possibly diabetes, renal tuberculosis, or other serious conditions.
12 Passing much urine in the night may indicate kidney disease, diabetes, or a heart or other condition that needs medical investigation.
13 Dribbling escape of urine may be caused by urinary tract infection, severe constipation or (in men) enlarged prostate.
14 In women, stress incontinence can suggest the presence of a cystocele (the bladder base bulging into the vaginal canal). Treatment is by vaginal support or surgery.
15 Urge incontinence is also sometimes due to cystocele.
16 Incontinence of urine may be due to impaired nerve or muscle function, bladder infection, or fright. Temporary incontinence may follow a stroke or unconsciousness.
17 Blood in urine could be due to kidney stones, bleeding tumors, or infection or injury affecting the urethra, ureter or kidney.

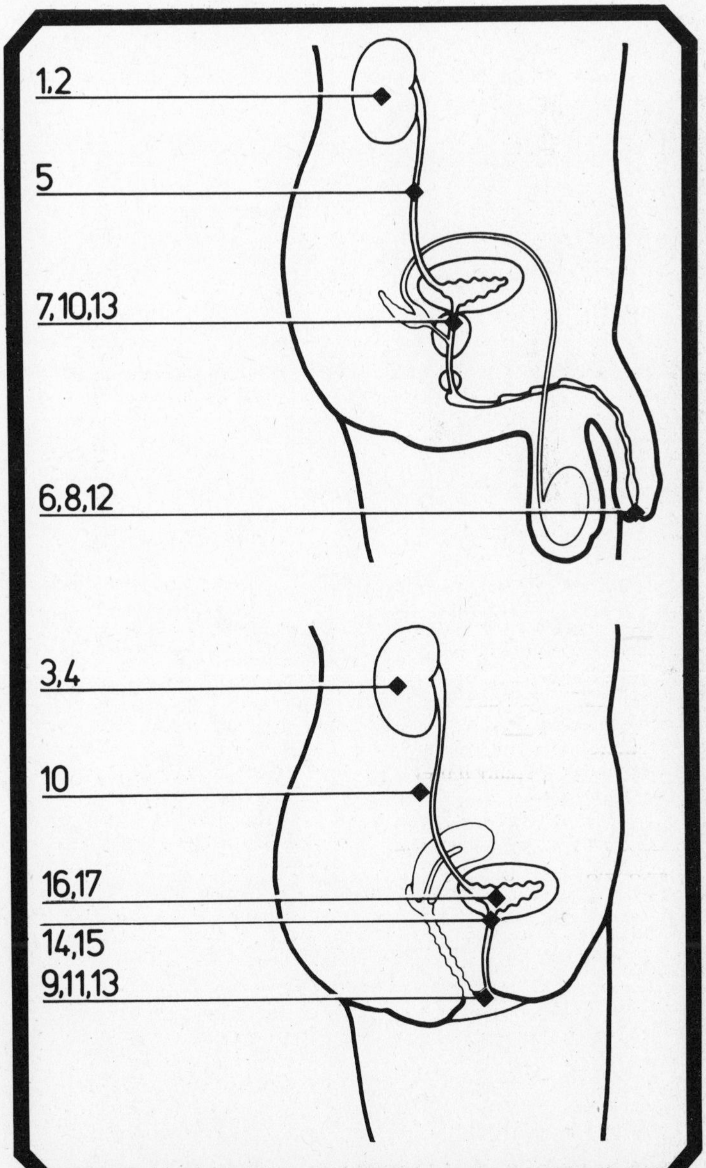

Liver, pancreas and gallbladder

The liver, the largest of all glandular organs, is a reddish mass weighing 3-4lbs, situated under the rib cage on the right of the body. Its functions involve making blood proteins and antibodies; storing proteins, vitamins, minerals and glycogen; and ridding the body of poisons, drugs and spent hormones. The liver sends bile, a liquid that aids fat digestion, to the gallbladder, which stores it and feeds it to the small intestine. Juices from the pancreas also flow to the small intestine and aid in the digestive process. Insulin, which helps the body to utilize sugar, is passed directly into the bloodstream from the pancreas.

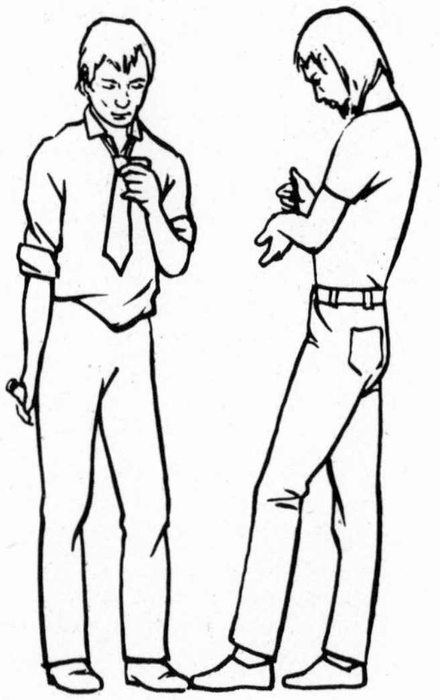

People at risk
Hepatitis type A can be caught from food or water contaminated by blood or stools; hepatitis B, from infected blood or syringes; and alcoholic hepatitis from years of heavy alcoholic drinking. Cirrhosis of the liver is usually due to long-term alcoholism, but may be a complication of other medical conditions. Pancreatitis often occurs in alcoholics, and individuals with bile tract disease. White overweight women aged over 40 seem most liable to gallstones, although the reasons for gallstone formation are still unclear. Diabetes among adults may be linked with excessive carbohydrate intake.

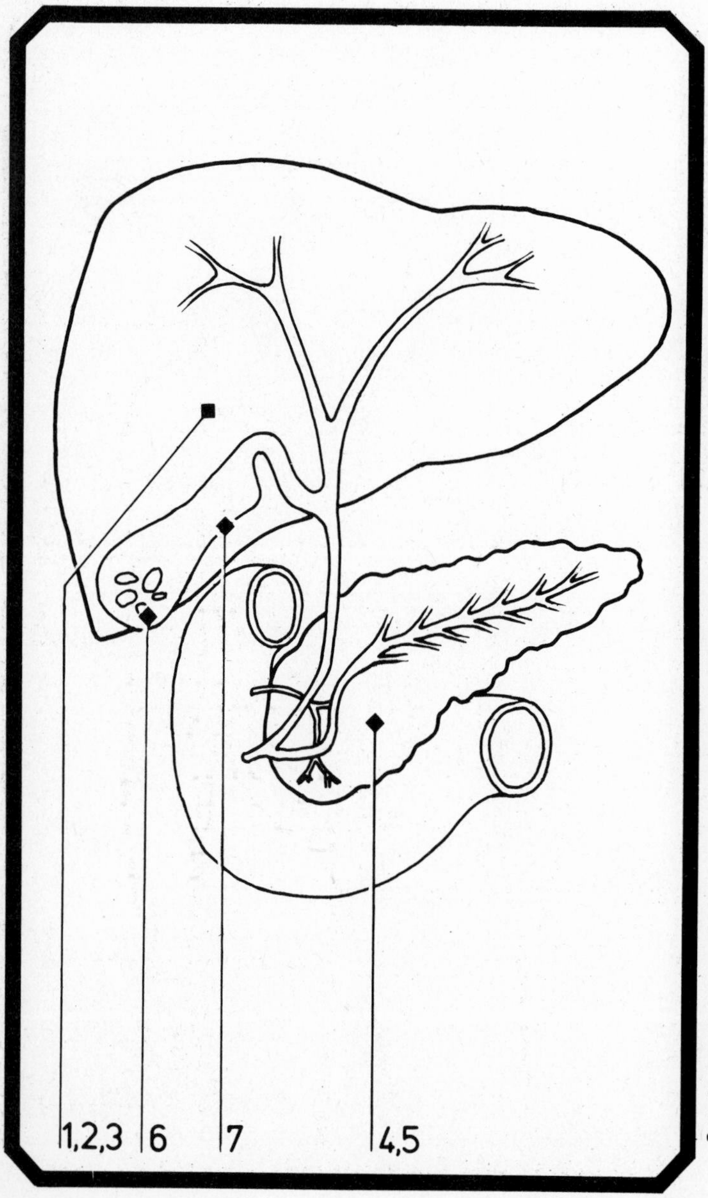

Sites of problems
The illustration shows the sites of some liver, pancreas and gallbladder problems.

1 Alcoholic hepatitis; the liver grows inflamed, and damage allows yellow bile pigment to enter the bloodstream, causing jaundice. The spleen is enlarged, fluid collects in the abdominal cavity, and there is usually fever.

2 Hepatitis A and hepatitis B also feature an inflamed liver but are due to viral infection. Abdominal discomfort and fever occur, and jaundice develops. In rare cases the liver is destroyed and the patient dies.

3 Cirrhosis is a chronic liver disease that destroys liver cells, replacing them with fibrous material; the liver may enlarge and harden. As it stops working properly, there may be internal bleeding, or blocked blood flow. Accumulating fluid may stretch the abdomen, and jaundice and kidney failure are likely.

4 Pancreatitis is inflammation of the pancreas, when pancreatic enzymes build up inside it, for instance if a gallstone blocks its outlet. It may occur in association with disease of the gallbladder. Steady, severe upper abdominal pain and vomiting after excessive alcohol intake may signal an acute attack. In chronic pancreatitis people suffer recurrent but milder attacks. Swift medical aid is essential; treatment includes bed rest, and at first only intravenous nourishment.

5 Diabetes occurs when the pancreas fails to make any or enough of the hormone insulin which the body needs for using sugar and starches. Juvenile onset diabetes usually involves the complete failure of the parts of the pancreas that make insulin (the islets of Langerhans); in these cases insulin injections are needed at regular intervals. In late onset diabetes the islet failure is often only partial, and if this is the case the patient can be treated with diet regulation and oral medication. Complications of diabetes may include arterial degeneration, heart disease, kidney disease, gangrene of the feet, and retinopathy (hemorrhages in the retina). Untreated severe diabetes can produce coma and death.

6 Gallstones are small lumps, usually of cholesterol, forming in people who tend to over-concentrate cholesterol in the bile. They may occur in the gallbladder without causing discomfort, but can also lodge in the bile duct, causing pain and jaundice.

7 Cholecystitis is inflammation of the gallbladder. An acute form may be due to bacterial infection of the gallbladder. Chronic cholecystitis is usually due to gallstones; if they block the bile duct there may be severe liver damage.

Diabetes
Diabetics must curb their intake of carbohydrates (foods containing sugars and starches). A doctor or dietician prescribes a daily allowance of carbohydrate foods, taking into account the person's age and level of activity. Many diabetics also need medication; tablets may suffice, but people incapable of making insulin must be given it by injection (usually self-administered). Regular meals help to keep the sugar and insulin in balance – too much or too little sugar can cause coma. Keeping the feet clean and dry and wearing well-fitting shoes is very important for diabetics as the blood supply to the legs can be poor.

Gallbladder troubles
An inflamed gallbladder will produce severe right-sided upper abdominal pain, spreading to the right shoulder blade. This usually happens within an hour after eating, and lasts several hours. Analgesics help to dull the pain, but doctors sometimes remove the gallbladder to avoid possibly fatal bile blockage. Where symptoms occur only after eating fats, a low-fat weight-reducing regime, perhaps supplemented with vitamins, may suffice. This means avoiding fried foods and such foods as butter, eggs, cheese and fatty meats. Cucumbers also may precipitate attacks.

Hepatitis
Both main forms of hepatitis are technically preventable. Alcoholic hepatitis is a serious risk in people drinking the equivalent of one half pint of spirits a day, especially when the alcohol is taken instead of food, since sufficient intake of nutrients helps to protect the body against alcohol abuse. Viral hepatitis can be guarded against by washing the hands thoroughly after bowel movements, and never sharing a razor or toothbrush. Victims of viral hepatitis are usually treated at home with bed rest, and allowed no alcohol or physical exertion. Alcoholic hepatitis calls for medication and a high-calorie diet.

Cirrhosis
To avoid cirrhosis of the liver, make sure that you drink no more than one quarter pint of spirits daily (or its equivalent), and that you eat a nutritious diet. Over-indulgence in alcohol is the commonest cause of cirrhosis. If the condition does develop, complete rest, a high-protein diet enriched by mineral and vitamin supplements, and total abstinence from alcohol may improve the patient's condition. Doctors are likely to prescribe drugs to alleviate fever if present, and a diuretic to release surplus fluid that may collect in the body, but the disease must be caught early if the patient's health is to be completely restored.

Signs and symptoms
This illustration locates the sites of some of the signs and symptoms produced by certain ailments affecting the liver, pancreas and gallbladder. Some of the conditions plainly show disease needing urgent medical aid; others hint at trouble less dramatically. Many symptoms are common to various ailments, some slight and some serious, and a doctor's diagnosis of liver, pancreas or gallbladder disease will often depend on the presence of several or many of these signs and symptoms. See a doctor immediately if you experience any of these severe symptoms, or if you exhibit several of the slighter ones simultaneously.
1 Excessive fatigue and lethargy are common signs of juvenile onset diabetes. Coma may result if the condition is left untreated.
2 Fever occurs in hepatitis and pancreatitis.
3 Sweating and shock may be caused by pancreatitis.
4 Yellowing of the whites of the eyes and the skin indicates jaundice, which is a common symptom of hepatitis and gallstones.
5 Insatiable thirst strongly suggests diabetes.
6 Breath that smells fruity and sweet is another common sign of diabetes.
7 Belching associated with upper abdominal pain may occur in gallstone troubles.
8 Nausea and loss of appetite, perhaps with vomiting also, occur in hepatitis, cirrhosis and pancreatitis.
9 Thin, spider-shaped blood vessels suddenly showing up on the face, upper trunk and arms are often caused by cirrhosis.
10 Severe pain below the right shoulder blade may be a symptom of gallbladder inflammation.
11 A swollen and tender liver often indicates early cirrhosis; the liver may become shrunken as the condition progresses.
12 A painful sensation of fullness in the stomach is one sign of pancreatitis.
13 White nails are a common sign of cirrhosis, and the ends of the fingers may become clubbed in shape.
14 Severe pain in the upper right part of the abdomen may be caused by hepatitis or gallbladder inflammation.
15 Clay-colored stools are one symptom of gallbladder inflammation and indicate that the bile duct has been blocked; an emergency operation is necessary. Soapy, foul-smelling stools are one symptom of hepatitis.
16 Heavy urine output may well indicate diabetes; in women, intense itching of the vulva may also occur. Dark brown or yellow urine may be indicative of gallbladder or liver disease.
17 Weight loss is often associated with diabetes, cirrhosis and hepatitis.

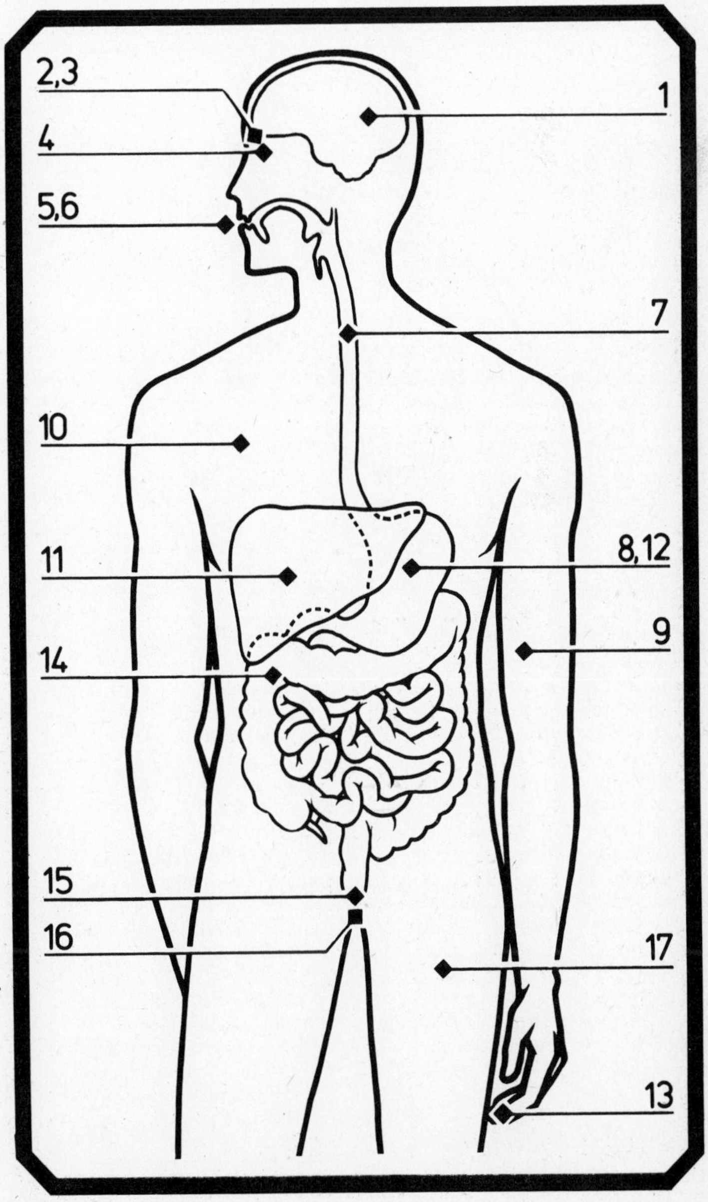

Breasts

The mature female breast is a milk-producing organ formed of many lobes, each with a tree-like system of milk ducts. Clustered nodules feed into small ducts that lead into a main milk duct opening into the nipple. Each lobe is embedded in fat and separated from neighboring lobes by fibrous tissue. On these pages we look at some common breast problems. Sometimes one breast develops before the other, giving grounds for needless worry. Variations in fat content (which largely gives a breast its bulk) can cause cosmetic problems. Breast infections, cysts and tumors can threaten health and so always deserve medical attention.

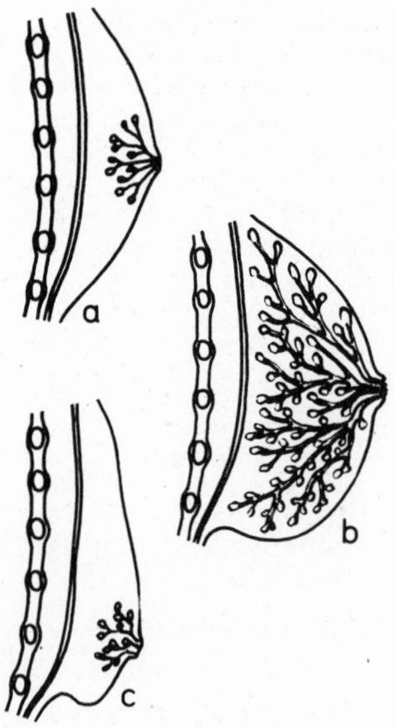

Changes in breasts
Breasts remain undeveloped before puberty.
a About age 11, breasts start to grow: grape-sized nodules beneath the nipples make the surrounding pigmented areas (the areolae) bulge outward. Often one breast starts to grow before the other. By 16 growth of milk ducts and fat makes breasts prominent and firm.
b In pregnancy the milk ducts grow until the breasts are one-third larger than usual. After childbirth, breasts may remain larger than they were.
c About the time of the menopause the breasts shrink and may begin to droop, although some women's breasts gain increased fat deposits.

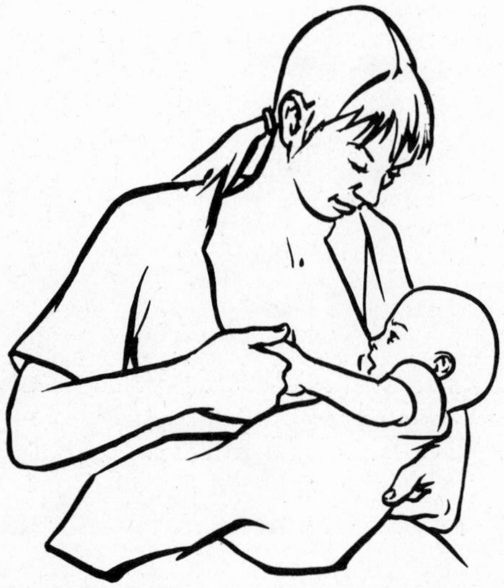

Nursing mothers
Whenever possible a mother should breastfeed rather than give formula, since human milk and the fluid preceding it (colostrum) confer immunity to some diseases, and breastfed babies are less liable to convulsions, diarrhea and vomiting than bottlefed babies. The mother should prepare her breasts and nipples during pregnancy (see page 133). It is important to keep breasts and nipples supple, and to learn to express colostrum when this appears. Wearing breast shields under the brassiere helps feeding if nipples are small or not prominent enough.
Soon after a birth, the mother should put her baby to each breast for a few seconds, then again 12 hours later, letting the baby suck each breast for 2–3 minutes. After a day her breasts may feel painfully swollen, and a week may pass before full milk supply arrives and feeding becomes free from discomfort. Before each feeding the mother should wash her hands, breasts and nipples. To feed her baby she should take up a comfortable sitting position, with her back well supported, and perhaps use a footstool. Sometimes the mother's milk output is insufficient, or vigorous sucking by the baby makes a nipple sore, cracked and infected. Then bottlefeeding is temporarily required.

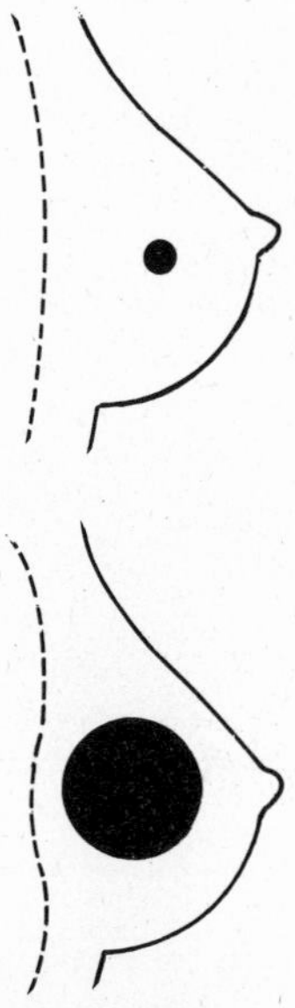

Cysts and benign tumors
Most lumps in the breast are harmless cysts or tumors. Cysts are small sacs comprising blocked milk ducts filled with fluid made by breast cells. All women's breasts contain scores of cysts too tiny to be noticed. Doctors can sometimes collapse a large cyst by inserting a hollow needle and drawing off the fluid. Benign tumors are growths that develop in a slow, orderly way (unlike malignant tumors). But if a benign lump in the breast keeps growing it may press hard enough on nearby nerves and other tissues to cause pain (a painful lump in the breast is usually benign). A surgeon will then remove the tumor.

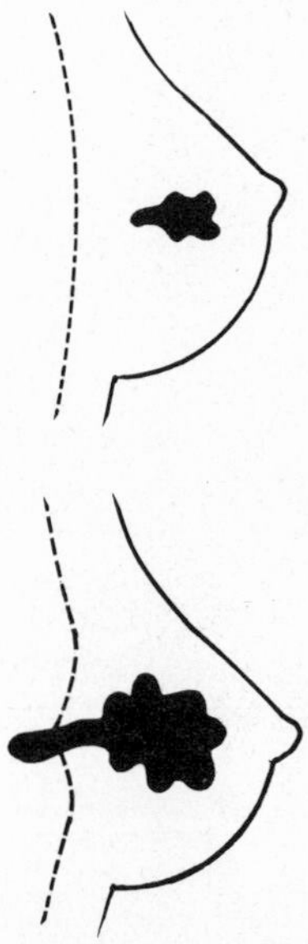

Breast cancer
This may show up as a change in nipple size, shape or color; bloodstained nipple discharge; a painless lump in the breast with dimpled skin above; or a hard lump in the armpit. Detection within a month of onset may be vital for survival, so monthly self-examination is essential (see p.166). Some groups of women tend to be more at risk than others. They include those with a relative who has had the disease; those with benign breast tumors; those who have had no children, one child, or a first child when they were over 35; and women experiencing the menopause in their 50s.

Support
Some women tend to decry the use of brassieres as pandering to the male desire for a stereotyped female form, but there is no doubt that there are times when brassiere support can prove extremely useful. Wearing a brassiere during vigorous exercises not only helps synchronize movements of breasts with those of the body as a whole; it makes activity feel more comfortable. Brassieres are also useful during pregnancy and while breastfeeding. At these times the breasts tend to be large and even pendulous. Wearing a firm brassiere helps to prevent supporting tissues becoming stretched.

Breast tenderness
Hormonal changes causing breast tenderness occur during the days leading up to menstruation and during pregnancy. All women are liable to suffer breast tenderness together with premenstrual tension. The cause is hormonal change which allows water to accumulate in cells within the breasts. This water makes the cells swell, and so increases local pressure. Drinks that encourage urination may help reduce discomfort; but do not drink more than usual. (See p.114.)

Acute mastitis
Acute mastitis (inflammation of the breast) happens mainly in breastfeeding mothers. The cause is normally bacteria that invade milk ducts or cracks in the nipple. The breast becomes tender, painful and enlarged, its skin grows hot and maybe reddened, and the woman may feel feverish. (All these symptoms mimic those of an advanced breast cancer.) In its early stages, acute mastitis may respond to cold packs and abandoning breastfeeding. Sulfa drugs or penicillin should kill the germs responsible. Applying heat may help localize any abscess, which can then be opened up and drained.

Chronic mastitis
This is the popular, misleading name for a longstanding non-inflammatory breast condition mainly found in women who are aged between 40 and 55. The cause is increase in the gland content of the breast, and the affected part or parts feel hard and enlarged (although softer than cancers), but unattached to skin or muscle. Nodules may make the whole breast seem rubbery or lumpy (both breasts may be involved). A woman may feel local pain and tenderness, especially after lifting heavy loads or before menstruating. There may be no need for medical treatment, but anyone with a lump in the breast should see a doctor.

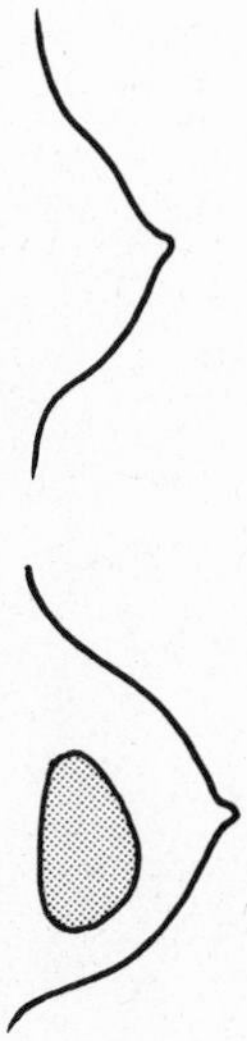

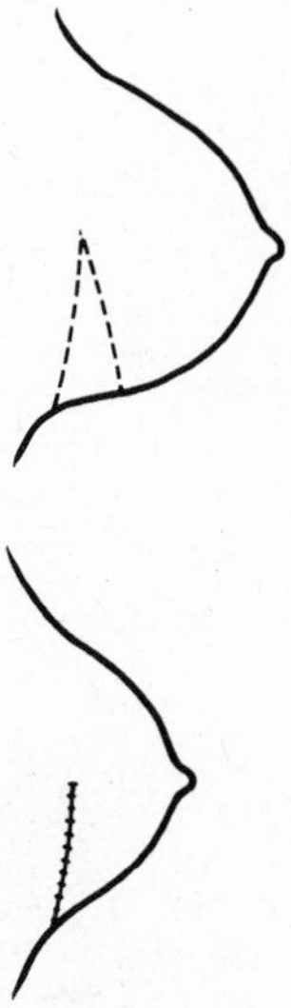

Augmentation
There are several options open to the girl or woman who wants larger breasts. The simplest course is wearing a padded brassiere. Keeping an upright posture and enlarging the underlying muscles by exercises are important aids. If the cause is lack of hormone stimulation, rubbing estrogen creams into the breasts at puberty may help, but this has only a limited effect. A more drastic course is undergoing cosmetic surgery to have the breasts augmented. Surgeons insert fluid-filled bags or silicone between breasts and the underlying pectoral muscles, as shown *above*. A disadvantage is risk of subsequent infection.

Reduction
Some slim women have very large breasts. Breasts may grow larger after a woman reaches her mid 30s. Abnormally large breasts may result from too much hormone stimulus, fluid retention or obesity. All that is needed may be the support of a firm brassiere, or exercise and a weight-reducing diet. But doctors may use hormone therapy to reduce enlargement gross enough to be embarrassing. Another possibility is cosmetic surgery as shown *above:* a surgeon removes some of the pads of fat that give the breasts bulk.

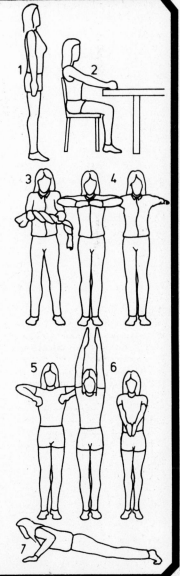

Bust improvement
Swimming and other exercise can lift and firm the bust, but because the breasts contain no muscle, improvement stems from developing the chest muscles that support the breasts and the muscles of the back and upper arms.

1 Stand so that your breasts rise clear of your diaphragm. Hold your head up and back and keep your shoulders back and down. This position should feel relaxed.

2 Sit with your outstretched arms resting on a table. Push your clenched fists hard down onto the table, counting 5. Repeat at least 20 times.

3 Gripping a big towel in both hands, twist for 30 seconds as if wringing out water.

4 Stand with your arms level with your shoulders, your elbows bent and your hands in front of your chest with the palms facing outward and the thumbs down. Thrust your arms back and straighten them. Repeat 20 times.

5 Raise your arms as in **4** but with your fists clenched and drawn in under armpits. Make big, backward circling motions with the elbows for 30 seconds.

6 Stretch your arms upward. With your palms pressed together, slowly lower your arms level with your waist. Repeat 5 times.

7 If you are fit enough try push-ups, lie on your stomach and press down with hands until you are supported on your hands and toes.

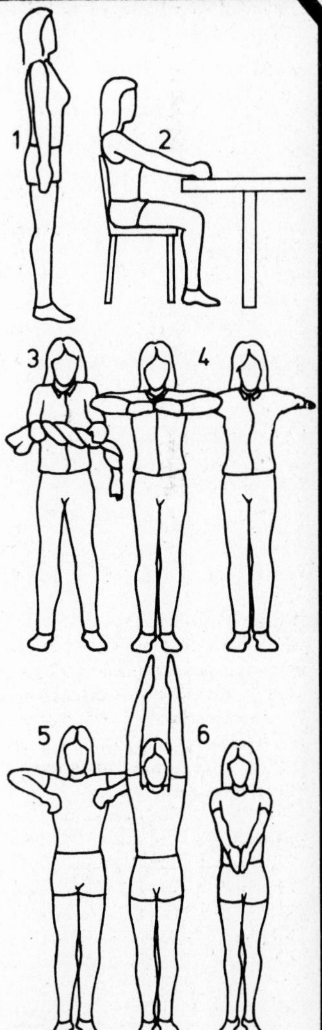

Reproductive system 1

A man's main sex organs are the penis and two bean-like testes suspended in the scrotal sac, visible below the base of the penis. Testes produce the male hormone testosterone, and sperm for fertilizing a woman's ova. Tubes carry sperm through the reproductive tract, where glands lubricate and nourish them. At orgasm muscular contractions force the resulting semen (a sticky white fluid) through the urethra and from the tip of the penis, which is then stiff and hard.
The main problems afflicting the male reproductive system are infections, congenital malformations, and benign and malignant prostate gland conditions. Most sexual conditions can be helped and anyone with a reproductive system problem should see his doctor. (See also pp.172–177.)

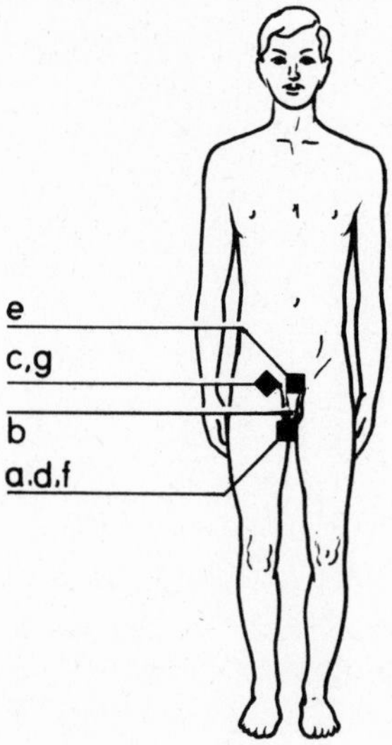

Onset of puberty
This varies from boy to boy but usually starts about 12, soon after the so-called adolescent growth spurt has set in.
a By age 12 the testes are growing noticeably (two years earlier they were only a fraction of their adult size).
Between 12 and 15:
b the penis starts to grow and undergoes spontaneous erection more often than before;
c pubic hair begins to grow around the base of the penis;
d testes begin secreting immature sperm, and nocturnal emission may start occurring;
e the prostate gland grows.
Between ages 15 and 18:
f mature sperm are produced;
g pubic hair coarsens.

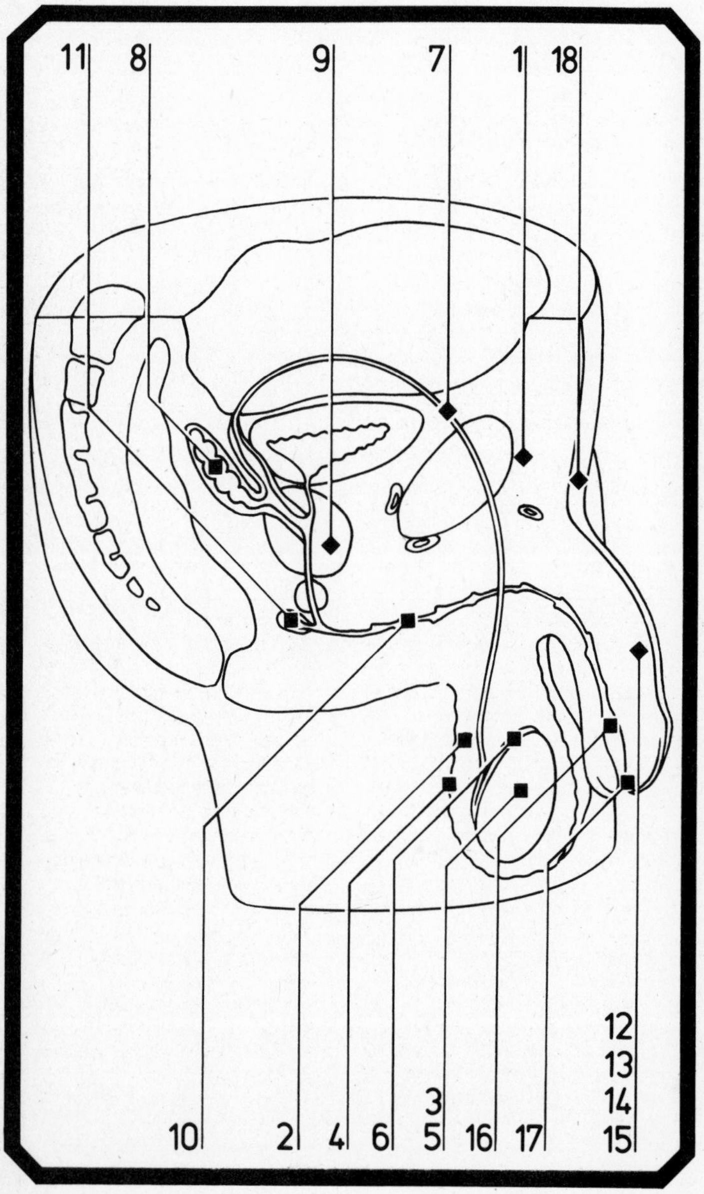

Male reproductive system and its problems
The two testes hang below the body in the scrotum where they are cool enough to produce fertile sperm. Testes secrete testosterone, a hormone producing male sex characteristics.
1 Testes that remain inside the abdomen fail to produce fertile sperm (see p.176), and may also develop cancer.
2 Scrotal swelling may be due to accumulated fluid, hernias (see p.99), cysts or tumors.
3 Inflammation of testes (orchitis) is usually due to mumps but can be caused by gonorrhea. Either way the consequence may be infertility, although this is a rare complication of mumps.
4 Varicose veins around the scrotum produce the condition varicocele, sometimes causing infertility. Regularly bathing the testes in cold water may help, or veins can be removed.
5 Billions of tiny, tadpole-like sperm cells develop in tiny tubes inside the testes each month. But if a high proportion is misshaped or lacks mobility a man may be infertile.
6 Epididymes are convoluted tubes on and behind the testes. They store sperm until these are ejaculated or disintegrate. In gonorrhea, epididymes may grow inflamed and painful.
7 The vas deferens tubes take sperm from the epididymes to the seminal vesicles. Tubal blockage by venereal disease can cause infertility, possibly treatable by bypass surgery.
8 Seminal vesicles store sperm and secrete fluid for it. They seldom get infected.
9 The prostate gland produces fluid to feed and stimulate sperm. It is liable to suffer inflammation or enlargement.
10 The urethra carries sperm and urine from the body. It sometimes suffers inflammation or blockage due to infection or kidney stones.
11 Cowper's gland adds lubricating fluid to semen.
12 The penis encloses the outer end of the urethra. When erect, the penis can be inserted into a woman's vagina during intercourse.
13 Congenital penis problems include a misplaced urethral outlet.
14 Acquired penis deformations include crooked erection due to injury; and nonsexual erection (priapism) with various possible causes.
15 Inability to achieve an erection may occur from psychological or physical causes (see p.174).
16 A painful penis may be due to inflammation or obstruction elsewhere in the urinary tract.
17 Some sexual infections show as sores on, or discharge from, the penis tip (see p.177).
18 Pubic skin troubles include sores, ulcers, warts, and mite and louse infestations – all results of sexual contacts.

Hygiene
Poor penis hygiene encourages accumulations of white smegma under the foreskin in uncircumcised men, causing inflammation of foreskin and penis tip with an offensive discharge. Accumulating smegma is also linked with certain cancers in men and in women with whom they have intercourse. Good penis hygiene stops smegma from collecting and so prevents such troubles. Uncircumcised males should take care to wash beneath the foreskin regularly. To do this they should first retract the foreskin; if inflammation prevents this, a doctor may prescribe ointment to clear up the infection producing the inflammation.

Urethritis
As its name implies, urethritis involves inflammation of the urethra. There may be discharge from the penis and urinating can be painful. If untreated, prostate, bladder and testes may all become involved, with local pain and swelling. The cause may be gonorrhea, or bacteria invading the urinary system. Nonspecific urethritis (the most common type) can be due to unidentified germs or reaction to chemicals in the vagina of the sexual partner. Patients should drink 8–10 glasses of water daily. Analgesics may relieve pain, and antibiotics kill most kinds of urethritis-causing germs.

Prostate problems
Prostatitis is inflammation of the prostate, due to urinary tract infection, and occurs in younger men. There may be pain, local tenderness, and difficulty passing urine. The acutely ill need bedrest, antibiotics, analgesics and 8–10 glasses of water daily. Weekly prostatic massage for 6–8 weeks may help. Avoid alcohol and sex. Benign prostate enlargement occurs mainly in men over 60. It may be symptomless. But if you pass urine little and often, with difficulty or discomfort, and your stools are very thin, you may need surgery. Cancer of the prostate has similar symptoms and requires surgery or hormone treatment.

Impotence
This means being unable to gain or maintain an erection and so have sexual intercourse. Many men are impotent at some time. Nine-tenths of cases are due to fear of failure, dislike of sex, or other psychological causes. Most temporary bouts of impotence can be cured by the restoration of good communication between the partners, so that misunderstandings, fears and unreal expectations can be removed; if the man has a warm, loving and understanding partner his confidence, and potency, will soon return. Cases of long-term impotence may need psychological counseling, and many respond to therapy (see p.174).

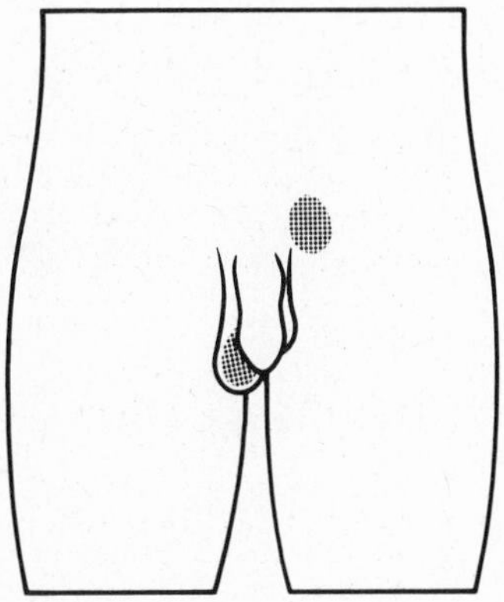

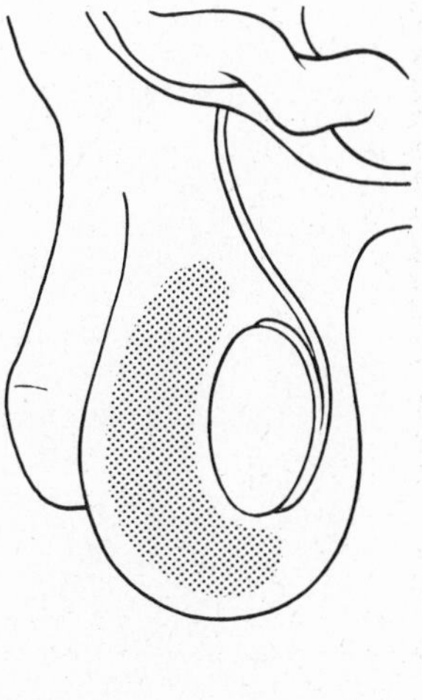

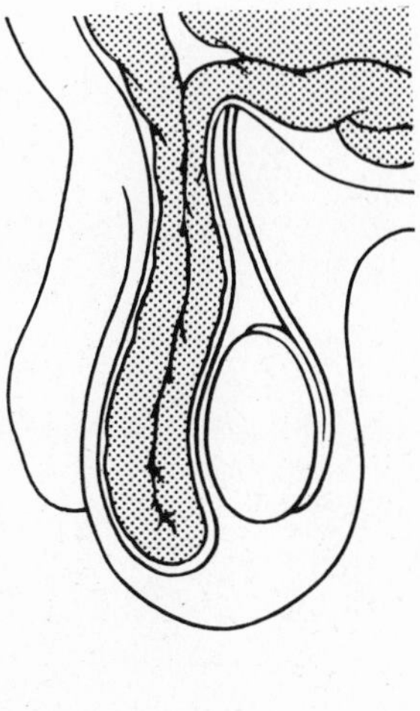

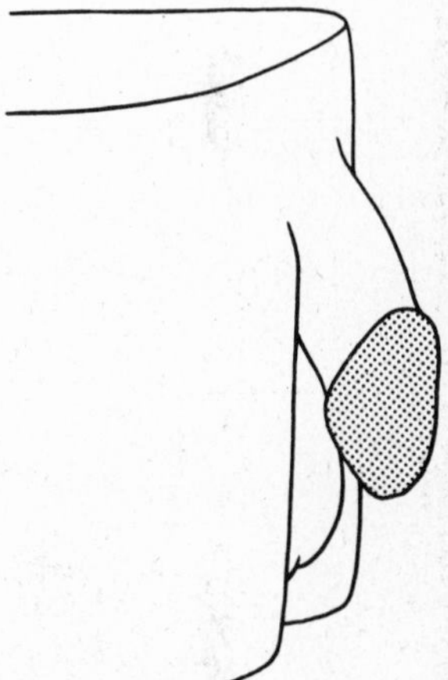

Undescended testes
Testes develop in the abdomen and normally descend into the scrotum about 8 weeks before birth. Sometimes they are only in the groin by birth but fall soon afterward. Even normally descended testes temporarily rise into the groin. If in any doubt whether testes have descended examine the baby after a warm bath, but avoid handling the testes. If both have not descended by the age of 2 your doctor may advise surgery if only one testis is involved, or hormone drugs if both are undescended. Patients must be treated before puberty. Otherwise, testes and sperm may not develop properly, causing infertility and a risk of cancer.

Hydrocele
This is a soft swelling in the scrotum, produced by a larger than normal accumulation of the fluid that helps protect the testes and leaves them free to move about. One side or both sides of the scrotal sac may be affected. A hydrocele is present in many newborn male babies and the condition usually corrects itself within the first two years of life. But if a loop of intestine herniates down into the scrotum through a channel, this may also fill with fluid, producing swelling in groin as well as scrotum. When this happens surgery is called for. Any swelling in the scrotum or groin should be investigated by a doctor.

Inguinal hernia
An inguinal hernia occurs when part of the intestine bulges down into the inguinal canal – the channel through which, in men, the testes drop into the scrotum before birth. Because this canal is larger in men than in women, more males than females suffer inguinal hernias. In men, inguinal hernia results from weak inguinal muscles; in boys it may be linked with a small developmental defect. A hernial sac may disappear while the patient lies down if the intestine slips back into the abdomen. Inguinal hernias are usually corrected by surgery to avoid the severe complications that may arise if they are left untreated.

Circumcision
This practice involves cutting off the foreskin, a loose fold of skin that covers the penis near its tip. Circumcision is a religious requirementof Jews and Moslems. This operation has the practical benefit of preventing build-up of smegma beneath a man's foreskin. However, circumcised babies are liable to get ulcers at the penis tip. Provided males maintain good penis hygiene there is no purely medical reason for circumcising routinely; rare emergency circumcision may be needed if the foreskin swells and blocks the urethral outlet.

Reproductive system 2

Inside the female reproductive system, ovaries produce eggs and the female sex hormones estrogen and progesterone. A ripe egg from an ovary passes through a Fallopian tube to the uterus. Meanwhile a penis inserted into the vagina may eject sperm that travel up through the cervix and then through the uterus, to fertilize the egg. The fertilized egg travels down the Fallopian tube and becomes implanted in the uterine wall until it has grown into a full-term baby and is forced by muscular contractions through the vagina and out of the mother's body. Sexual or other infection can affect all parts of the female genital tract, and some parts are liable to damage or displacement. Some ailments are merely irritating, but others can cause infertility or chronic illness, and occasionally even death if not diagnosed and treated early enough.

Women can do much to prevent problems by simple hygiene. This includes: wearing clean cotton panties daily (not nylon ones, as these promote fungal infections); washing the vulva daily with mild soap; wiping the genitals from front to back after a bowel movement; remembering to remove tampons after a period; avoiding chemicals that irritate the vagina; and ensuring that the sexual partner is clean and disease-free. Ideally a woman should learn to use a speculum, an instrument that enables her to see her internal genitals clearly; she will then be able to notice any unexplained change. Abdominal pain or swelling, or pain during or after intercourse, should always be investigated medically.

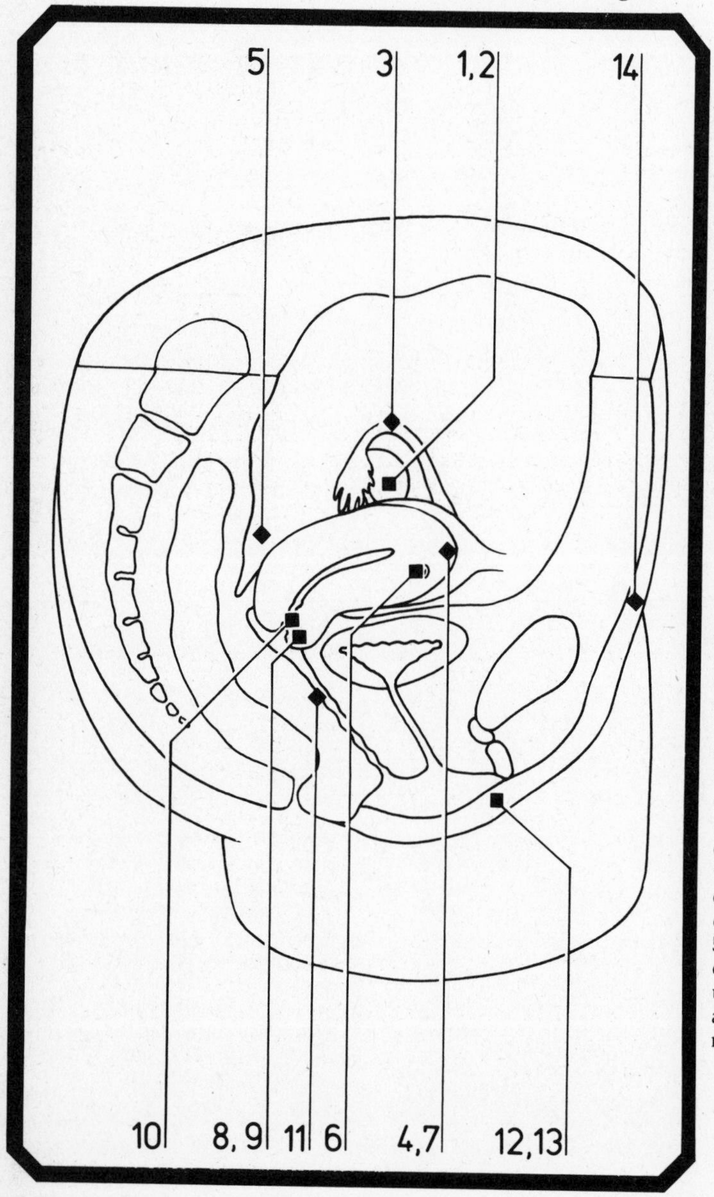

Female reproductive system and its problems

1 Ovarian cysts are sacs of mucus or fluid that grow in the egg-shaped ovaries, and which may be tiny or enormous. Some cysts become twisted, producing sudden severe pain, nausea and even shock; troublesome or large cysts need removal.

2 Solid ovarian tumors may be benign or malignant. Some produce female hormone, causing precocious sexual development or postmenopausal bleeding; a few produce a hormone which deepens the voice, shrinks the breasts and produces facial hair.

3 Salpingitis is inflammation of the Fallopian tubes caused by bacterial infection – frequently gonorrhea. Pain in the lower abdomen and cervical discharge occur, and infertility and peritonitis may be complications if the condition is left untreated.

4 The uterus in a non-pregnant woman is a small, pear-shaped organ; during pregnancy the fertilized egg imbeds itself in the endometrium (the rich lining of the uterus) and the uterus enlarges to make room for the developing fetus.

5 Endometriosis is the growth of endometrial cells outside the uterus, causing backache and abdominal pain, particularly at menstruation.

6 Fibroids are benign tumors of the uterus; they are present in 20% of women aged 35–40 and range from the size of a pinhead to the size of an unborn baby. Large fibroids disturb normal menstruation and bladder action and require surgical removal.

7 The uterus occasionally becomes tilted or drops downward in some women.

8 Cervicitis is inflammation of the cervix, the neck of the uterus. Cervicitis is caused by infection and produces thin, clear mucus, perhaps streaked with blood or pus.

9 Cervical erosion is a rough, reddened area lining the os (cervical opening) and needing electric cauterization if it causes persistent trouble.

10 Cervical polyps are benign tumors in the cervix, sometimes producing bleeding, discharge, pain and infertility. They should be removed surgically.

11 Vaginitis is inflammation of the vagina, the muscular passage between the cervix and the external genitals.

12 Vulvitis is inflammation of the vulva, the external genitals.

13 Syphilitic sores and some other venereal lesions may show up on the vulva.

14 Pubic skin troubles include sores, ulcers, warts, and mite and louse infestations – all a result of sexual contact.

Douching
This involves squirting water into the vagina through a tube from a douche can. Douching gently in early morning with 1 teaspoon of common salt per pint of water may help wash out troublesome mucus or discharge. Never douche forcefully, insert the nozzle in the neck of the womb, or use disinfectants or other irritants. Carelessness can irritate or even damage reproductive organs, especially in pregnancy. If it is advised by your doctor, douching with warm water and bicarbonate of soda before intercourse may improve chances of conception. Douching afterward may reduce risk of sexual infection but has no contraceptive value.

Discharge
Being able to distinguish normal from abnormal vaginal discharge is an important part of monitoring the health of the female body. Between menstrual periods, normal discharge includes watery mucus from the cervix, clear fluid sweated from the vaginal walls (notably in sexual excitement) and a clear or milky, slippery fluid from the vaginal entrance. Abnormal discharge is often smelly and discolored. Thus it is a foamy greenish-yellow in trichomoniasis; thick and white in candidosis (a yeast infection); creamy, yellow and blood-streaked in nonspecific vaginitis.

Irritation
Irritation of the genital tract may be due to infection or have chemical or mechanical causes. Yeast and Trichomonas infections cause soreness and itching. (See also symptoms of venereal diseases, p.177.) Chemical causes include antiseptic soap, cosmetic powders, deodorants, detergents applied to the vulva and mouth of the vagina, perspiration or urine trapped by nylon panties, and smegma secretion if it accumulates near the clitoris. Contraceptive caps or tampons left in the vagina for longer than the recommended period cause irritation and infection.

Endometriosis
This is a condition where some of the cells that form the mucous membrane lining the inside of the uterus get misplaced, for instance in uterine muscle or in the ovaries. In time they grow into cysts. At menstruation the cysts bleed and swell, with pain in the rectum, bladder or abdomen. Intercourse is also sometimes painful. Cysts blocking ovaries or Fallopian tubes can cause infertility. Doctors may give hormone treatment or advise surgery for cyst removal. In some instances endometriosis requires hysterectomy. But the condition may vanish permanently when pregnancy begins and it usually causes no more symptoms after the menopause.

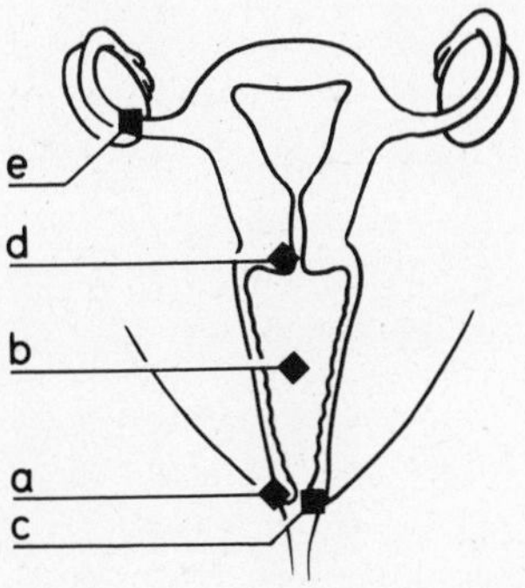

Infection
Between puberty and the menopause estrogen hormone helps to protect the vulva and vagina against many infections. But illness, injury, overdouching, or intercourse with a sexually infected partner may cause trouble. Yeast infection or trichomoniasis of the vulva (**a**) and vagina (**b**) produce irritation and discharge. Cuts or abrasions (**c**) may give rise to infection by streptococcal bacteria. Various microorganisms can infect the neck of the womb (**d**), causing cervicitis, or the Fallopian tubes (**e**), causing salpingitis. If you suspect any infection of the genital tract consult your doctor.

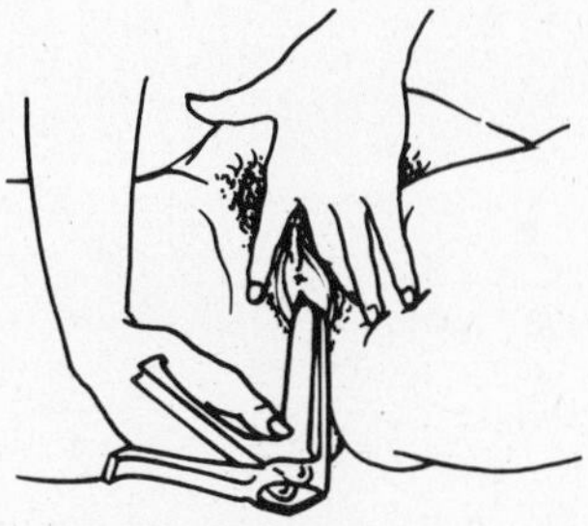

Self-examination
A woman who regularly inspects and so grows familiar with her own internal sex organs quickly notices if something is amiss, and can seek early treatment. Self-examination involves inserting a speculum with closed blades, handles uppermost as shown *above*, inside the vagina (which may be lubricated first). Locking the blades open, examine the vagina with a mirror and flashlight. The cervix will show at the upper end of the vagina as a smooth, pink dome with central opening (the os). Note normal changes in the cervix, os, vagina and vulva, and learn to recognize abnormal discharge or other changes.

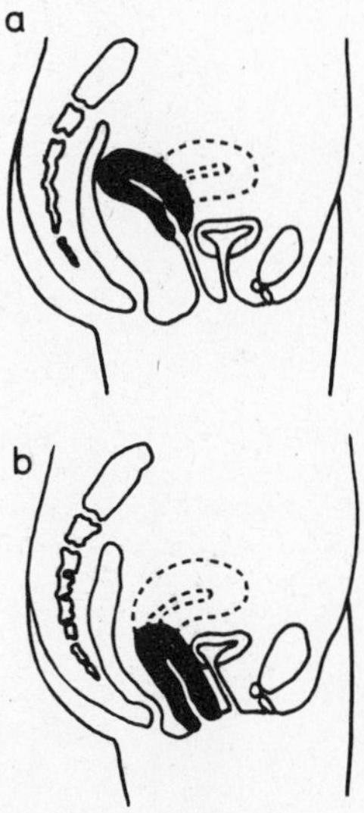

Displaced uterus
Some women suffer retroversion or prolapse of the uterus.
In retroversion (**a**) the uterus is always tilted backward, causing urine retention in pregnancy, maybe with cystitis or even a miscarriage. Doctors can often treat it by manually repositioning the uterus, though surgery is sometimes needed. In prolapse (**b**) weakened muscles let the uterus sag down into or even beyond the vagina, causing discomfort, discharge, backache, and urination that is frequent and difficult. Doctors may insert a supportive pessary but usually prefer surgical repair.

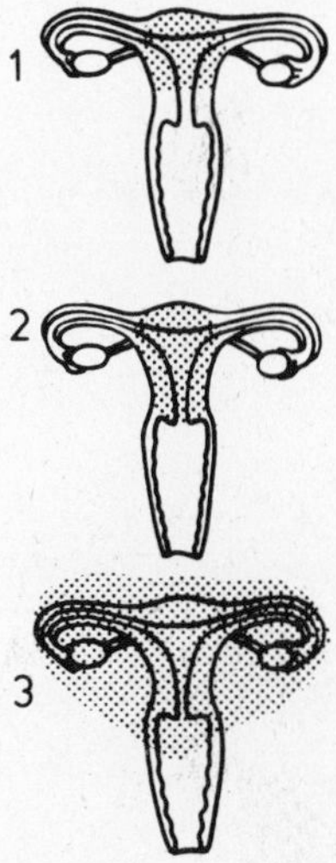

Hysterectomy
This is an operation to remove the uterus. It may be subtotal, involving uterus alone (**1**); total, involving uterus and cervix (**2**); or radical, involving uterus, cervix, part of the vagina, local lymphatic ducts, ovaries and Fallopian tubes (**3**).
Conditions that may require hysterectomy include fibroids, endometriosis, metropathia hemorrhagica (a condition arising from impaired ovarian control of menstruation), cancer, and precancerous changes. If the ovaries have to be removed, hormone treatment can prevent menopausal symptoms and most women can enjoy a normal sex life.

Reproductive system 3

About once every 28 days, females between the ages generally of 12 and 47 experience a flow of blood and mucus from the vagina. This regular flow indicates that several things have happened. First, hormones have helped thicken the womb lining to receive a fertilized egg. Next, an ovary has released an egg. When this has remained unfertilized, hormone action has helped to break up the womb lining, which has leaked out with some blood – a process called menstruation. Women wear pads or insert tampons in the vagina to absorb the menstrual flow. But many have to cope with other problems, ranging from premenstrual tension to period pains and abnormal periods. Here we look at common problems associated with menstruation.

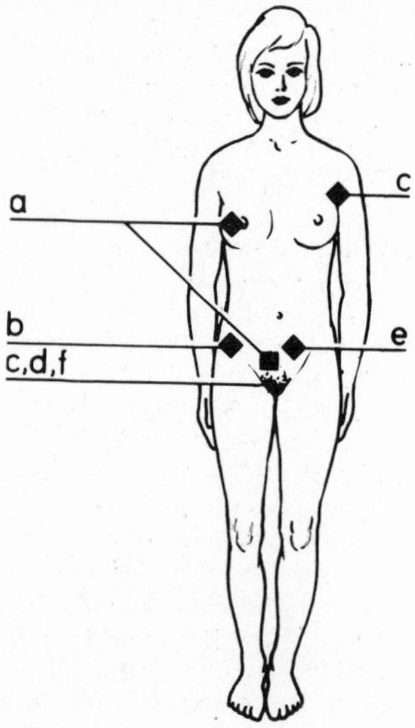

Onset of puberty
This can start as early as 9 or as late as 15, but usually begins about 11 in the Western world. Thus girls tend to reach puberty ahead of boys. Time of onset has grown earlier this century as diets and living standards have improved.
a By 11 nipples are becoming prominent and breasts, uterus and ovaries are growing.
b Pelvis broadens and pads of fat develop on the hips.
c Body hair increases.
d Menstruation may begin between ages 11 and 13.
e Ovulation usually starts about the age of 14.
f Later, genitals mature and menstruation becomes regular.

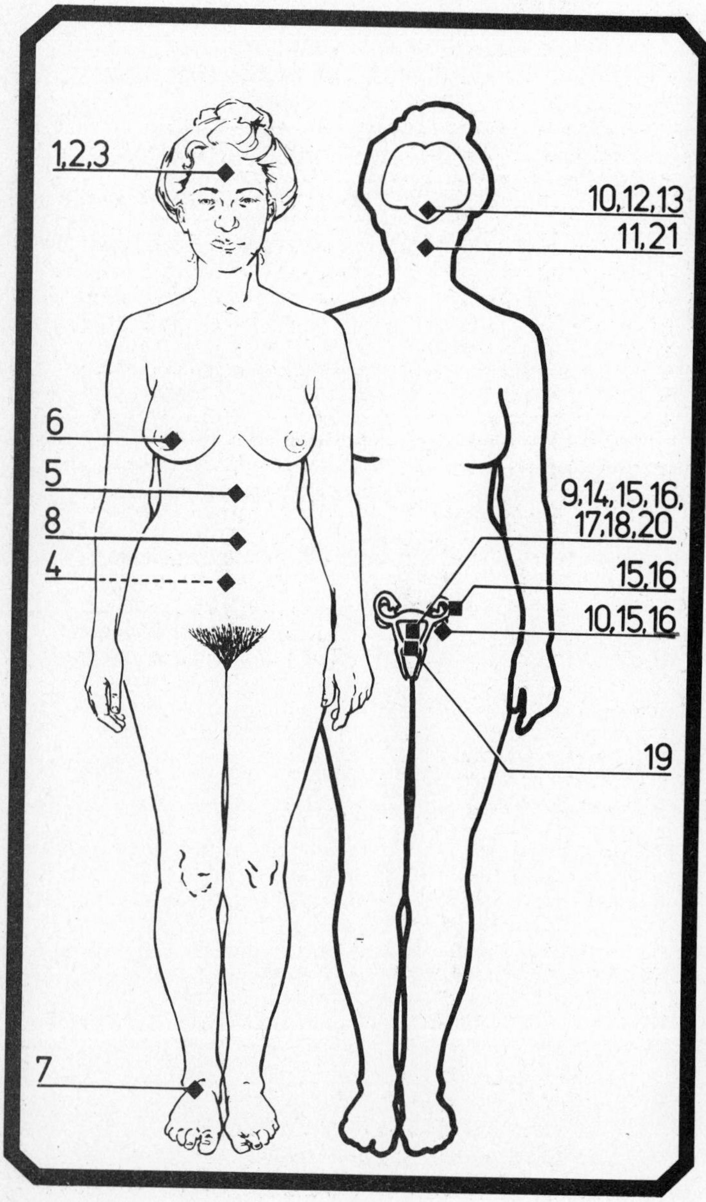

Premenstrual problems
The body's overreaction to the hormonal changes triggered by the menstrual cycle produces premenstrual problems – notably premenstrual tension – in about half of all women. Discomfort sets in about a week before the menstrual flow starts, and stops when the flow begins. On the far left half of the illustration we show common sites of problems, which are both physical and psychological.
1 Headaches (migraine sufferers get their very worst headaches at this time).
2 Psychological tension, making a woman tend to feel nervous and irritable.
3 A tired, depressed feeling.
4 Low backache.
5 Nausea.
6 Painful, tender, swollen breasts.
7 Puffy feet and ankles produced by fluid collecting in the tissues. Thumb pressure drives it out, leaving the skin temporarily pitted.
8 Bloated abdomen (also due to fluid retention).

The symptoms of premenstrual tension may be alleviated in several ways. Doctors may prescribe progesterone or modify the hormonal changes of the menstrual cycle. A mild analgesic should help to stop discomfort, and limiting salt intake some days before menstruation helps to reduce tension. Coffee, tea or cola drinks raise urine output and reduce fluid retention.

Menstrual problems
The near half of the illustration shows sites of major menstrual problems.

Lack of menstrual discharge may be caused by:
9 Abnormality of the uterus.
10 Failure of the ovaries to stimulate the adolescent uterus, perhaps through malfunction of the hypothalamus gland.
11 The nervous disorder called anorexia nervosa (see p.28).
12 Malfunction of the pituitary gland: overproduction of prolactin, interfering with another hormone in the ovaries.

Irregular periods may be caused by:
13 A malfunction of the hypothalamus gland.

Painful periods may indicate:
14 Normal hormonal changes that affect the uterine muscle.
15 Pelvic damage caused by inflammation of the ovaries, Fallopian tubes and uterus, sometimes following abortion or childbirth. These internal organs may become "glued" to bowel and pelvic walls.
16 Similar damage caused by endometriosis, gonorrhea or syphilis.

Heavy periods may suggest:
17 A troublesome intrauterine device.
18 Some type of tumor, notably (benign) uterine fibroids.

Postmenopausal bleeding has many possible causes. The three commonest are:
19 Cervical cancer.
20 Endometrial cancer.
21 Estrogen medication.

Absence of periods
Absence of menstruation is called amenorrhea. Girls who have never menstruated by 16 may have womb or ovary problems needing medical help. Women who stop having periods before the menopause (average onset: 48) may be pregnant or breastfeeding a young baby. But amenorrhea is also linked with ill-health, drug-taking, traveling and emotional stress including fear, shock, depression or tension, especially when there is loss of appetite and weight. Amenorrhea is often treatable with drugs, stimulating glands to produce the right hormones at the right time, or preventing hormone overproduction.

Irregular periods
At certain times in life and among some women it is quite common for menstruation to be somewhat irregular. In the first months after the menarche (onset of menstruation) a girl may find she misses one or two periods (but of course if there has been intercourse she should have a test for pregnancy). Even adult women may find that their menstrual cycle varies from month to month: cycles may be as short as 21 days or as long as 35. However, disorders of the hypothalamus gland in the base of the brain sometimes make periods become irregular or even cease. Many women also find that periods grow irregular as the menopause approaches.

Heavy and light periods
Most women shed 2-4 tablespoons of blood during each period. Some lose more, some less. At menarche (first onset of menstruation) vaginal discharge may redden only gradually. Women on contraceptive pills have light periods; periods may grow lighter or heavier as the menopause approaches. Heavy or prolonged bleeding may occasionally occur at menarche, or in women with intrauterine contraceptive devices, or it may occur for psychological reasons. But heavy bleeding and bleeding between periods or after the menopause may indicate disease, so your doctor should be told.

Painful periods
Dysmenorrhea (painful periods) may be primary or acquired. Primary (spasmodic) dysmenorrhea is due to hormonal changes in the womb; it may cause a day's discomfort or severe, cramping pain in lower abdomen or back with nausea and headaches. It is often worst in nervous, tense girls and women, who suffer least when on vacation. Taking more, not less, exercise may help and doctors may prescribe analgesics, iron pills and even a course of contraceptive pills. Acquired dysmenorrhea is due to internal disease and features one-sided pain in the lower abdomen. Treatment may be by medication or surgery.

Exercising
Doctors believe there is a close link between exercise and lack of period pains. They point out that healthy, active women and girls suffer least, and some athletes claim they feel fittest while menstruating. On the other hand many women suffering period pains perform sedentary work: this encourages constipation which is a factor that helps to promote dysmenorrhea. Leaving school to take up a sedentary job often coincides with the onset of painful periods, at least partly because the individual may stop sports activities. Instead of taking to your bed with hot blankets and analgesics to relieve mild pains, many doctors suggest eating an iron-enriched diet (to combat loss of iron in menstruation) and exercising. The following types of exercises are among those considered suitable.
a Walking. This should be brisk and done for a fairly extended period. It provides a rhythmic exercise yet does not strain individual joints.
b Swimming. This is a fine all-round activity, exercising heart, lungs and muscles and helping keep joints flexible. Aim for at least 10 minutes' vigorous swimming per session.
c Cycling briskly for several miles provides useful exercise, though some people complain it accentuates back problems.
d Dancing is also helpful, but again only vigorous activity counts as useful exercise.

a
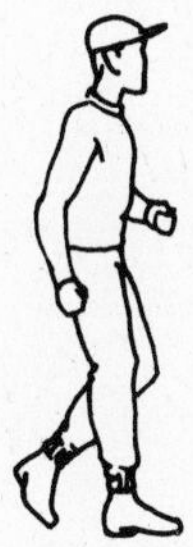
b
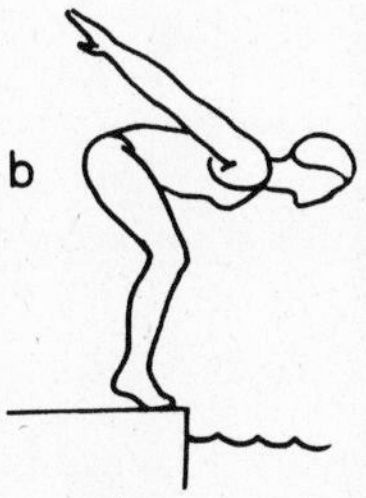
c
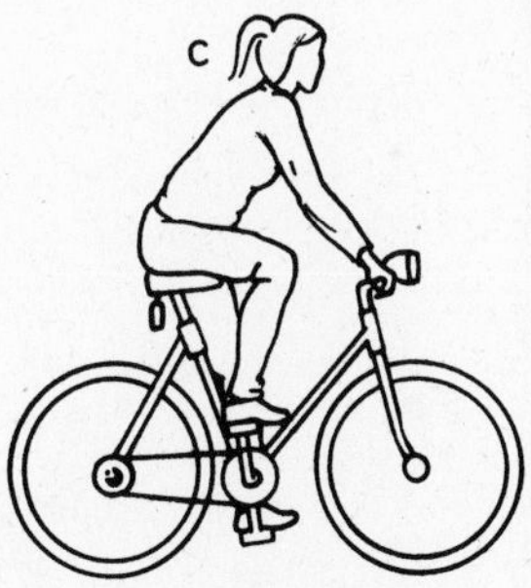
d
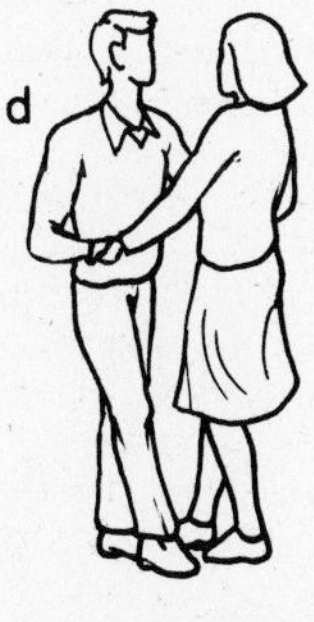

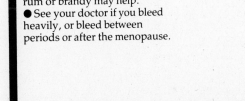

Do
- Prepare young girls for the onset of menstruation – otherwise their first flow of blood can be quite frightening.
- See a doctor if menstruation has not started by age 16.
- Drink coffee or tea to help combat fluid retention, but keep to normal fluid limits.
- Try a mild analgesic for acute premenstrual discomfort.
- Cut down salt intake (try a salt substitute) for some days before menstruation starts.
- Take exercise. This helps to reduce the discomfort that many women feel while menstruating.
- Seek medical help if you suffer severe period pains, especially one-sided, lower abdominal pain.
- Take extra iron in your diet if menstruation makes you anemic.
- Avoid constipation (exercise and bran in the diet help): it may worsen period pains.
- Get plenty of sleep and nourishing food to help to minimize period pains.
- Try a warm bath and half a day's rest with a warm electric pad and a mild analgesic if you suffer severe attacks of period pains. A sip of rum or brandy may help.
- See your doctor if you bleed heavily, or bleed between periods or after the menopause.

Don't
- Ignore severe premenstrual symptoms.
- Stand for long periods while suffering premenstrual tension.
- Drink more liquids than usual during the few days before each period begins.
- Automatically cope with period pains by "giving up" (ie simply taking time off work or going to bed).
- Become dependent on analgesics or tranquilizers to help you cope with premenstrual tension and period pains.
- Lead a life that lacks regular vigorous exercise.
- Allow yourself to become constipated.
- Ignore heavy, irregular or postmenopausal bleeding, or more than a few months of missed periods. The longer you leave it the more difficult it may become to treat the underlying cause.

Arms and hands

The complex interplay of joints, muscles and tendons in the arm and hand make them capable of a wide variety of movement. The shoulder swivels, the elbow and wrist are levers, and the many joints in the hand allow the brain to control very complicated maneuvers. The arm is also strong; the biceps and triceps muscles in the upper arm are large and powerful, and added strength for lifting comes from the shoulder muscles. Since the arms and hands are used constantly, from pushing back the bedding in the morning to switching off the light at night, problems such as injury or illness can cause great inconvenience as well as discomfort. Here we look at ways of preventing or minimizing the effects of some common arm and hand problems.

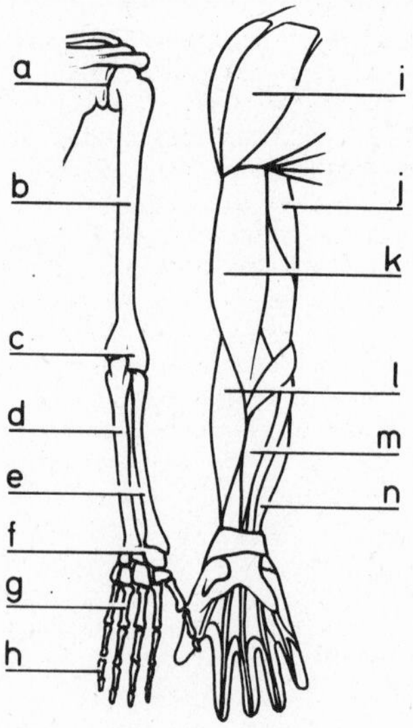

Structure of the arm and hand
The diagrams here show the main bones and muscles of the arm and hand.
a Shoulder joint.
b Humerus.
c Elbow joint.
d Ulna.
e Radius.
f Wrist joint.
g Metacarpals.
h Phalanges.
i Deltoid muscle.
j Triceps muscle.
k Biceps muscle.
l Brachioradialis muscle.
m Flexor carpi radialis muscle.
n Flexor digitorum superficialis muscle.

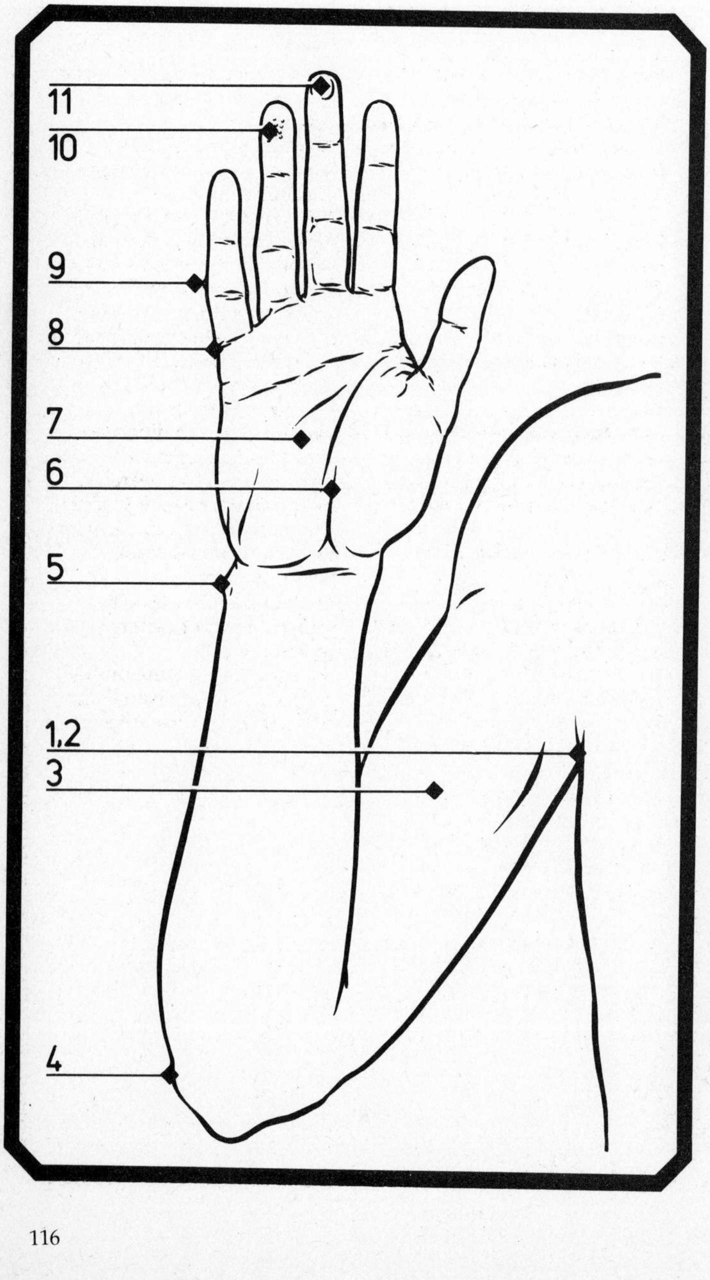

Common arm problems
1 Excessive underarm perspiration; this embarrassing problem may be relieved by using an antiperspirant and by wearing loose-fitting clothes made only of natural fibers. If the trouble is severe your doctor may be able to prescribe a long-lasting antiperspirant, but if these measures do not work surgery may be required to remove the overactive sweat glands.
2 Underarm odor; this can usually be prevented by washing regularly — several times a day if necessary — to prevent the build-up of bacteria, and by using an underarm deodorant.
3 Rupture of the bicep; this problem can occur at any age, but may be seen particularly in middle-aged men who tend to strain flabby muscles by lifting or pulling heavy objects.
4 Tennis elbow; any repeated rotary forearm action combined with a strong handgrip may lead to this pain on the outer side of the elbow. Massage and immobilization of the joint may ease the condition.
5 Ganglion of the wrist; the sac-like swelling encloses fluid around a tendon. Traditional treatment is to burst the ganglion by hitting it with a heavy book, but in fact if left alone the swelling often disappears spontaneously.

Common hand problems
6 Chapped skin; this often occurs in people with dry skin, but may be prevented by using a protective cream before exposure to cold or wind.
7 Sweaty palms; the sweat-producing mechanism is often triggered off by fear or excitement, but washing the hands regularly and dusting them with talc may keep the problem under control.
8 Dermatitis; this condition may be caused by contact with an irritant, such as washing soda, or by over-sensitivity to certain substances. Avoidance of the irritant is the main treatment.
9 Warts; common warts are probably caused by a virus, and often disappear spontaneously. Your doctor may recommend a suitable caustic solution to dissolve unsightly warts, and severe cases may have to be removed surgically.
10 Chilblains; these painful swellings are the result of circulation problems. You may be able to avoid chilblains by keeping your hands warm in cold weather and by avoiding excessive smoking.
11 Mallet finger, an injury often caused by a hard blow to the fingertip.

Hair removal
Many women consider underarm hair superfluous and choose to remove it. One of the most common methods used is shaving, either with an electric shaver or with a conventional razor and lather or talc. Hair-removing creams and lotions, known as depilatories, are also in common use; the hair is loosened at the skin's surface by a chemical action and wiped off with the depilatory. The regrowth after depilation is smoother and sometimes slower than after shaving, but depilatories are expensive and rather messy; they also tend to have strong chemical smells, and can cause allergic reactions.

Circulation
The arms and hands are quite frequently affected by circulatory problems. The arms become mottled when the circulation is poor, and if the hands are affected they may become numb and possibly develop chilblains. Massage of the hands will help to improve their circulation, and they should be protected from extremes of heat and cold. If your hands become cold and you don't have any protection for them, keep moving them and flexing your fingers so that the blood supply is maintained. Excessive smoking reduces the blood supply to the hands and so should be avoided.

Trembling hands
The tremors most commonly noticed in the hands are those experienced by elderly people; as they become more unsteady in general, they may also find that they have a weaker grip and tend to fumble over such tasks as threading a needle or fastening a button. In most cases this is a natural part of the aging process, and develops only very slowly. Trembling hands in younger people can often occur during illness, especially if there is a fever, and during times of stress, nervousness or excitement; an overactive thyroid gland can also cause trembling hands.

Tingling hands
A tingling sensation in the hands is often a perfectly harmless occurrence, and is frequently experienced in the late months of a pregnancy; the tingling should disappear after the baby is born. If it does not, or if you experience tingling in your hands while you are taking the contraceptive pill, or if you have other apparently causeless symptoms as well as tingling hands, you should see a doctor so that the possibilities of blood disorder or rare diseases of the nervous system can be ruled out. Tingling hands may occur as a result of nervous overbreathing (see p. 91), or of median nerve compression.

Splinters
If the end of the splinter protrudes from the skin, wash the area well and pluck out the splinter, as shown *right*, with a tweezer or needle that has been sterilized in boiling water. Press the skin so that a spot of blood comes from the wound; this will help to wash out any bacteria and also any parts of the splinter that may have been left behind. Apply a mild antiseptic and a sterile dressing. Deeply embedded or inflamed splinters will need medical attention. Never try to remove a splinter from the eye; go straight to a hospital for treatment.

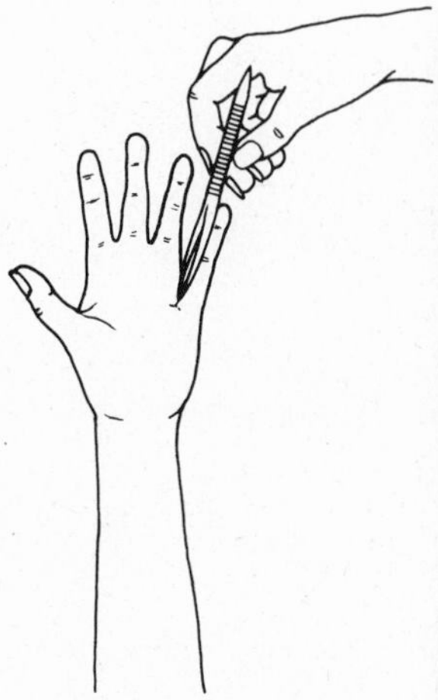

Rings
If you wear a ring or rings permanently, you should make sure that you wash the part of the finger that is usually covered by the ring; if this is neglected, localized dermatitis often results. If a ring becomes stuck on a finger that has grown or swollen, try removing it by lubricating the finger with soft soap. If this does not work, bind some thread round the finger just above the ring, as shown *right*; slide the ring up, remove the thread, and bind again above the ring's new position. Do not leave the thread on for more than a minute or so as it cuts off the blood supply to the finger.

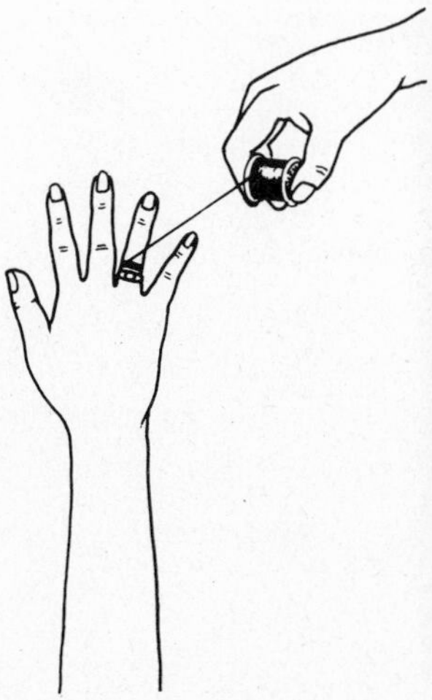

Do
- Exercise your arms regularly to avoid flabby muscles.
- Wash your underarms at least once a day.
- Use an antiperspirant if you are prone to excessive perspiration.
- Use an underarm deodorant daily if necessary.
- Massage any aching arm muscles to relieve the pain.
- Seek medical aid for any inexplicable tingling in your hands.
- Flex your hands and fingers in cold weather to help prevent frostbite and chilblains.
- Keep your hands protected against extremes in temperature and against wind.
- Sterilize any instruments used to extract splinters.
- Seek medical help for embedded or infected splinters.
- Make sure that you wash any parts of your fingers usually covered by rings.
- Use a hand cream after dishwashing, gardening and cleaning.
- Immobilize your arm in a sling if you damage your elbow, shoulder or wrist joint until you can seek a doctor's advice; this will prevent any further damage until the condition can be diagnosed.

Don't
- Wear man-made fibers if you are prone to excessive perspiration.
- Pull, push or lift heavy weights if your arm muscles are out of condition.
- Allow depilatory chemicals to remain on the skin for longer than the recommended time, as they have a caustic effect and will make the skin very sore.
- Continue to use your arm for any strenuous activity if you develop tennis elbow or joint problems; activity will aggravate the condition, and should not be resumed until the problem has disappeared.
- Expose your hands to potent chemicals or to strong solutions of washing powder; use protective gloves.
- Allow your hands to be exposed to wind, severe cold or severe heat.
- Allow the moisture in your hands to dry out; use a hand cream if your hands are prone to chapping.

Nails

The fingernails are rigid structures formed from dead cells filled with keratin, a tough protein. Because the cells are dead there is no feeling in the fingernails, although damage to the lower part of the nail will cause pain in the nerves to which it is attached. Each nail grows from a matrix, or nail bed, protected by the cuticle at the base of the nail; full nail care involves nurturing the nail from the time it takes shape in the nail bed, and keeping it healthy, well-shaped and undamaged as it grows. Uncared-for nails are unattractive and also unhygienic; if the nails are not cleaned properly they can harbor, and encourage the growth of, many kinds of bacteria. Caring properly for your nails does not take much time and will enhance your hands whether you are male or female.

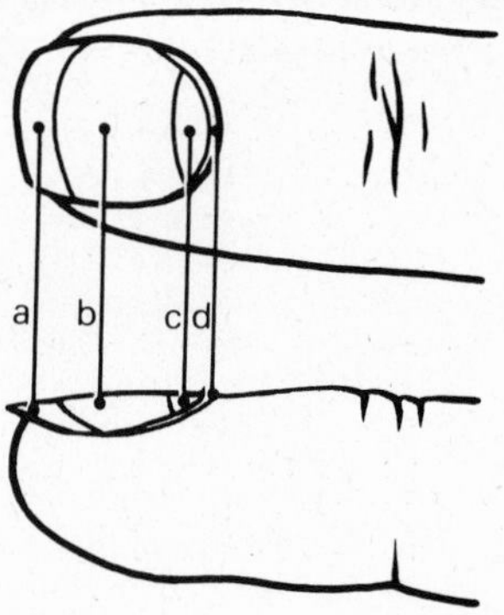

Parts of the nail
a Hardened part of the nail; this extends over the fingertip and is not attached on the undersurface.
b Attached fingernail.
c Half moon; this is the top of the matrix or nailbed, and is most easily seen on the thumbnails.
d Cuticle; this fold of skin protects the bottom of the nail.

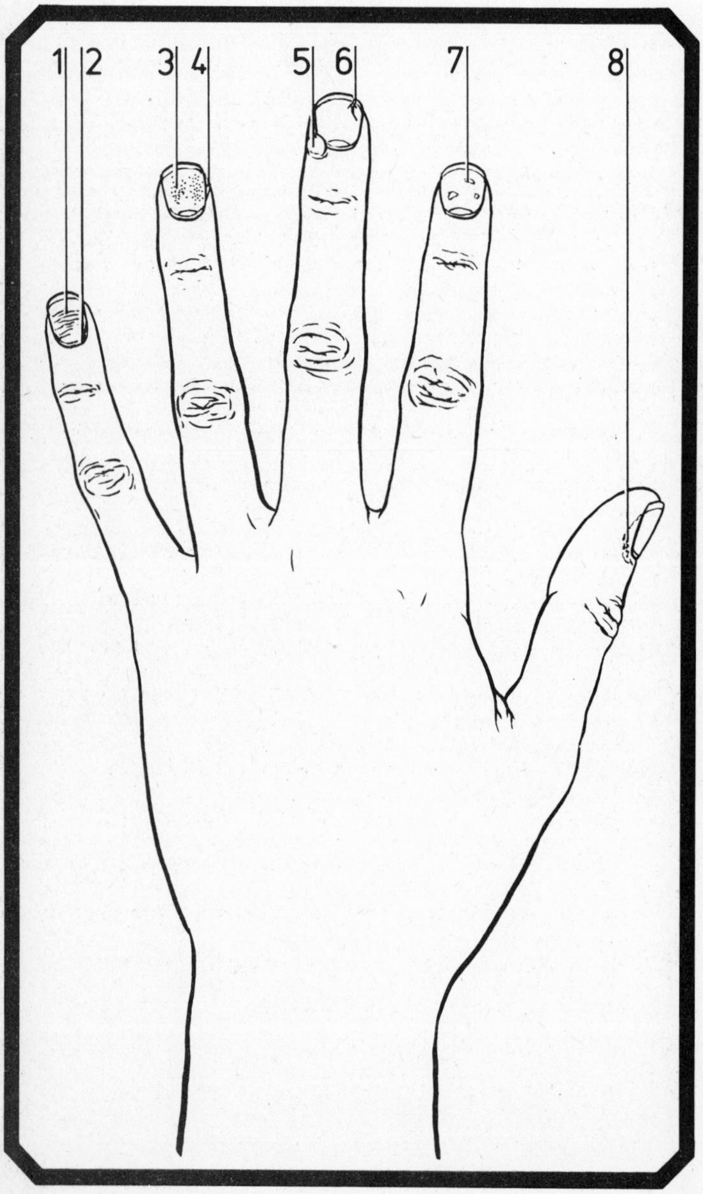

Fingernail problems
The illustration *left* shows some of the common problems that affect fingernails and which can be prevented or alleviated by good nail care.
1 Ridges on the fingernails can occur as a result of damage to the matrix, for example if the fingers have been crushed in an accident or through heavy manual work. Ridges can also occur if the matrix is damaged by over-enthusiastic shaping of the cuticles, especially if this is done with a metal instrument.
2 Damaged cuticle caused by attempts to shape it with a sharp instrument such as a scissor blade.
3 Cloudy nail; this may occur if nail polish is left on the fingernails for too long, or if an alcohol-based polish remover is frequently used. The condition can be alleviated by massaging the nails with one of the over-the-counter nail preparations – these usually contain lanolin and protein – and polishing them with a soft buffer.
4 Hangnail, a sliver of nail or hard skin that projects beyond the rest of the nail and causes snagging. It can be removed by clipping carefully with scissors.
5 Whitlow, an extremely painful boil-like infection that grows under or near the fingernails. Whitlows can be bathed and poulticed to soften them but will generally require lancing by a doctor.
6 Broken nails should ideally be filed down immediately. If the break is very close to the skin a special liquid can be painted over the break, so strengthening the nail at that point.
7 White spots can appear on the nails as a result of damage to the matrix during growth.
8 Sore skin around the nails is often caused by picking at rough edges of the nails or at uneven cuticles. Keep the nails well trimmed, and make sure that the cuticles are softened and shaped so that they do not become ragged.

Weak and brittle nails
Weak and brittle nails may simply be a constitutional fault in nail growth that is difficult to change, but various measures can be taken to strengthen them as much as possible. Frequent immersion in water or contact with turpentine, paint stripper etc can soften and damage the nails, so rubber gloves should be worn for household tasks. Gloves should also be worn for gardening so that the nails are not chipped by sharp stones. Preparations can be bought that claim to harden the nails, but their efficacy varies.

Diet and the nails
Although it is not usually possible for healthy people to improve the state of their nails significantly by changes in diet, it is true that poor nails can show up severe dietary deficiencies; once these are remedied, the state of the nails will inevitably improve. Calcium is necessary for the formation of healthy nails as well as for bones; also severe vitamin deficiency, such as rickets, causes damage to the nails. Gelatin can only improve the condition of the nails if taken in impractically large quantities.

Nail biting
This is a nervous habit that usually dates from childhood but can continue into adulthood. In severe and prolonged cases, the shape of the nail is so damaged that normal growth is never resumed even if the habit is stopped. Nail biting in children may be a result of boredom, anxiety, insecurity, unhappiness or other nervous problems. Painting the nails with bitter aloes or other foul-tasting substances may discourage the nail-biting, but the parents should also be alerted to look for psychological reasons behind the habit.

Nail polish
Nail polish varies in popularity with changes in fashion and custom. There is no harm in wearing nail polish as long as certain precautions are taken to protect the nails. The polish should never be left on the nails for too long, otherwise it will prevent air from reaching the nails. Dark colors should be applied over a clear or pale base coat so that they do not require extra solvent and rubbing to remove them. Polish remover often has a drying effect on the nails, so hand cream should be rubbed into them regularly.

Home manicure
A home manicure will help to keep the nails in good condition and makes them more attractive in appearance.
a Cut your nails with a short-bladed pair of scissors. Nail-clippers are not recommended as they do not give a good shape to the nail. The nails should be cut in a gently sloping curve; do not cut them down at the sides.
b File the nails into the exact shape required with an emery board or a nail file coated with diamond slivers. Metal nail files are too coarse and tend to split the layers of the nail. File each nail from the sides toward the center, holding the file toward the underside of the nail rather than the top.
c Trim any ragged cuticles close to the nail. Soak the hands in warm soapy water for a few minutes, and then gently push down the cuticles with an orange stick to expose the "half moon" area at the base of the nail.
d Polish your nails with a chamois buffer or a wool pad. Rub the buffer over the entire surface of the nail until a sheen appears.

a
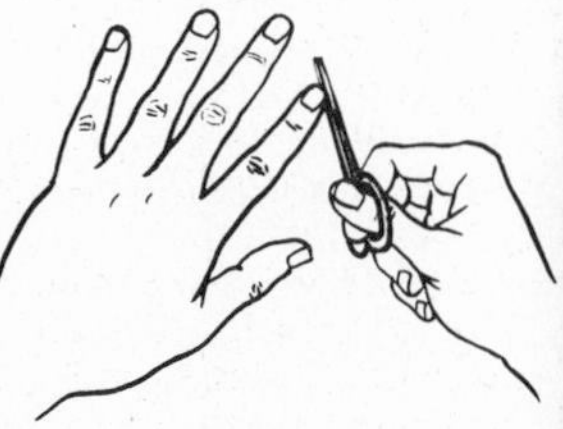

b
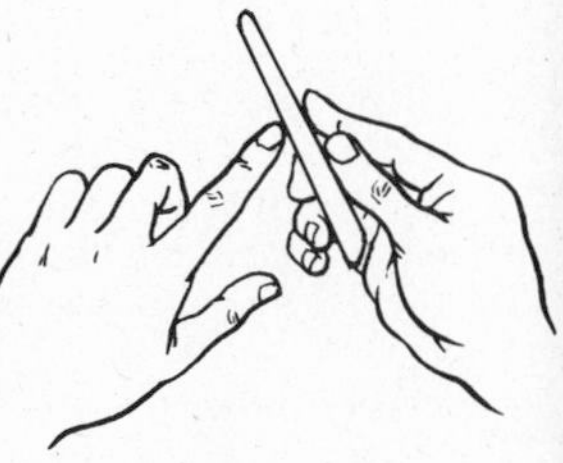

c
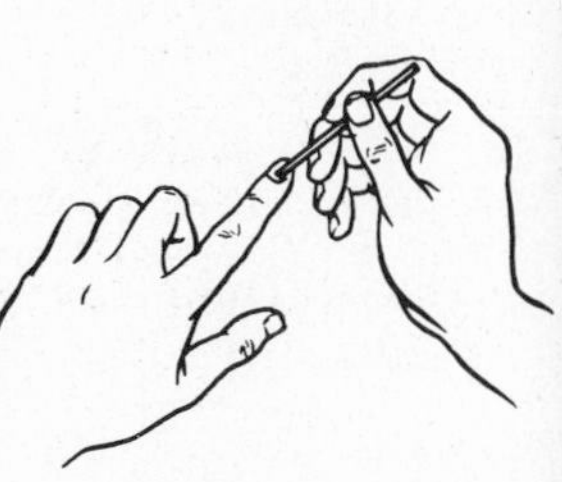

d
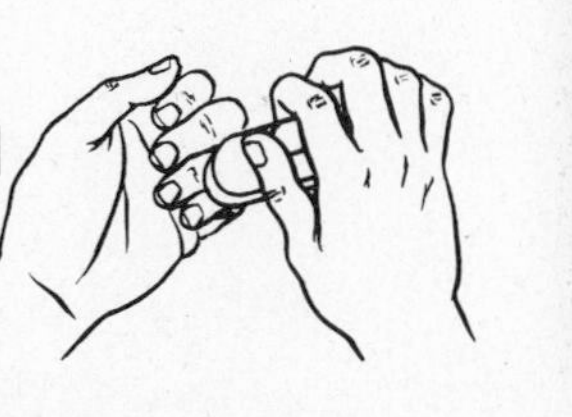

Do
- Clean your nails daily to prevent dirt from building up underneath the nails.
- Give yourself a regular manicure.
- Use an emery board or a diamond nail file for shaping your nails.
- Keep your nails carefully trimmed so that they do not split or crack.
- Treat your cuticles and nail beds very gently, as the entire nail can be damaged by rough handling of this area.
- Wear gloves for work that might chip the nails.
- Protect the nails against frequent immersion in water or contact with solvents.
- Use a pair of small scissors for trimming your nails.
- Use a pale nail polish as a base under darker colors.
- Use an oily nail polish remover.
- Go without nail polish entirely for several weeks once or twice a year, to allow the air to your nails.
- Remove nail polish every night.

Don't
- Dig under your nails when you clean them; this can drive dirt further under the nails and set up an infection.
- Try to cut away your cuticles, unless they are very ragged.
- Use a metal nail file.
- Push your cuticles back roughly, or by using metal instruments.
- Cut or file down at the corners of your nails; this tends to weaken them and make them more likely to chip.
- Wear nail polish if your nails have a tendency to become brittle.
- Use an alcohol-based nail polish remover.
- Paint dark nail polish onto your nails without using a pale base coat first.
- Scrub at your nails with polish remover.
- Use a nailbrush; this can drive dirt further under your nails.
- Allow dirt to remain under your nails; remove it with an orange stick.
- Bite or chew your nails, or suck your fingers.
- Pick at your nails or the skin around them.
- Allow the nails to become too long; this weakens them and makes them more likely to break.
- Use your fingernails for opening cans, bottle tops etc.

Legs

Legs are generally robust parts of the human body, but are nevertheless prone to many problems because of the various strains imposed by their functions. The knee is the largest joint in the body, and takes the strain of almost all of our body weight, and consequently its wellbeing can be affected by bad posture, by poor walking habits, and also by the state of the thigh and calf muscles. Whenever one part of the leg is injured or troublesome, it tends to affect the rest of the leg adversely and the problem is multiplied. On these pages we look at some of the common leg problems and show you how to avoid them, or their effects, as much as possible.

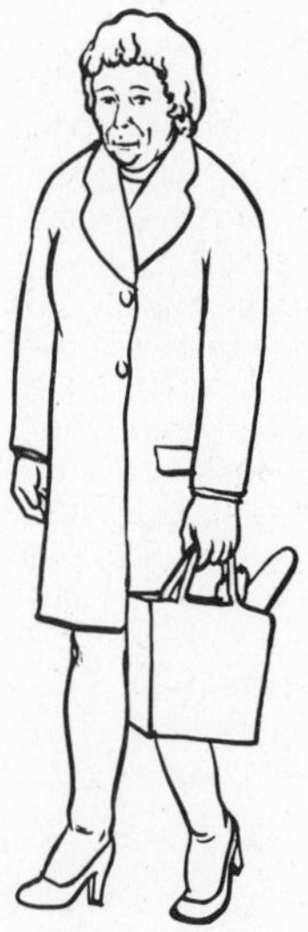

Aggravating situations
Certain occupations or habits have a tendency to increase the likelihood or the severity of leg problems. Overweight people increase the strain on their knee joints, and this is also true of women carrying extra weight because of pregnancy. Poor posture also strains the knees, and high-heeled shoes place an unnatural strain on the legs and should not be worn for long periods. Standing occupations, such as serving behind a counter or cooking, increase circulatory problems as the calf muscles sometimes do not work hard enough to pump the blood back up to the heart.

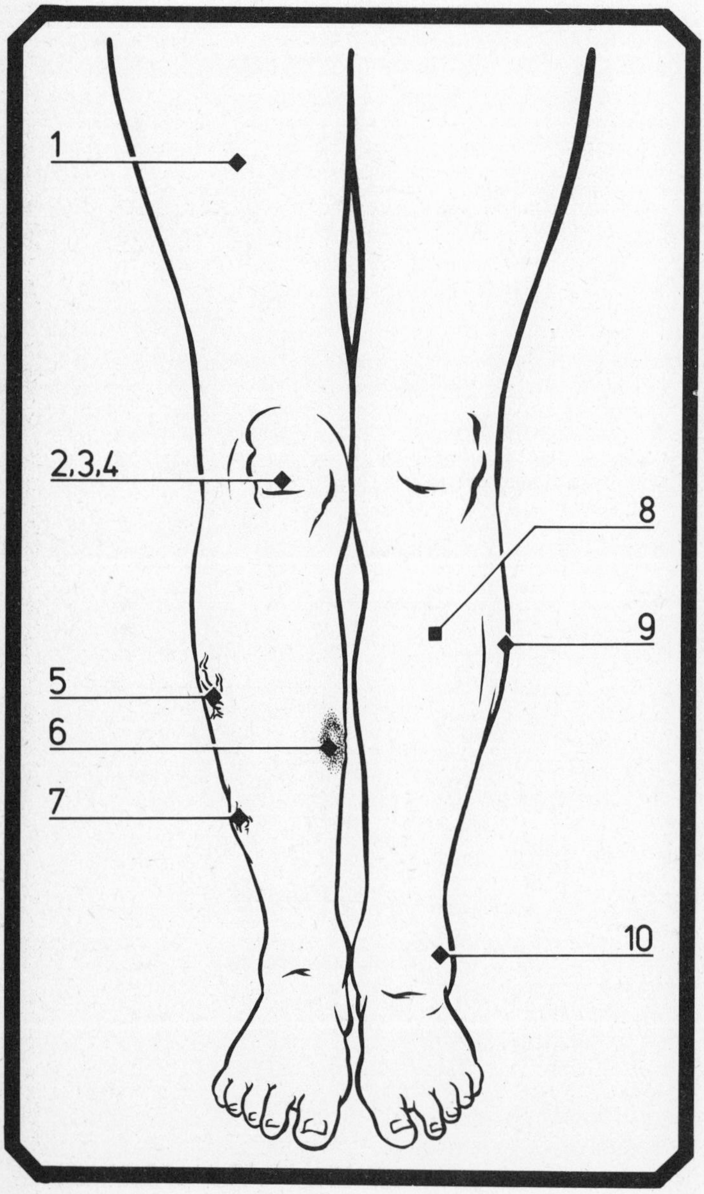

Common leg problems
The illustration *left* plots the sites of some of the problems that commonly affect the legs.
1 Sciatica; this severe pain down the leg is caused by pressure on the sciatic nerve.
2 Housemaid's knee; this condition is an inflammation of the knee joint, and may be caused by frequent kneeling.
3 Runner's knee; this condition often affects joggers and long-distance runners, and consists of pain and strain caused by insufficient foot support during running. Soft supports in the running shoes usually ease the problem.
4 Degenerative arthritis; this problem occurs more often in the knee than in any other joint because of the weight-bearing function. Obesity often precipitates the problem, especially in women.
5 Varicose veins; these are engorged blood vessels that have lost their elasticity and are no longer capable of helping to pump the blood up the leg.
6 Phlebitis; this condition is caused by the clotting of blood in the surface veins of the leg, and can have serious complications.
7 Varicose ulcer; ulcers of this type are usually caused by varicose veins, and involve breakdown of the surrounding tissue and often intense itching.
8 Shin splints; this condition may be suffered by runners, and takes the form of pain over the shin area. It is often caused by running on hard surfaces, such as roads or sidewalks, or may be another condition caused by inadequate support from running shoes.
9 Cramp; the intense pain of cramp is often experienced in the calves, and is caused by the muscle going into spasm (see p.73). This may be because of an insufficiency of salt, or the legs may have been exercised earlier without allowing them sufficient time to warm up and cool down.
10 Swollen ankles; the accumulation of fluid in the ankles causes them to swell and feel tender and heavy. Obesity, pregnancy, excessive water retention, lack of exercise and heart failure are all contributing factors.

Varicose veins
These develop when valves in the veins become faulty and allow the blood to pool in the veins, causing them to swell and become engorged. The blood flow around the legs is disturbed and the problem is increased unless the faulty valves are removed or normal flow can be established by exercise. Standing occupations, although they do not cause varicose veins, do increase any inherent tendency to them because the blood is not being circulated around the legs efficiently. Any measures that improve the blood flow away from the legs will help, such as walking, leg exercises, and sitting with the feet raised.

Other circulatory problems
Many circulatory problems in the legs are associated with or complications of varicose veins. Varicose eczema is caused by scratching the inflamed skin over the veins. Varicose ulcers appear when the tissue degenerates as the circulation deteriorates. The ulcers are open wounds and need dressings until they are healed. Phlebitis, clotting of the surface vessels, can be eased by extensive bandaging of the leg until the condition subsides and the underlying causes can be treated.

Sciatica
Sciatica is the term used to describe pain that is spinal in origin but that is felt in the sciatic nerve in the leg. The diagram shows the usual place of origin of the pain, in the lumbar region of the spine (**A**), and the part of the legs where the pain is generally felt (**B**). The pain results from pressure exerted on the sciatic nerve when it is squeezed or pressed by one of the vertebrae or by an intervertebral disk. The condition is usually cured by resting in bed, followed by physical therapy, but surgery may be needed in severe cases. Avoiding back strain by good posture and exercise may help prevent sciatica.

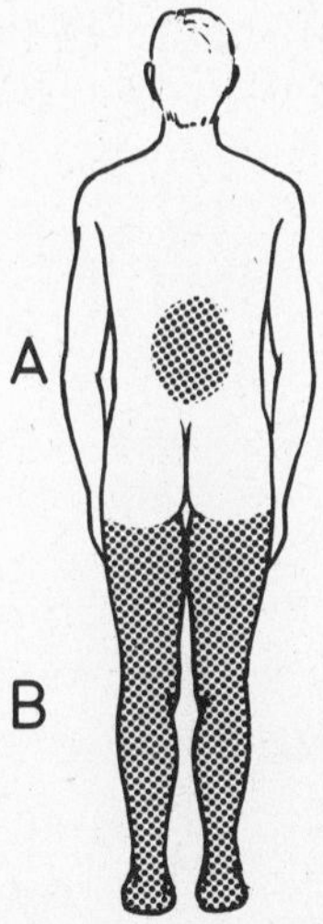

Bow legs
This condition is an outward bowing of the knee joints, as shown in the diagram *right*. The condition is often seen in children of early school age, and occurs because the bones are still pliable and because the child is still developing his or her particular style of walking; there is no need for concern unless the problem persists into later childhood, when surgery may be required. Many mothers wonder whether their toddlers are going to be bow-legged, but all babies learn to walk with their legs bowed out as they find it easier to balance; this does not mean that they will have later problems. One cause of bow legs is lack of vitamins A and D in infancy and childhood.

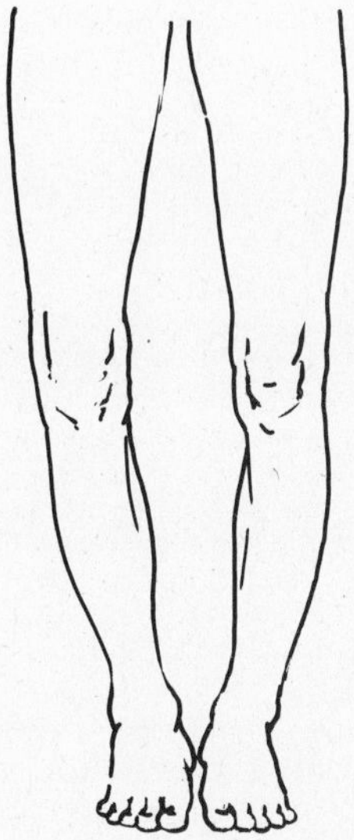

Knock knees
This condition is caused by an inward bending of the knee joint, as shown in the diagram *right*. In the same way as bow legs, and for similar reasons, knock knees often occur in children of early school age and are a cause for concern only if they continue into later childhood. Shoe wedges may be fitted to encourage the child to walk with a more conventional gait, but if the problem has not corrected itself by age 9 or 10, surgery may be performed to correct the joints.

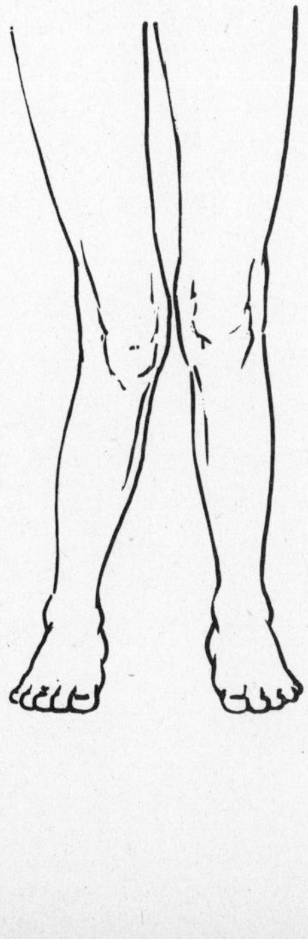

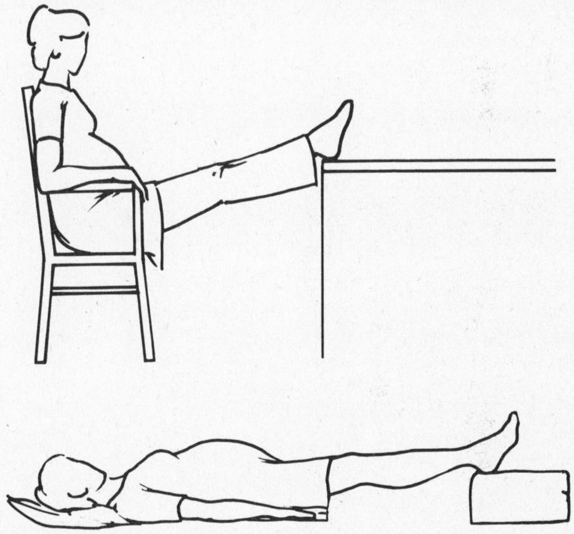

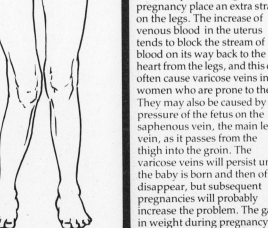

Pregnancy
Various physiological changes that take place during pregnancy place an extra strain on the legs. The increase of venous blood in the uterus tends to block the stream of blood on its way back to the heart from the legs, and this can often cause varicose veins in women who are prone to them. They may also be caused by the pressure of the fetus on the saphenous vein, the main leg vein, as it passes from the thigh into the groin. The varicose veins will persist until the baby is born and then often disappear, but subsequent pregnancies will probably increase the problem. The gain in weight during pregnancy adds to the load to be borne by the legs, and usually means that the legs will become tired more easily and need more rest. The increase of fluid in the body during pregnancy, especially if it is associated with circulatory problems in the legs, may cause swollen ankles. For all these problems, one of the best solutions is to sit or lie with your feet higher than your head; this eases the pressure on tired feet and blood vessels, and enables blood and other fluids to flow away from your legs with the aid of gravity. If you are pregnant you should try to rest this way for at least 30 minutes every day; if the trouble is very severe, tilting your bed by raising its foot slightly may help.

Feet

The feet are very complex structures, as their tasks require combinations of balance, movement, rigidity, maneuverability, strength and flexibility. Each foot contains 26 bones, 19 muscles and over 100 ligaments to help it carry out these diverse functions. Problems with the feet can affect a great deal of the rest of the body, causing leg pain, back pain, poor posture and fatigue. Foot problems may affect the muscles or bones, or may be viral, fungal or bacterial infections; other foot problems may simply be caused by poor foot hygiene or a lack of general care. Here we show you ways in which you can help to prevent many of these problems by giving your feet a little extra attention.

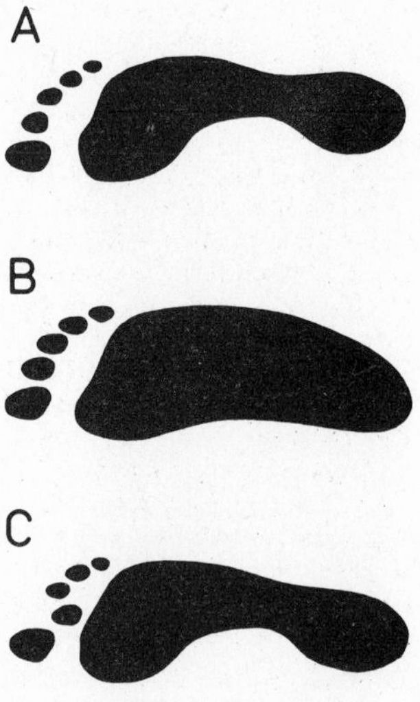

Footprints
The state of health of the foot is often reflected in the shape of its footprint. The top diagram here (**A**) shows a foot that is structurally sound; the print is well-formed and doesn't show any unnatural bumps or hollows. The middle footprint (**B**) shows a foot with a fallen arch; the sole of the foot is flattened out, and this is apparent in the print. The print at the bottom (**C**) shows a foot with a hammer toe; one of the toes is drawn up out of the natural line.

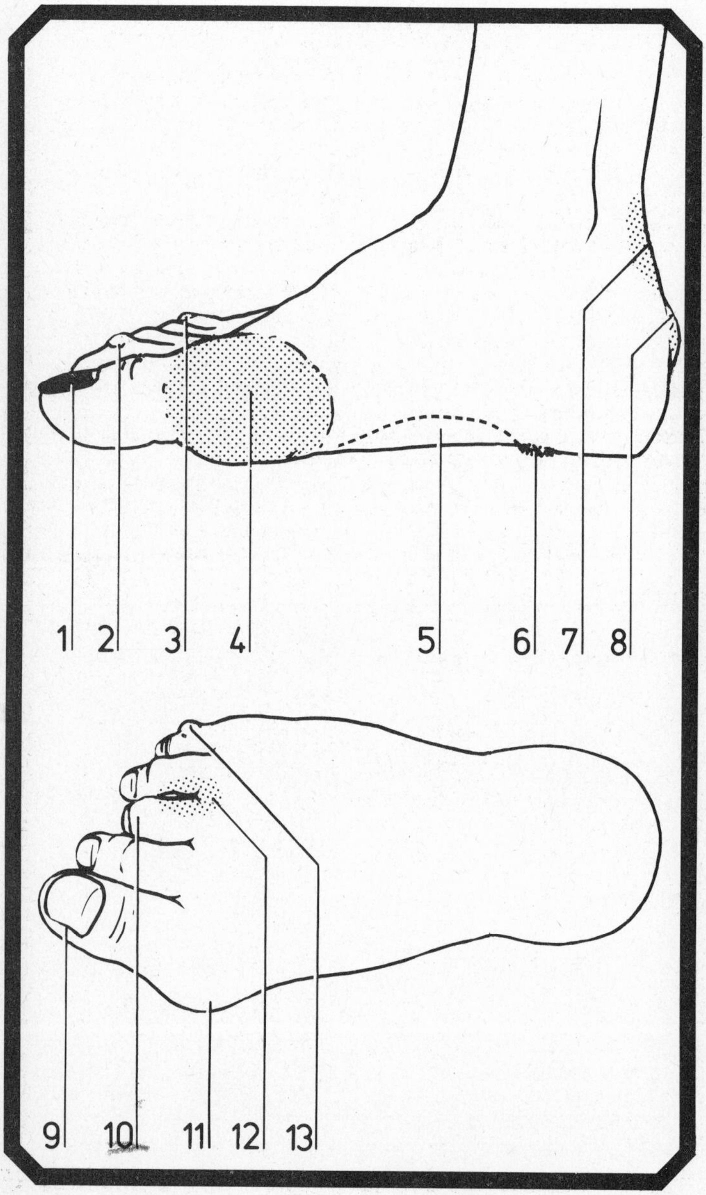

Common foot problems
The illustrations *left* show the sites of some of the most common foot problems.
1 Black nail; this is caused by a tiny hemorrhage under the nail, often the result of a blow from a heavy object.
2 Callus; friction against any part of the foot may cause a hard patch of shiny yellow skin known as a callus.
3 Corn; this is a condition that often develops from a callus.
4 Bunion; a bunion may develop as the underlying joint becomes swollen and deformed usually as a result of poor footwear.
5 Fallen arch or flat foot; this condition is not always problematic, although arches that are in the process of falling may cause pain and a chiropodist should be consulted.
6 Verruca; this is a wart that usually appears on the weight-bearing areas of the foot, including the toes.
7 Achilles tendinitis; inflammation in this area is usually caused by poor footwear that places strain on the heel.
8 Blister; friction between the skin and ill-fitting footwear may cause a fluid-filled blister. Small blisters can be covered with surgical tape and will probably disappear; larger ones should be lanced with a sterile needle and then pressed with a sterile swab to release the fluid.
9 Ingrown toenail; this very painful condition occurs when the side of the toenail begins to grow down into the tender pulp of the toe.
10 Hammer toe; this is often the result of pinching the toes into tight or pointed shoes. The toe finally becomes permanently bent up at the joint.
11 Gout; deposits of uric acid around the joint cause this condition, sometimes called the most painful condition known to man. The big toe is the joint most often affected. Although overeating and overdrinking do not cause gout, excesses of this kind increase the body's level of uric acid and may well precipitate an attack.
12 Athlete's foot; this fungus infection thrives between the toes, especially if the skin is moist.
13 Chilblain; this circulatory problem can often be prevented by giving the feet alternate hot and cold baths to stimulate the circulation.

Young feet
From babyhood to late childhood, the feet are slowly hardening from cartilage into bone, and mistreatment of the feet when they are young can result in permanent deformity or foot problems. Babies should be allowed to wear one-piece baby suits only if the feet of the suits are stretchy enough to fit without causing the toes to curl up, and they should not wear shoes until they are walking unaided. Babies often appear to have flat feet, or fallen arches; in fact the flatness is caused by a pad of fat, and the baby's feet are probably perfectly healthy.

Shoes and socks
The fit of shoes and socks is important throughout life, since the feet can be pushed out of shape by constant mistreatment at any time of life. Socks should always be long enough to fit over the foot when unstretched, and after laundering the socks should be pulled back into shape to prevent shrinkage. Shoes should be comfortable and should fit well in length and in width; in shoes for children there should be ¾in growing room beyond the big toe. Fashion shoes should only be worn occasionally; everyday shoes should have relatively low heels that are broad enough to spread the body's weight evenly.

Corns
Corns are impacted and thickened dead cells that have not been shed from the skin normally but have been hardened by friction from ill-fitting shoes. Corns have nuclei, often mistakenly called roots, and any cure must remove the nucleus as well as the dead skin. Wearing correctly-fitting footwear is an important corrective measure, and professional treatment from a chiropodist will remove the corn. Do not try to remove it yourself, as you may damage the foot. Numerous corn preparations are sold over the counter, but most of them do nothing more than soften the skin.

Verrucae
Verrucae are warts that form on the feet; they are unsightly, and can cause considerable pain. They are transmitted very rapidly in damp conditions, so anyone who develops a verruca should refrain from using swimming pools and communal shower rooms until it has gone. Like ordinary warts, verrucae often disappear spontaneously, but if they are large or painful they usually have to be removed. Treatment may involve applying softening chemicals, cutting out the wart, or destroying the infected tissue by heat or cold.

Home pedicure
It is worth spending the time every few weeks to give your feet a complete home pedicure; this will rejuvenate them and help to prevent many of the common foot problems.
a Bathe your feet in alternate baths of hot and cold water; this stimulates the circulation, and also helps to relieve tired feet.
b Rub down any calluses or hard skin patches with a wet pumice stone smeared with soap. Do not try to pare or cut any skin away.
c Dry your feet thoroughly with a towel, particularly between the toes. This will help to discourage fungus infections such as athlete's foot.
d Dust your feet very lightly with talcum powder; a little powder will help prevent sweaty feet, but too much will aggravate the problem.
e Cut your toenails straight across; do not be tempted to shape them or cut them down at the sides, as this will encourage ingrowing.
f Exercise your feet by trying to pick up a pencil with your toes. This will keep the muscles well toned and help the circulation.

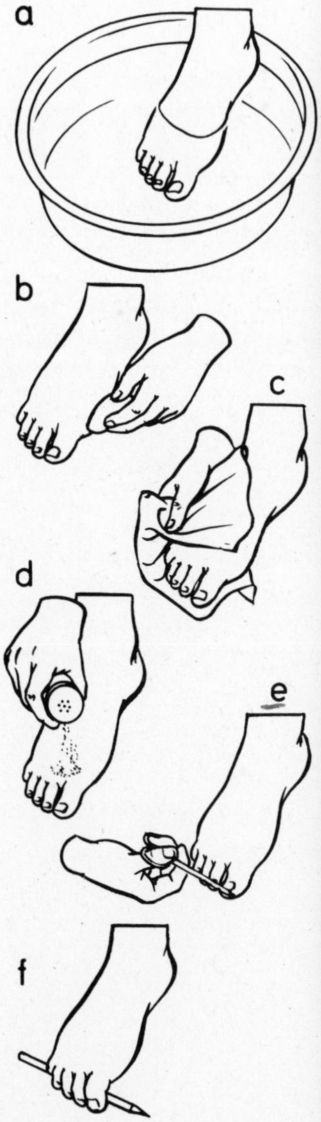

Do
- Use correct posture so that you are not putting an undue strain on your feet.
- See a chiropodist if you experience pain in one or both feet.
- Bathe and exercise your feet to stimulate the circulation.
- Wash your feet regularly to remove dirt and perspiration.
- Dust your feet lightly with talcum powder to discourage perspiration.
- Wear shoes that fit comfortably in length, width and depth.
- Have a child's feet measured each time he or she needs a new pair of shoes.
- Ensure that new shoes for a child have roughly ¾in growing space beyond the big toe.
- Wear clean socks or stockings each day.
- Pull socks back into shape after laundering to avoid shrinkage.
- Cut your toenails straight across.
- Use a pumice stone gently on calluses and hard skin each time you wash your feet.
- Check your shoes for rough patches if you often develop blisters or calluses.

Don't
- Dress babies in one-piece suits that constrict their toes.
- Put a baby's feet in shoes too early.
- Tuck the covers in tightly over a baby's feet.
- Hand shoes down from one child to another; shoes conform themselves to the shape of the owner's feet, and may damage a different pair of feet.
- Wear shoes that pinch.
- Wear high heels for everyday work; keep them for occasional wear.
- Wear socks that are too short in the feet.
- Dust your feet thickly with talcum powder, or sprinkle it into your shoes and socks.
- Force your toes into pointed shoes.
- Eat or drink excessively if your doctor warns you that you are prone to gout.
- Cut your toenails down at the sides.
- Dig under your toenails to clean them; soak them in a warm bath instead.
- Use public swimming baths or showers if you have a verruca or athlete's foot.

CHAPTER 3

Different phases of life present various health problems. Children react differently from adults to the same disease, and certain illnesses or conditions are more likely in children or adolescents than in adults. Momentous changes take place in the body during puberty and adolescence, and also in women during pregnancy, and each of these times has its own possible health problems. Middle age and later life bring about slow changes in the body and its functions, and an understanding of these natural changes will help the older person to spot any unusual or worrying changes. In this chapter we look at the various phases of life and the health concerns particularly associated with them.

TIMES OF LIFE

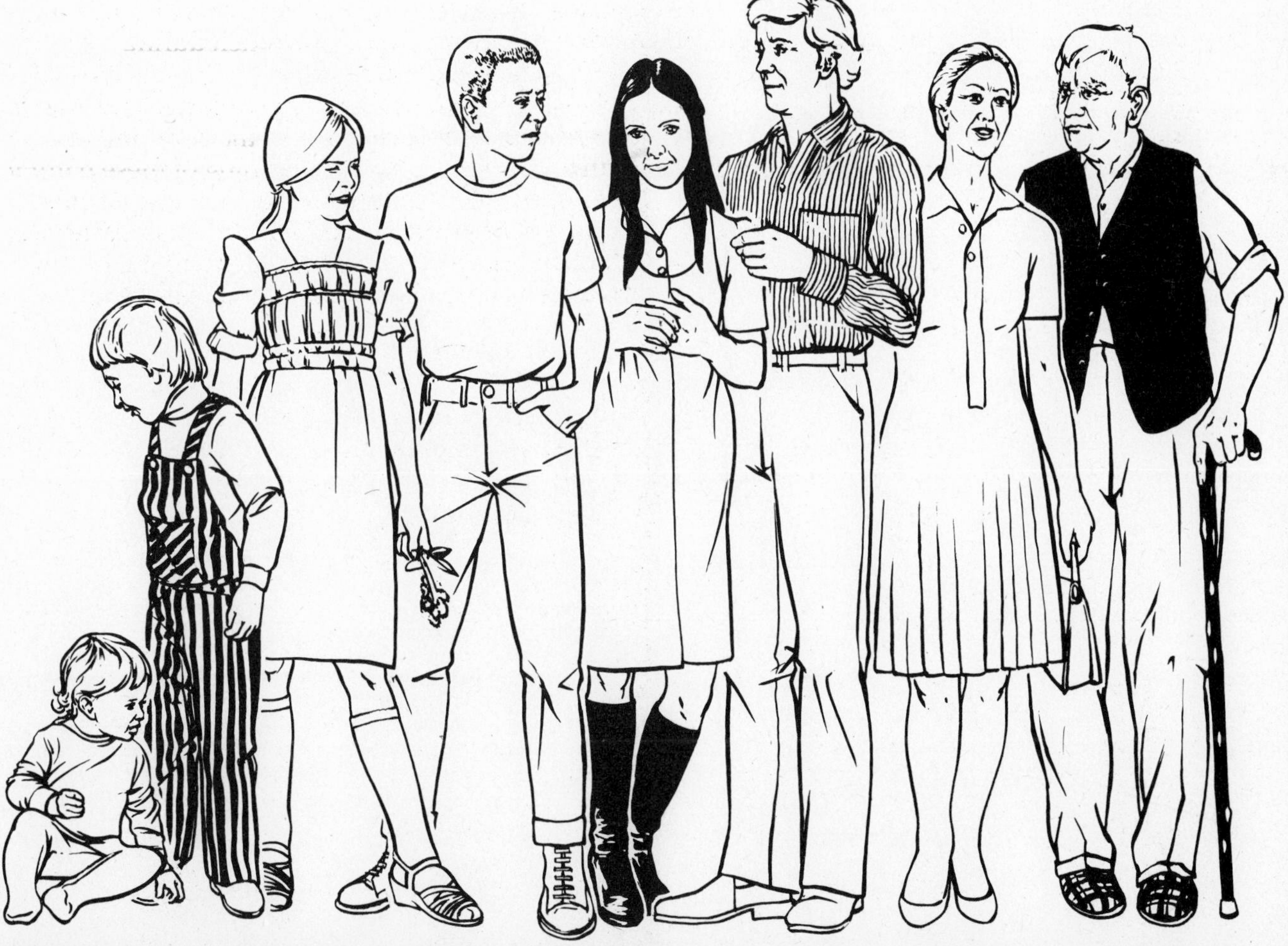

Childhood

Parents have a great deal of control over the physical, mental and emotional development and wellbeing of their children. Teachers, friends and siblings may exert powerful influences, but the parents in particular have the potential to produce positive feelings (such as love, security, trust and respect) or negative feelings (such as resentment, distress, distrust and rebellion) in their children. On these pages we look at some of the needs of young children, from babyhood through the first 10 years, and talk about various ways in which parents can provide stable, safe and happy environments for their children and help them toward their goals of maturity, self-respect and independence.

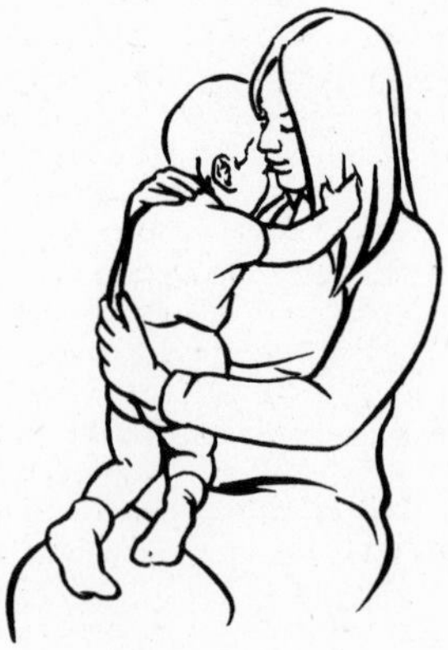

Accidents and mishaps
Active children can be expected to be involved in many minor accidents as they explore, climb, play, fight and develop new skills. Of course play areas should be as safe as possible, but scrapes, scratches, bruises and bumps are inevitable parts of childhood and will usually require only a cuddle and a piece of adhesive tape as treatment. Minor falls are also common, but if the child loses consciousness at all, or if you suspect a sprain or a fracture, contact a doctor for advice. Don't be tempted to overprotect your child; minor mishaps are an important part of growing up and learning about the world outside the home.

Babies
Much conflicting advice is given to the mothers of small babies, but these points cover some of the common problems and their remedies. Feeding is an all-important issue; breast-feeding is better for the baby nutritionally and also cheaper, but bottle-feeding may be more convenient in a busy schedule. In the first few weeks of life babies form a strong emotional bond with the person who supplies them with their greatest sources of pleasure – food and physical contact – and bottle-fed babies should be held closely during feeding so that they receive the same physical contact as breast-fed babies. Wind is a common babyhood problem, and is best dealt with by holding the baby over your shoulder or across your lap after a feeding and gently rubbing its back until it burps up the excess air. Wind that remains in the stomach may cause colicky pains and distressed crying, but it will eventually pass through the digestive system. Diaper rash occurs when urine remains in prolonged contact with the baby's skin, and can usually be cleared up by using a medicated cream and allowing the air to reach the baby's bottom for 10–15 minutes at least once a day.

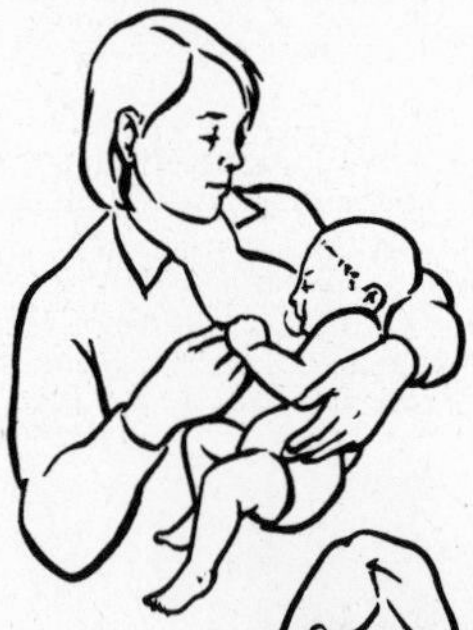

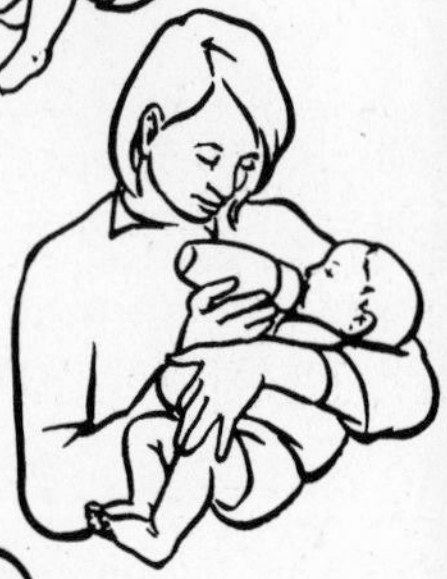

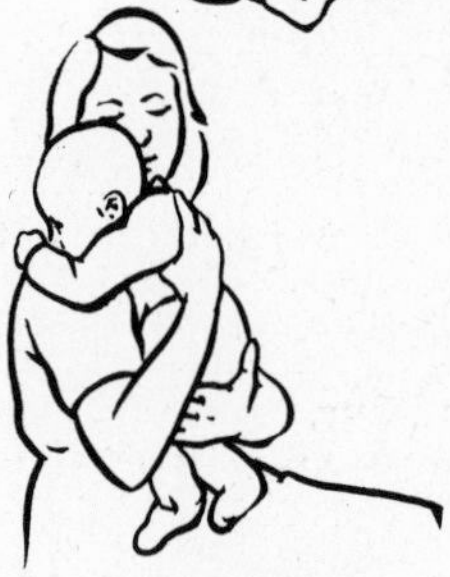

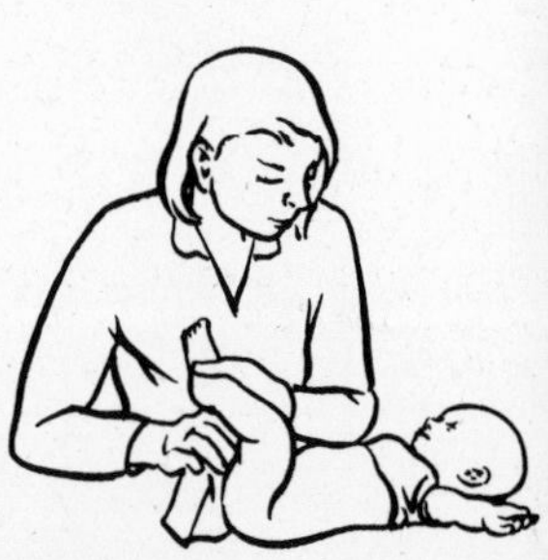

Medical care
For the first year or two of its life, your baby will be seen regularly by your pediatrician. It is important to develop a good family relationship with your pediatrician, so that the child trusts him and also so that he can be aware of family circumstances that may affect your child's behavior, progress or health. If a baby becomes ill it is easier to take its temperature rectally, with a special thermometer, rather than orally; medicine can be given by squeezing it into the side of a baby's mouth from a dropper. Age 2 is a good time to take your child to the dentist for the first time, to familiarize him or her with the procedure. Children of 2–5 who are ill can develop a very high temperature very quickly, but this can usually be reduced by giving them aspirin. Medicine can be given mashed up in a favorite food if the child is reluctant to take it plain. When your child starts school at around age 5, he or she should be given a thorough medical examination, including tests of eyesight, hearing and balance. Problems such as knock knees or bow legs should have resolved themselves by age 9 or 10; if they have not, the child should be taken to a specialist.

Immunization
Many of the most unpleasant infectious diseases cause the body to produce antibodies against the agent of infection (bacteria, virus etc), which for the rest of the person's life grant him or her immunity from further attacks of the same disease strain. Immunization consists of harmlessly stimulating this antibody production so that immunity from even one attack results. Immunization programs against serious diseases will begin shortly after birth and will continue at intervals throughout childhood. In general your baby will be given DPT (diphtheria, pertussis or whooping cough, and tetanus) vaccine and polio vaccine at 2–3 months, with booster shots of each later in childhood. From 12 months onward, the child can be given vaccines against measles, mumps and German measles. Immunity against mumps can be particularly helpful for boys, who may develop serious complications if they contract the disease after puberty, and German measles vaccine is recommended for girls before they reach childbearing age since babies in utero can be severely damaged if their mothers contract the disease during pregnancy. Influenza vaccine can be given to children with respiratory problems, to whom the disease would be dangerous, and other immunizations may be needed if traveling abroad.

Babies' needs
Many of a baby's needs are physical. It needs to be fed, to be kept comfortable by having clean clothes and dry diapers, to be warm, and to feel a great deal of physical contact. In the womb the baby has been surrounded by warmth, darkness, gentle noises and security; out in the world it has to grow used to fluctuations in the environment that we take for granted, and in the early months should be shielded as much as possible from loud noises, sudden movements, bright lights and rapid temperature changes. Babies have little resistance to infection; sterilizing feeding bottles and pacifiers will help to destroy germs.

Children's needs
As children grow, their needs become less purely physical and more emotional. As well as food, warmth and physical affection, older children need to have security, continuity in their lives, leadership that they can look up to, and praise and encouragement for their efforts. Discipline of some sort is necessary in a child's life, so that he can be sure that people care for him and want him to learn self-control. Self-respect in childhood will help him toward maturity and independence later, and this is best achieved by making sure he knows he is loved and valued as an individual.

Routines
Structure is an important element in a child's life no matter what his age, and also makes life easier for the rest of the family. Although it is not desirable for a child to live by a strict timetable, he needs to know what is expected of him, so fairly regular mealtimes and bedtimes are important. Your child should learn hygiene routines, such as washing his hands after visiting the bathroom, as early as possible, and acceptable social behavior such as politeness and sharing is also more easily encouraged the earlier it begins.

Diet
The food children eat, or don't eat, is often the cause of a great deal of parental worry. Some children will try as many foods as they are allowed; others will eat only two or three types of food. As long as the child has a daily portion of fruit or vegetables, a serving of meat, fish, cheese or eggs, some carbohydrate such as bread or cereal, and a helping of yoghurt or milk, you can be sure that he is getting enough vitamins, roughage, calcium and protein to remain healthy. Don't be tempted to offer him candy or snacks between meals if he will not eat at mealtimes, as he will come to expect such treats.

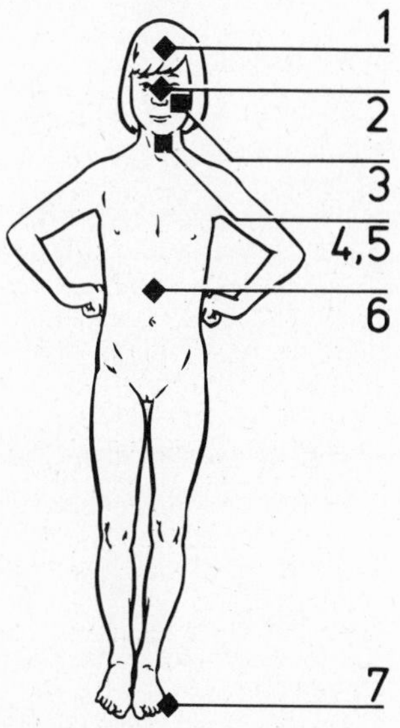

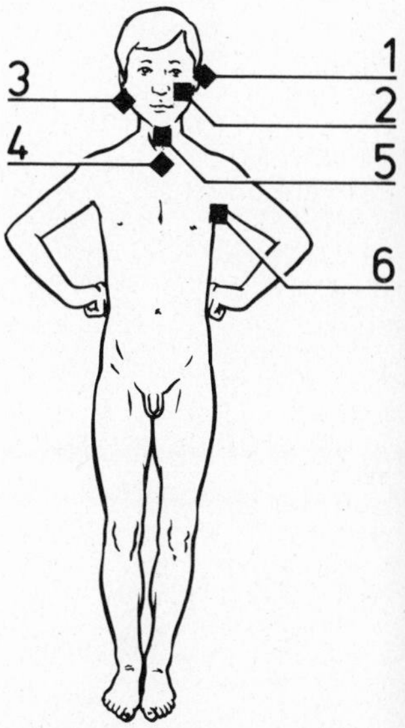

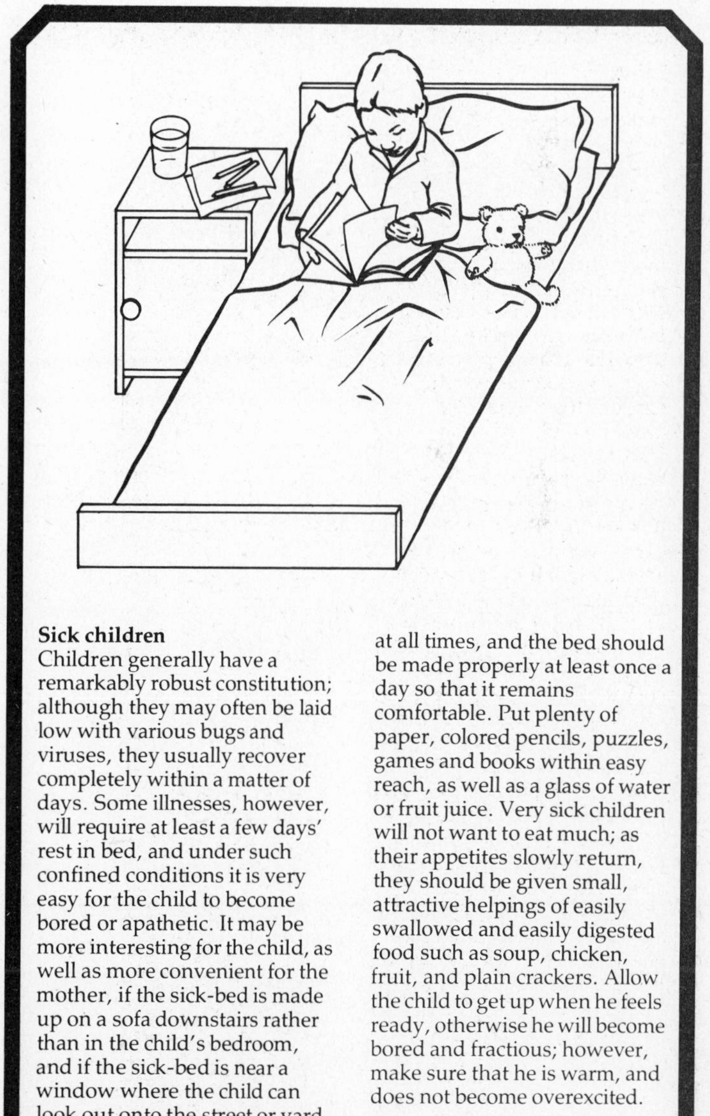

Starting school
Once the child is at school, he will come into contact with the health problems of many other children, and will tend to develop minor illnesses much more frequently than he did at home. The diagram *above* shows the sites of some of the common complaints your child may develop as a result of such close proximity to other children.
1 Lice and nits.
2 Cold.
3 Impetigo.
4 Sore throat.
5 Cough.
6 Upset stomach.
7 Verruca.

Infectious diseases
The diagram *above* shows the sites at which some of the infectious diseases associated with childhood begin.
1 Measles; this rash begins behind the ears and spreads over the body.
2 German measles; this rash begins on the face and neck.
3 Mumps; the glands of the neck swell painfully.
4 Chicken pox; this rash begins on the face, neck and chest.
5 Whooping cough; wheezy breathing and coughing are symptomatic of this disease.
6 Scarlet fever; this rash spreads from the armpits and groin.

Sick children
Children generally have a remarkably robust constitution; although they may often be laid low with various bugs and viruses, they usually recover completely within a matter of days. Some illnesses, however, will require at least a few days' rest in bed, and under such confined conditions it is very easy for the child to become bored or apathetic. It may be more interesting for the child, as well as more convenient for the mother, if the sick-bed is made up on a sofa downstairs rather than in the child's bedroom, and if the sick-bed is near a window where the child can look out onto the street or yard. The child should be kept warm at all times, and the bed should be made properly at least once a day so that it remains comfortable. Put plenty of paper, colored pencils, puzzles, games and books within easy reach, as well as a glass of water or fruit juice. Very sick children will not want to eat much; as their appetites slowly return, they should be given small, attractive helpings of easily swallowed and easily digested food such as soup, chicken, fruit, and plain crackers. Allow the child to get up when he feels ready, otherwise he will become bored and fractious; however, make sure that he is warm, and does not become overexcited.

Puberty and adolescence

Puberty is the time of life that marks the end of childhood and the beginning of adolescence; the adult hormones begin to work in young teenagers and produce the characteristic growth spurts, bodily changes and altered outlooks that are part of the preparations for adulthood. Puberty usually begins at a certain body weight, so boys and girls who are tall or heavy for their age are likely to begin the changes of puberty before their smaller or slighter contemporaries. Puberty takes place over several years, and is well established by the time a boy has his first ejaculation or a girl her first menstrual period; during adolescence the changes in height and body shape may continue as late as age 18 in girls and the early 20s in boys.

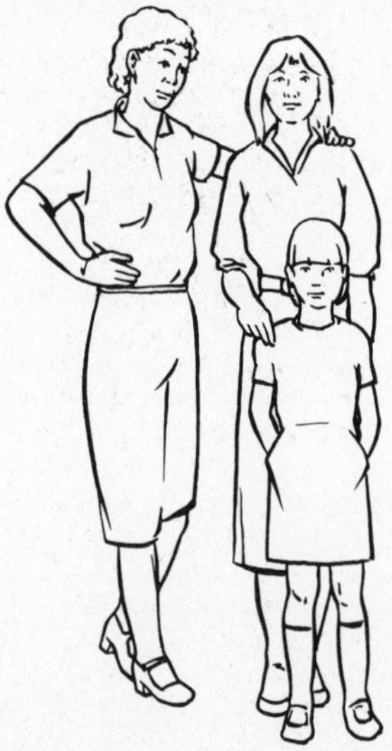

Transition period
Puberty and adolescence are difficult times, because the boy or girl is caught between two phases of life. Childhood has the benefits of security, dependence, and the knowledge that other people are in charge of your welfare; adulthood has the benefits of social and financial independence, sexual relationships, and free choice over your own lifestyle. The adolescent exhibits behavior from both categories, and is also disturbed by physical and hormonal changes; the combination of these factors produces the characteristic mood swings of adolescence.

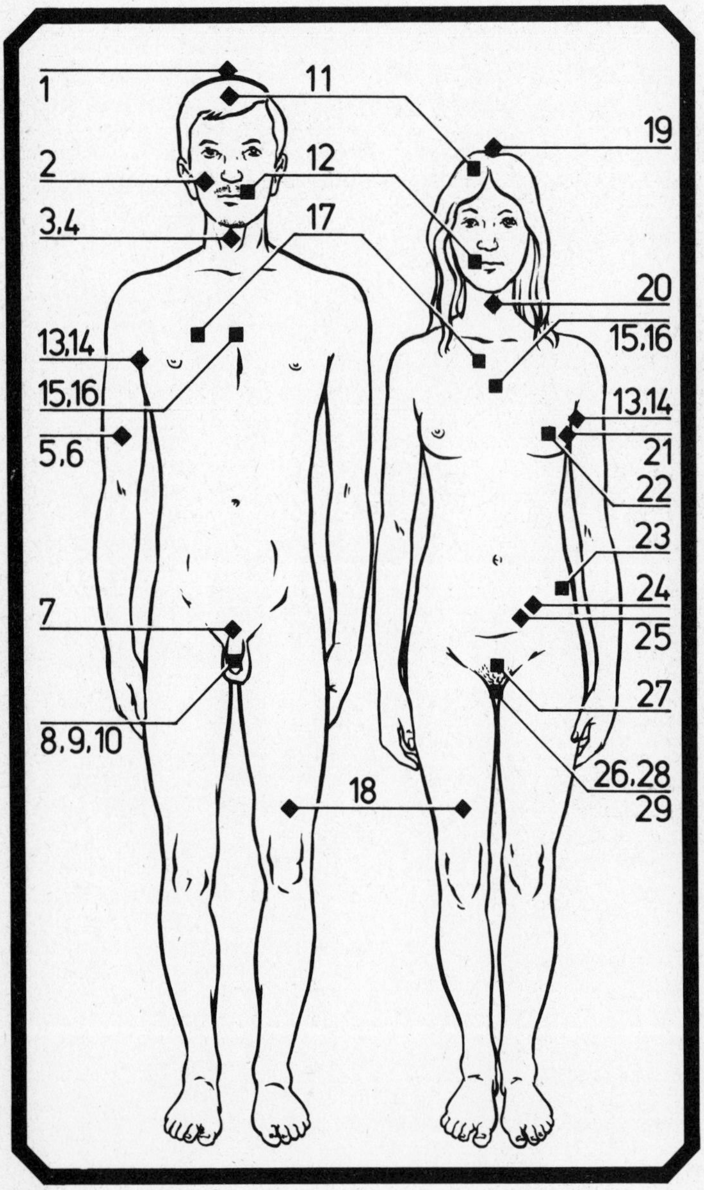

Changes in boys
The diagram *far left* shows the sites of major physical changes in boys at puberty.
1 Body height increases considerably.
2 Hair begins to grow on the chin, cheeks and upper lip.
3 The voice deepens as the larynx grows.
4 The Adam's apple enlarges.
5 Muscles over the whole body develop and become more noticeable.
6 Bodily strength increases greatly.
7 Pubic hair grows around the base of the penis.
8 The prostate gland enlarges.
9 The genitals increase in size.
10 Ejaculation often occurs during sleep.

Changes in both sexes
11 The hair and skin become more greasy as a result of hormonal action.
12 Body temperature falls slightly.
13 Underarm hair grows.
14 Sweat glands under the arms and in the groin produce more perspiration than before.
15 Blood pressure and blood volume increase.
16 Heart rate slows.
17 Breathing rate slows.
18 Bones harden and change their proportions.

Changes in girls
The diagram *near left* shows the sites of major physical changes in girls at puberty.
19 Body height increases, although not as markedly as in boys.
20 The voice deepens slightly.
21 The breasts enlarge.
22 The nipples stand out from the surrounding skin.
23 Fat pads form on the hips and thighs.
24 The pelvic girdle widens to prepare the girl for childbearing.
25 The ovaries begin to release eggs in a monthly cycle.
26 The vaginal walls thicken.
27 Pubic hair grows around the vulva and over the pubic bone.
28 Menstruation occurs monthly as the uterus sheds its lining.
29 The genitals increase in size.

Conformity
Being thought the "odd one out" can cause an enormous amount of suffering for a teenager during a period when he or she is perhaps deeply disturbed by the relentless changes in physique and mood. The teenager, especially in the years 12–16, usually satisfies his or her need for security at a time of emotional turmoil by conforming to the habits, dress, appearance and tastes of the peer group. Later in adolescence the mature teenager will develop enough security in personal views to make an independent stand away from the masssed views of his or her friends.

Rebelliousness
The challenging of authority is an inevitable part of the life of a healthy adolescent. By tackling the values held by parents, teachers etc, the adolescent both discovers whether those values are worthwhile, and also affirms his or her own newly-acquired independence. In most cases, this rebelliousness covers fairly minor offenses such as truancy, indolence at work, rudeness, or staying out late; in these cases, parents can be reassured that the phase will eventually pass. More severe rebellion, such as criminal activity, usually requires analysis of the emotional disturbances behind the actions.

Relationships
After puberty the full sexual nature of the individual develops, and the adolescent becomes very sensitive and responsive to sexual stimuli. Hero-worship of an older person of the same sex is often based on admiration of that person's sexuality, and is later replaced in many cases by an attraction to a particular film star or other cult figure of the opposite sex. This kind of fantasy heterosexual interest usually moderates into attraction to friends of the opposite sex, and dating begins. Adolescence is often the time of the first full sexual experiences.

A sense of values
As the growth toward full physical, emotional and mental maturity progresses, adolescents are either consciously or subconsciously establishing the values, attitudes and tastes that they will probably hold for the rest of their lives. In childhood the standards of the parents have usually been accepted unquestioningly; adolescence gives the individual the opportunity and the motive to examine prevailing standards and decide whether to uphold or replace them. Political awareness usually develops during this time, and the adolescent adopts his own moral and social code of values.

Problems in adolescence
The illustration *right* shows the sites of some of the health problems that are common during adolescence.

1 Fatigue and lethargy often occur during adolescence, partly from physical causes such as hormone activity and partly from psychological reasons.
2 Sleep disturbances may occur, especially if the person is worried or fearful.
3 Mood changes are caused by hormone action, and are often confusing for the individual and those around him alike.
4 Acne is a frequent result of the increased greasiness of the skin; the pores become clogged and then form infected pimples.
5 The appetite may become increased or decreased during adolescence, and may lead to overeating or undereating.
6 Mononucleosis (glandular fever) is common among adolescents, and its effects may last for a month or more.
7 Body odor from the armpits and groin can occur when insufficient attention is paid to hygiene.
8 Clumsiness is a phase often passed through by adolescents who do not yet feel at home in their taller, heavier bodies.
9 Overweight in early adolescence may be a sign of rapid puberty, in which case the problem will disappear as the body's height catches up with its weight; or it may be a result of greatly increased appetite.
10 Stretch marks occur when the increase in weight during puberty has been very rapid; they begin as red lines and eventually fade to a permanent silvery-gray.
11 Menstrual pain may begin to occur in later adolescence. The possible reasons for menstrual pain are many, and if the girl is being greatly inconvenienced by monthly pain she should be seen by a gynecologist.
12 Genital problems such as vaginal discharge and "jock itch" may develop if the adolescent does not appreciate the need for genital hygiene.

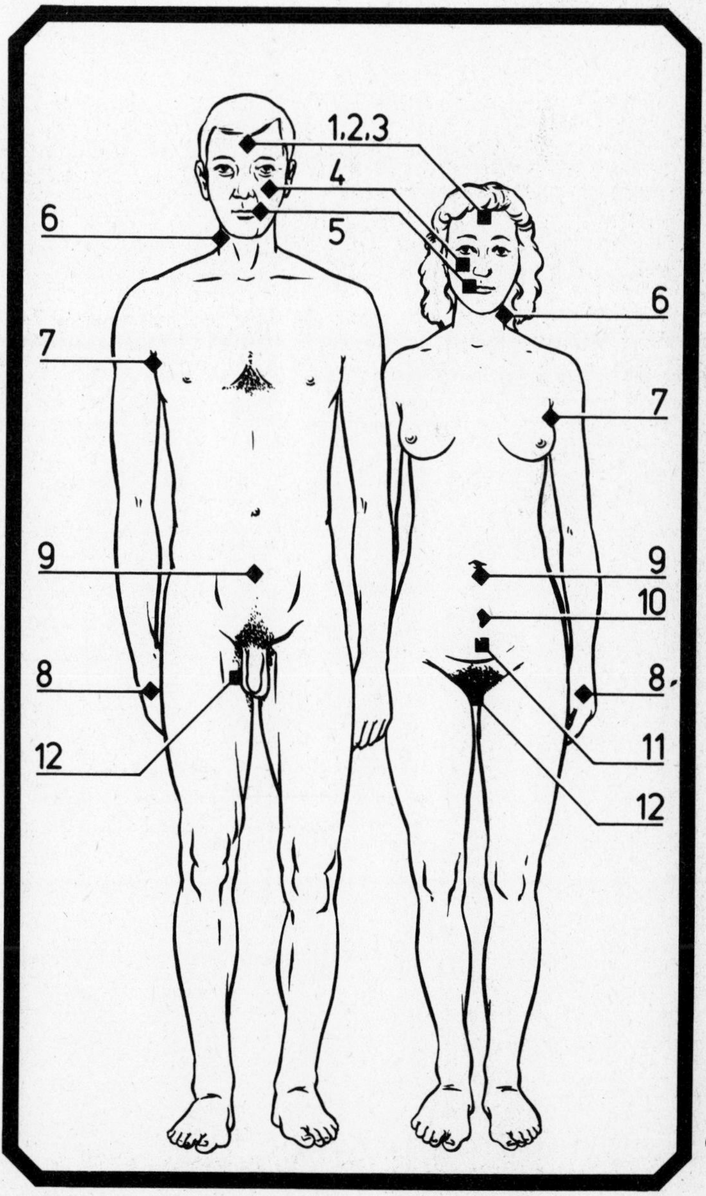

Pregnancy 1

The three main stages of a woman's reproductive life – puberty, pregnancy and the menopause – are all associated with changes in hormone levels, physical characteristics and behavior patterns. In pregnancy the hormonal changes cause the menstrual periods to stop, and re-program the body to provide for the development and growth of the baby inside the uterus. The physical changes involve not only the mother's enlarging abdomen, but also modifications in many of her body systems. Changes in her behavioral patterns may affect her sleep, her activity level, her emotions, and even her tastes in food or drink. On these pages we show you ways in which you can help to keep yourself in good condition through all the changes associated with pregnancy and birth.

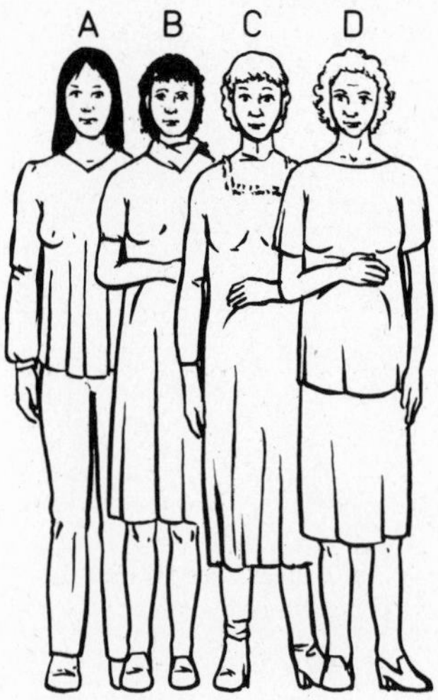

Age and pregnancy
The age of the mother may affect several factors in the pregnancy and birth, especially in a first pregnancy.
A Mothers under age 20 run a higher risk of anemia, toxemia of pregnancy, and congenital abnormality of the baby, but labor is usually easier.
B Mothers aged 20 to 30 have the lowest rates of stillbirth and early infant death.
C Mothers aged 30 to 40 have longer labors, a greater risk of twins, heavier babies, and more complications of pregnancy and birth.
D Mothers over 40 have a high risk of mongoloid babies and of complications, but may have very short labors.

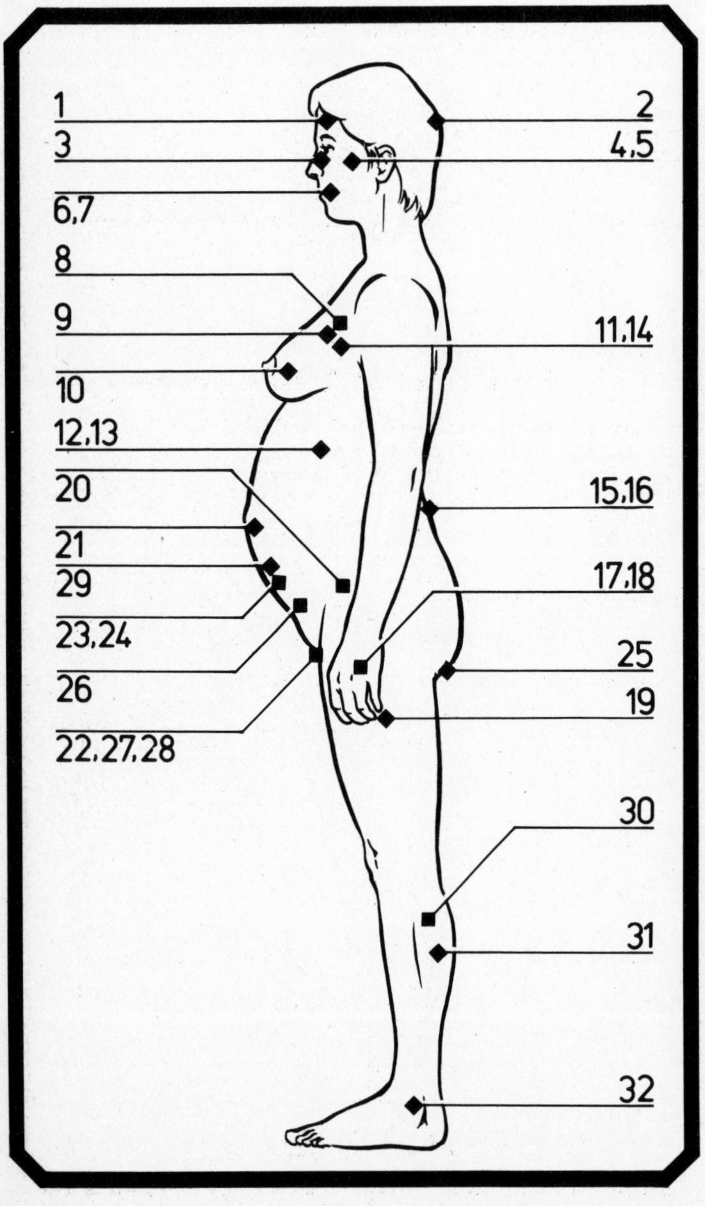

Changes in pregnancy
The diagram *left* plots the sites of many of the physical changes and minor physical problems that may be encountered during pregnancy.
1 Fainting.
2 Brittle hair.
3 Nasal congestion and nosebleeds; these result from an increased blood supply to the tissues.
4 Increase in skin pigmentation, especially in dark-haired women.
5 Aggravation of dry or greasy skin problems.
6 Slight rise in basal body temperature.
7 Bleeding from swollen and tender gums.
8 Heartburn.
9 Shortness of breath.
10 Increase in size and weight of the breasts, and possible tenderness.
11 Raised blood pressure.
12 Changes in appetite; these may take the form of cravings, distates for certain foods, or an increase or decrease in the amounts eaten.
13 Nausea and vomiting, especially in the morning during the early months of pregnancy.
14 Palpitations.
15 Postural changes as the body adapts to the extra load of pregnancy.
16 Backache caused by changes in the muscles and tendons of the back.
17 Clumsiness, caused by changes in the nerves and circulation and also by increased size and weight.
18 Tingling hands.
19 Brittle nails.
20 Congestion of the pelvis and abdomen caused by the increased blood supply.
21 Stretch marks, small red lines that develop over the abdomen during pregnancy and fade to silvery marks later.
22 Cessation of the menstrual periods.
23 Constipation.
24 Wind in the intestines.
25 Hemorrhoids.
26 Frequent urination, a result of the enlarging uterus pressing on the bladder.
27 Vaginal discharge.
28 Darkening in color of the vagina, from pale pink to dark pink or violet.
29 Weight gain, caused by: the baby itself; the fluid around it in the uterus; fluid retained in the mother's tissues; the placenta; the increase in volume of the mother's blood; and some laying down of fat.
30 Cramps in the calves.
31 Varicose veins.
32 Swelling of the ankles and feet.

Early signs of pregnancy
The sign most usually noticed first by a woman who has conceived is that her next period fails to arrive. She may notice a tingling, fullness or heaviness in her breasts or abdomen, or she may need to pass urine more often than usual. Morning sickness may appear very early in pregnancy, and she may notice a sudden distate for alcohol, smoking, or certain foods. The pregnancy is usually confirmed by a urine test, done with a home kit or arranged by a doctor, and as soon as the pregnancy is certain a doctor's advice on prenatal care should be sought for the welfare of both mother and baby.

Miscarriage
Miscarriage, or natural abortion, is the death of an embryo or fetus in the uterus or its expulsion before it is capable of sustaining life. As many as 20% of pregnancies may end in miscarriage, but many of these are very early and may be mistaken for a slightly overdue period. Most miscarriages take place in the first three months of pregnancy, but later ones may occur if there is a weakness of the cervix or if the mother has used violent bowel purgatives which initiate contractions. If a miscarriage is suspected, the mother should go straight to bed and call a doctor.

Digestive problems
Digestive problems are rife in pregnancy. One of the chief causes is pressure from the uterus, which presses the diaphragm upward and so exerts pressure on the stomach; this can cause heartburn and indigestion. Eating bland foods and avoiding strong spices and heavy meals may ease the problem. Constipation is also a frequent problem during pregnancy and is caused by the slowing down of the digestive system and the relaxation of the muscle walls. Constipation can usually be alleviated by drinking plenty of fluids and by eating sufficient roughage, but strong purgatives should never be used.

Nausea and vomiting
Morning sickness affects many women in early pregnancy; some may simply feel nauseous first thing in the morning, but others actually retch or vomit. Although this problem usually disappears by the third or fourth month it is miserable while it lasts. But with a little care its effects can be minimized. Drinking a bland liquid such as milk or water during the night or immediately on waking will help to allay much of the nauseous feeling, and so will eating something bland such as dry toast, cookies or an apple. Mothers prone to nausea should avoid all rich and fatty foods as much as possible.

Prenatal care
Prenatal facilities are designed to provide the best possible care for the pregnant mother and her baby. They provide frequent checks on the wellbeing of mother and baby, give advice on daily care and routines, and watch for any signs of conditions that may endanger the baby or complicate the birth. A detailed history of the present and all previous pregnancies is taken, and close attention is paid to all the following points.

1 Height; this is measured at the first prenatal visit. Body measurements provide clues as to whether the mother's physique will allow an easy birth.
2 Relaxation; the ability to relax fully aids labor, and so is usually taught during the prenatal period.
3 Diet; a good diet throughout pregnancy ensures that mother and baby are well nourished.
4 Blood pressure; this is a good monitor of the mother's circulation, and is taken at every prenatal visit.
5 Blood tests; these will be used to check for infection, anemia etc.
6 Breast care; the mother will be advised on how to keep her breasts in good condition during pregnancy and prepare them for breastfeeding.
7 Amniocentesis; a sample of the fluid around the baby may be taken to check for abnormal signs if this is thought necessary (for instance during an older woman's pregnancy). Amniocentesis occasionally causes some risk to the fetus.
8 Ultrasound; this method of checking the progress of the baby is used in many clinics, and involves bouncing sound waves off the fetus.
9 X-ray; this technique was once used to check the size and position of the baby, but is now avoided as much as possible and used only when complications occur that cannot be checked in any other way.
10 Weight; the mother's weight is checked at each visit to ensure that she is not gaining too rapidly or slowly.
11 Abdomen; an external examination of the abdomen is made at the first prenatal appointment.
12 Pelvic examination; this is done to establish the presence of the pregnancy and to check for abnormalties of the vagina or uterus.
13 Smear test; this is sometimes performed as an extra safety precaution.
14 Vaginal swab; the vaginal secretions are examined for any infection or abnormality.
15 Urine test; this is done regularly to test for diabetes or other irregularities.
16 Exercises; prenatal advisors recommend suitable exercises for the pregnant mother.

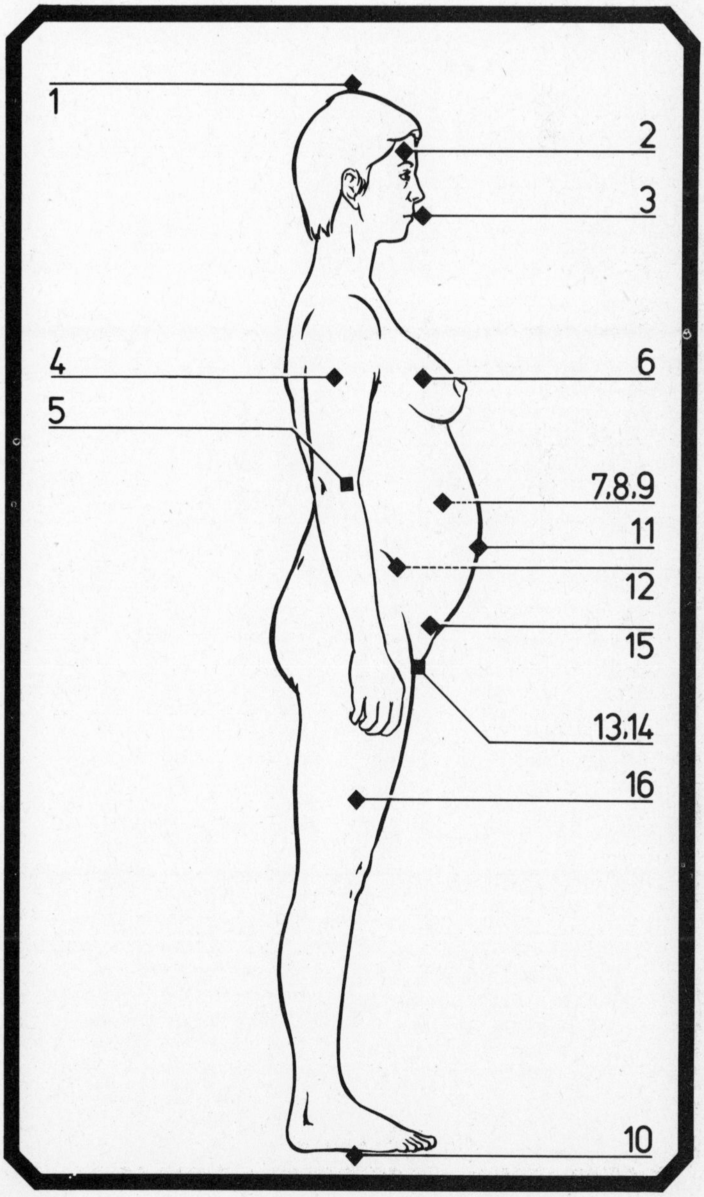

Pregnancy 2

A full-term pregnancy lasts approximately nine months, and for convenience this time-span is divided into three equal parts, or trimesters. Each trimester presents its own particular concerns and problems for the mother as the baby within her develops and grows and her body changes to accommodate it. As well as the physical changes during pregnancy, the expectant mother has to adapt her routine and her family life to prepare for the birth and homecoming of the baby. The mother's life will be altered radically, particularly with a first baby, by an extra member of the family, and much of the advice given during pregnancy is designed to help her make this transition as easily and healthily as possible.

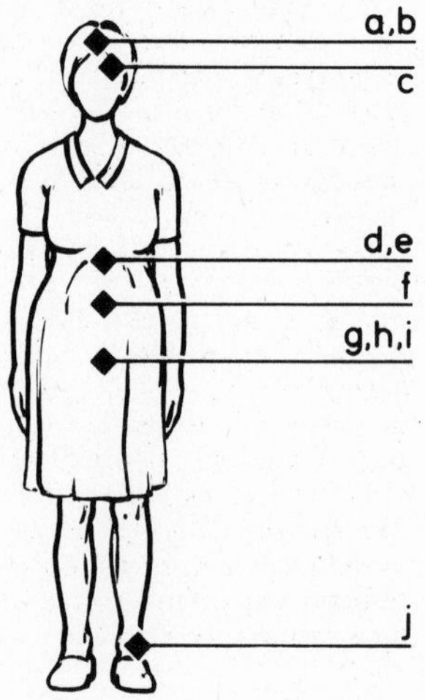

Danger signs
If any of these symptoms occur, a doctor should be seen immediately in case the mother or baby is in danger.
a Continuous severe headache.
b Frequent fainting.
c Blurred vision.
d Excessive vomiting.
e Severe, continuous abdominal pain.
f Absence of fetal movements for 48 hours or more in late pregnancy.
g Breaking of the waters of the uterus.
h Vaginal bleeding, other than small amounts at the times of the first missed periods.
i Pain on urination.
j Excessive swelling of the hands, face or ankles.

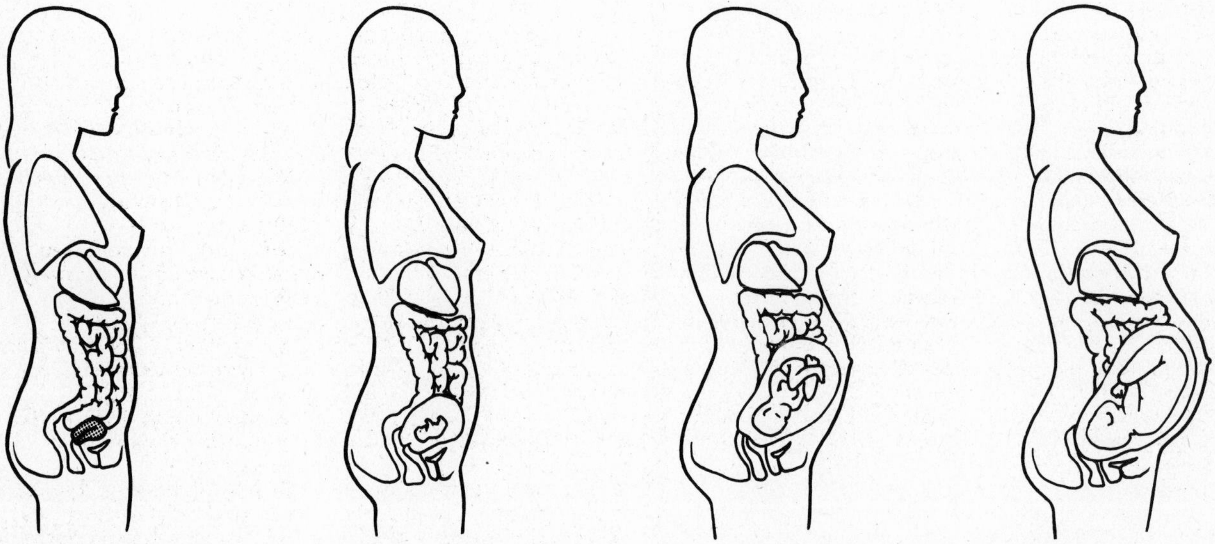

The first trimester
This period covers the first 3 months, or 13 weeks, of the pregnancy. By week 4, illustrated *above,* the fertilized egg is established in the uterus and the embryo is forming, but the uterus has not yet started to enlarge. Pregnancy can usually be confirmed at week 5 by a urine test and at week 8 by an internal examination. Drugs, alcohol and tobacco can affect the baby's development adversely in this trimester, and so should be avoided as much as possible. Morning sickness is common during this time, but usually disappears by the end of the trimester.

The second trimester
This period covers the second 3 months, weeks 14 to 26, of the pregnancy. By week 16, illustrated *above,* the mother's abdomen has begun to swell visibly; by the end of the trimester the swelling will be very marked. Early in the trimester the fetal heart can be heard through a stethoscope; by the end of the trimester the fetus will be about 13in long. By that stage its eyes will be open and it will be moving about in the uterus; these movements can be felt by the mother. The mother may develop food cravings during this trimester, but these should be indulged only if they are nutritious.

The third trimester
This period covers the last 3 months of pregnancy, from week 27 to about week 40. At week 28, illustrated *above,* the fetus is legally capable of supporting life; if born at this stage it has a 5% chance of survival. Babies born before week 38 and weighing less than 5lb 8oz are termed premature, and often require special care. During this trimester the baby increases rapidly in size and weight, and the mother's posture changes as she adapts to the increased load. Her navel flattens, and heartburn often occurs as the stomach is pushed upward by the displaced diaphragm.

At birth
By week 40, illustrated *above,* the baby's head is engaged in the mother's pelvic cavity ready for birth. If the baby is not in the correct position, it can sometimes be turned by careful manipulation of the mother's abdomen. The baby is about 20in long and weighs on average 7lb 8oz. When the mother's body is ready to give birth, the uterus contracts rhythmically, producing labor pains. The early contractions open the cervix, and later contractions push the baby out of the mother's body into the world.

Accidents
The baby is extremely well protected in the uterus, and it is very unlikely that it will be dislodged by minor accidents to the mother such as slipping over. As a precautionary measure, however, a doctor should be consulted if a mother in the second half of pregnancy feels no fetal movement within 3 or 4 hours of a minor accident; although the baby often stays still for far longer periods than this, it is wise to check on its welfare. If the mother has a major accident, such as a car crash or a fall from a considerable height, a doctor should be consulted immediately.

Breast care
Breast care during pregnancy is particularly important if the mother hopes to breastfeed, but all pregnant women should take care of their breasts to prevent them from becoming flabby and sore. Wear a good supporting brassiere as soon as the breasts begin to feel heavy so that the muscles are not stretched; the cup size required will increase as the pregnancy progresses. The nipples should be washed daily with mild soap and water, and massaged with lanoline cream to keep them soft and supple. Inverted nipples, which will make breastfeeding difficult, can often be corrected by wearing special nipple shields.

The father's role
The welfare of the mother and baby, as well as bonds within the family, will be increased if the baby's father takes an interest in the pregnancy and the birth. This will also help to prevent him from feeling jealous of the mother's inevitable attention to the baby's needs. A father who is willing to learn how to change a diaper or comfort a crying baby will take a lot of the pressure off the mother so that she has time to enjoy the baby and the other members of the family. With a doctor's permission, intercourse can continue until a few weeks before the birth.

Family problems
If the expectant mother already has one or more children, she will have to adapt their routines so that she has enough rest to attend to her own health and that of the baby when it is born. Older children should be encouraged to think of the baby as belonging to the whole family, rather than just to the mother, and they will probably enjoy helping in the baby's everyday care. Jealousy of a new baby is inevitable, and older children may revert to infantile habits such as sucking a bottle or wetting the bed in order to receive the same attention as the baby; these phases eventually pass.

Diet in pregnancy
As soon as the pregnancy is confirmed, the mother should begin to pay careful attention to what she eats (and drinks). The pregnant mother should not "eat for two"; she will need to make sure that she gets enough vitamins and calcium, but overeating will only produce obesity as it does in non-pregnant women. The main emphasis is on nutrition and digestibility; she should avoid pre-packaged and convenience foods as much as possible and eat wholesome fresh fruit and vegetables, cereals, and protein foods. Rich foods that may cause indigestion or constipation should be avoided.

Food in pregnancy
The lists *below* show different types of foods grouped according to their desirability in the diet of a pregnant woman. Protein foods such as meat, fish, eggs, cheese and milk should be eaten as much as possible, and so should fresh fruit and vegetables, as they contain many vitamins that are lost when the food is processed. Onions, peppers, spices, carbonated drinks etc are likely to cause digestive problems, and high-calorie foods such as cakes and candy will aggravate dental and weight problems.

Highly recommended	Recommended	Not recommended
Milk	Cereals	Processed meats
Cheese	Dried fruit	Pre-cooked foods
Fish	White bread	Canned fruit
Lean meat	Red vegetables	Canned vegetables
Offal	Orange vegetables	Pastries
Eggs	Other fresh fruits	Cookies
Leafy green vegetables	Nuts	Candy
Yellow vegetables	Yoghurt	Peppers
Citrus fruits		Leeks and onions
Wholemeal bread		Curry
		Carbonated drinks

Do
- See a doctor as soon as you suspect you may be pregnant.
- Follow any health care advice given by your doctor or clinic.
- Attend all your recommended prenatal visits and classes.
- Take a bland drink during the night or first thing in the morning if you suffer from morning sickness.
- Take extra care of your teeth and gums during pregnancy.
- Rest with your feet up at least once a day.
- Eat a diet rich in calcium and vitamins.
- Eat plenty of fruit and cereal to avoid constipation.
- Take regular gentle exercise in the fresh air.
- Wear comfortable, loose-fitting clothes.
- Wear shoes with low, wide heels.
- Wear a well-fitting brassiere.
- Wash and massage your nipples daily.
- Wear support stockings if you suffer from tired legs.
- See a doctor immediately if you develop any of the warning signs, or have any other cause for alarm.
- Avoid alcohol and smoking as much as possible.

Don't
- Use a vaginal douche at any stage of pregnancy.
- Use any drugs, including over-the-counter preparations and home remedies, without consulting your doctor.
- Use powerful laxatives to relieve constipation.
- "Eat for two."
- Put on more weight than recommended by your doctor.
- Eat a diet high in carbohydrates.
- Eat spiced or fatty foods if you suffer from morning sickness.
- Eat spiced foods or carbonated drinks if you suffer from indigestion, wind or heartburn.
- Have intercourse in the last few weeks of pregnancy.
- Have intercourse earlier in pregnancy if your doctor advises against it.
- Continue sports that include a high risk of falling, such as horseback riding, skiing, rock climbing.
- Travel in airplanes late in pregnancy, as the pressure changes can prevent sufficient oxygen from reaching the baby.
- Wear shoes with high, spindly heels.
- Wear tight-fitting clothes that may restrict the circulation.

Pregnancy 3

Careful attention to posture, relaxation and exercise will be invaluable to the expectant mother throughout her pregnancy and after the baby's birth. Muscles and tendons are prone to softening and sagging during pregnancy, and the mother's extra weight and increased size tend to aggravate the problem. Her posture alters as the pregnancy progresses, and she may experience aches and pains in her back and legs as a result. On these pages we look at some of the ways in which the expectant mother can use her body as efficiently as possible during pregnancy. These hints will help her to avoid strain and unnecessary health problems, and encourage her to give birth confidently and recover her figure afterward.

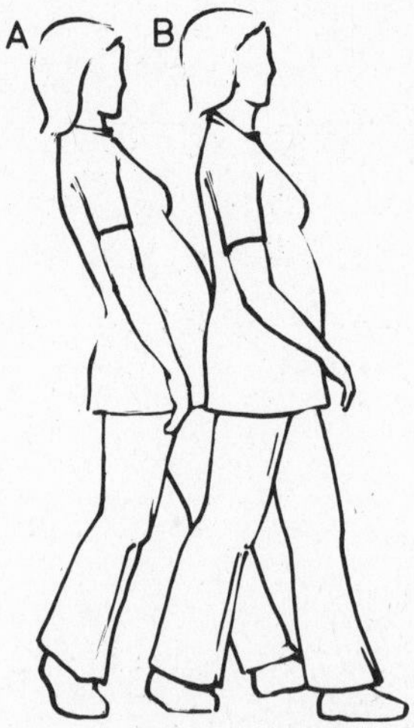

Posture
During pregnancy there is a great temptation to walk badly, with the pelvis tilted forward and the back hollowed (**A**). Wearing high heeled shoes increases this tendency as they throw the trunk forward and make the body off-balance. A hollowed back may be inevitable in the very late stages of pregnancy, when the abdomen is very large, but in the early and middle stages try to walk with the spine as straight as possible (**B**). The head should be erect, and the abdomen and chest supported by the muscles of your trunk. Wearing low-heeled shoes will help you to maintain the correct posture.

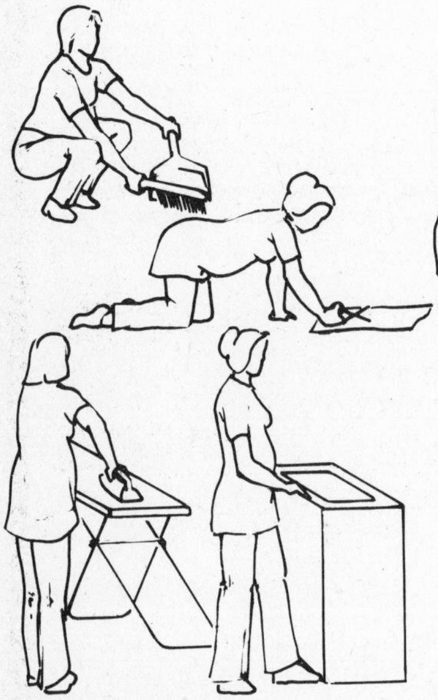

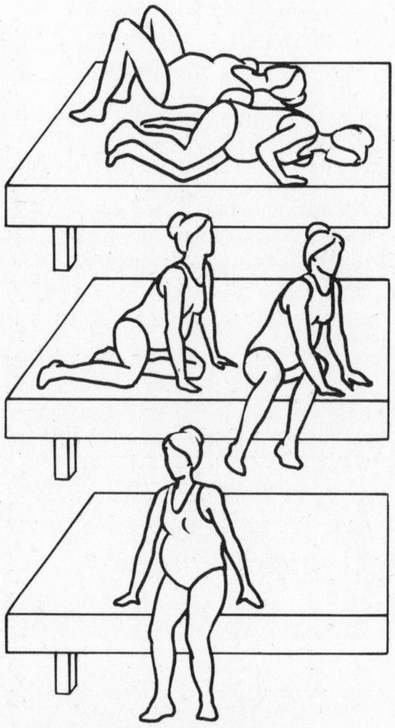

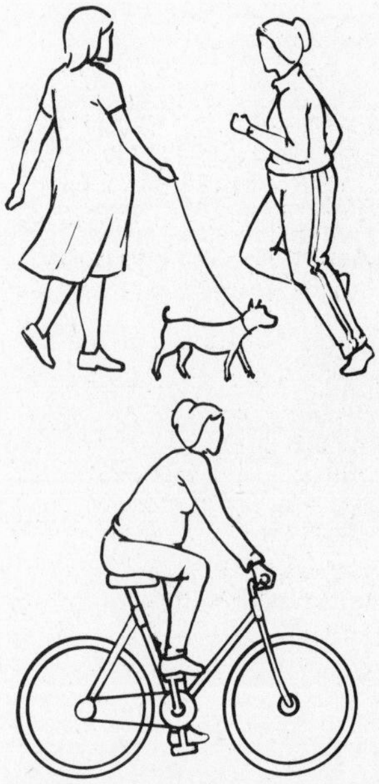

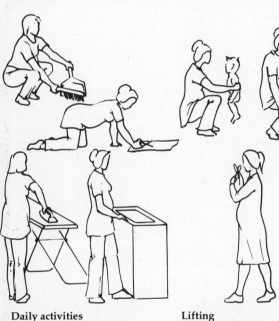

Daily activities
Because the back carries much of the burden of the extra weight during pregnancy, its muscles are very susceptible to undue strain imposed by bending at the waist. The illustrations *above* show the correct posture for various everyday activities; in all cases the back is kept as straight as possible and the strain is taken by the legs. Never stoop down by bending the spine; always bend at the knees instead. If your back aches at the end of the day, try kneeling on all fours and alternately humping and hollowing your back (see p.135) to ease the muscles.

Lifting
Avoid lifting very heavy objects during pregnancy, as this can cause unnecessary strain on the back and abdomen. If lifting is unavoidable, try using the methods shown *above*. A child can be lifted easily by squatting right down with your knees apart and your spine straight; hold the child close to your body and straighten up slowly. To lift an object from the floor, put your feet in a walking position and bend your knees, keeping your back straight, until you can reach it easily. Bags and parcels should be carried high in your arms, not in front of your abdomen or balanced on one hip.

Getting out of bed
As the abdomen enlarges it becomes increasingly difficult to rise from a lying position. Pregnant mothers should not bend forward to sit up as this places too much strain on the abdominal muscles. The method shown *above* is a safe and easy procedure for getting out of bed, and can also be modified for getting up from the floor. If you are lying on your back, bend your knees up and roll over onto one side; your arms can be used to raise your trunk from the bed, and it is then easy to swivel around so that your feet are over the side of the bed.

Sports
It is generally not wise to take up a new sport during pregnancy, but many sports can be continued if the mother was used to that kind of recreation before pregnancy. Swimming is an excellent activity for expectant mothers, but diving into the water should be avoided; scuba diving and water skiing are not recommended as they are too hazardous. Jogging, cycling, racket sports and dancing are all good exercise in moderation. Sports that include a risk of bad falls, such as gymnastics, climbing, trampolining, ice and roller skating and skiing, should be avoided. Walking in the fresh air provides excellent exercise.

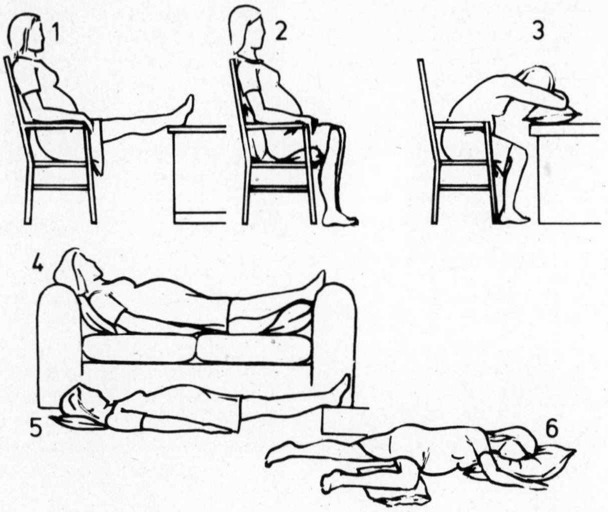

Relaxation
It is very valuable for pregnant women to spend some part of each day relaxing, especially in the later stages of pregnancy. Daily relaxation rests the mother's body, and also teaches her to relax at will; this ability will be very useful during the birth, when she needs to conserve energy between contractions. Raising the feet above the level of the head improves a sluggish circulation, and the mother should try to do this whenever she rests. Shown here are some recommended positions for relaxation.
1 Sit well back in a chair with your feet raised and a pillow in the hollow of your back.
2 Sit in a chair with pillows behind your back and under your thighs; this will help to relieve backache.
3 Sit in a chair and lean forward to rest your head and arms on a desk or table.
4 Lie on a sofa or bed with your head and feet supported by pillows.
5 Lie on your back on the floor with your head on a pillow and your feet resting on the edge of a low table or footstool.
6 Lie on your side on a bed or on the floor; bend the knee of the leg that is uppermost and support it on a pillow. Rest your head and one forearm on another pillow.

Pelvic floor muscles
The muscles of the pelvic floor work very hard during pregnancy to support the weight of the developing baby, and it is easy for them to become flabby and out of condition. Pelvic floor exercises will help to keep the muscles strong and supple.
7 While lying, standing or sitting, pull up the muscles of your vulva as tightly as possible. Hold this position for a count of 5, and then relax. Repeat up to 30 times per day.
8 Kneel on all fours, and slowly arch your back while you pull your abdomen in. Hold for a count of 5, and then relax.

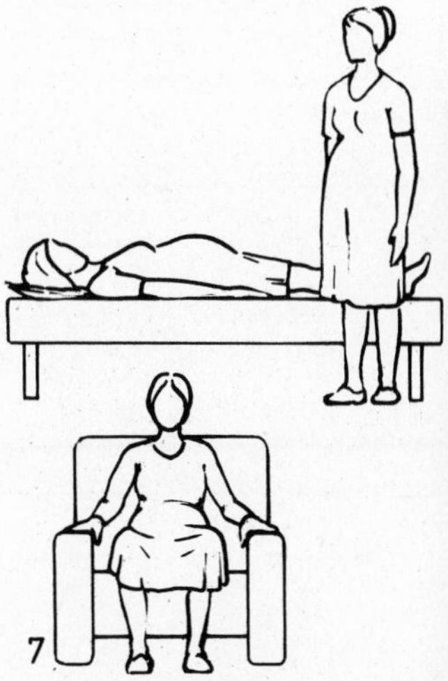

Postnatal relaxation
After the baby's birth, one of the most important considerations for the mother is rest. Try the following positions for relaxation.
12 Lie on your stomach with your head resting on your hands and a pillow under your stomach to prevent pressure on your breasts.
13 Lie on one side with one leg bent and your head resting on a pillow.
14 Lie on your back, with your head resting on a pillow and your arms at your sides.

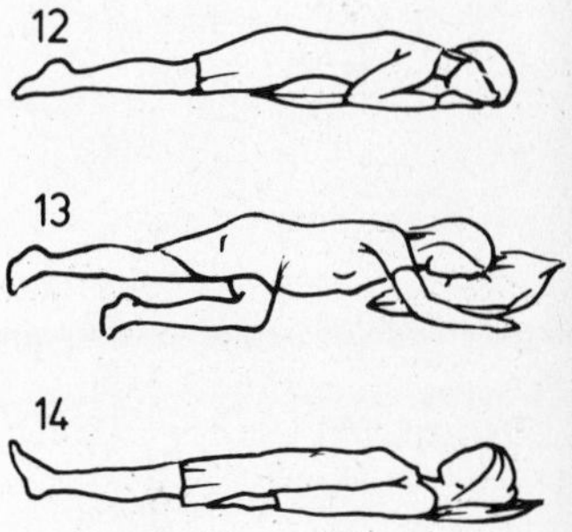

General exercises
These exercises will help to improve muscle tone and circulation during pregnancy.
9 Lie on your back on the floor with your knees bent and your feet flat on the ground. Slowly extend each leg in turn, and then slowly return them to the starting position.
10 Lie on your back with your knees bent and your feet flat on the floor. Tighten your buttock muscles, and hold this position for a moment before relaxing.
11 Sit in a chair with your heels resting on the floor. Bend your feet upward and then point them downward.

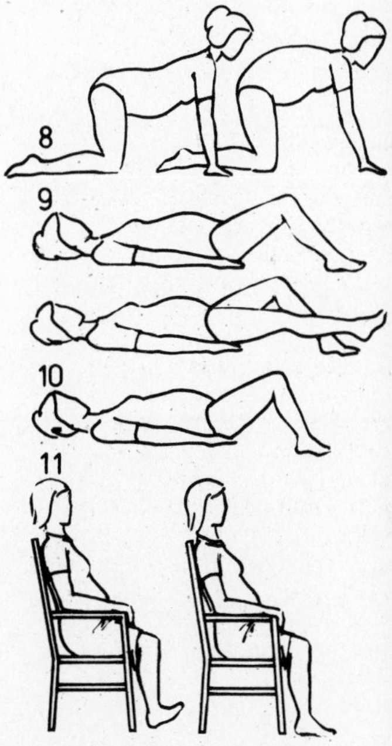

Postnatal exercises
Provided that your doctor approves, these exercises may be done from the third day after the baby's birth.
15 Lie on your back with your knees bent and your feet flat. Squeeze your buttock muscles together, draw in your abdomen, and try to press the small of your back onto the bed.
16 Lie on your back with your knees bent and your feet flat. Roll your knees over to the right, and then over to the left.
17 Lie on your back with your legs out straight. Tense your thigh muscles, hold for a moment, and then relax.

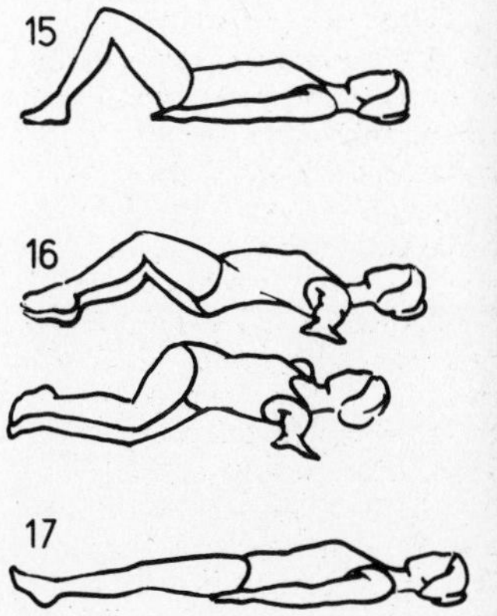

Middle age 1

The lengthened life-span of people in the Western world has made middle age out of the time of life that used to be considered old age. In 1850 the average life expectancy for both sexes was 40, whereas today it is just under 70 for men and just over 70 for women. Recent research has meant that middle age has received new emphasis as a time of growth, readjustment and self-assessment. Middle-aged people can sometimes pass through a time of emotional turbulence similar to adolescence, but used properly these turmoils can help to better the quality of your life and lead eventually to an old age as free as possible from dissatisfaction and regret.

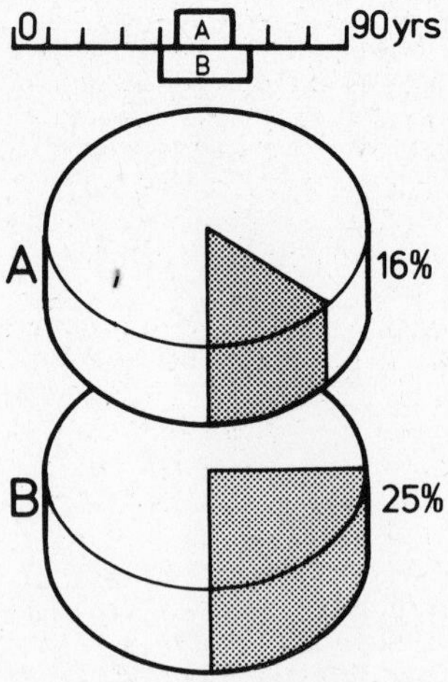

Middle age
The ages considered as the boundaries of middle age vary a great deal from country to country. Retirement, which could be seen as the end of middle age, can occur as early as 55 in some countries or as late as 68 in others, and of course many people continue working after the official retirement age. In the United States the middle-aged comprise 16% of the population if the boundaries of midle age are taken as 45 and 60 (**A**), but if middle age is considered as the years between 40 and 65, then 25% of the population falls into the category (**B**).

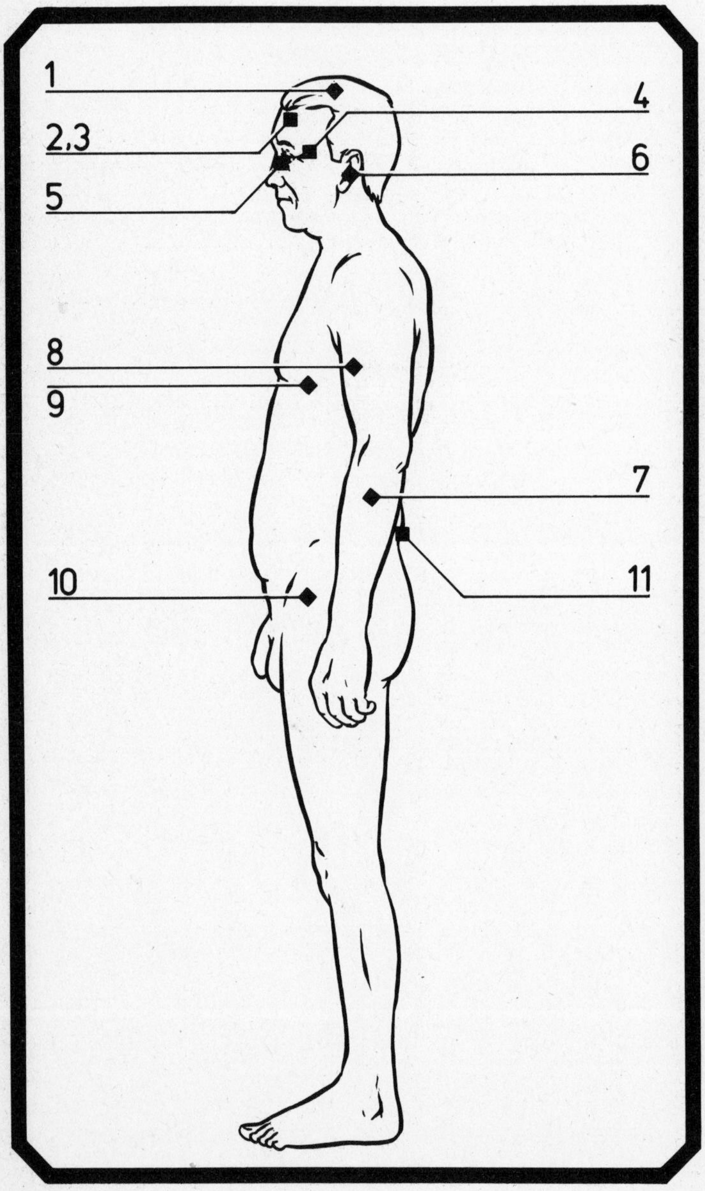

Changes in middle age
The illustration *left* shows the sites of some of the main physical changes experienced by both sexes in middle age.
1 Graying of the hair; this is caused by a decrease in the pigment produced by the hair roots, and is often well established by middle age.
2 Sleep; many people find that they need less sleep as they grow older. This is caused partly by decreased activity and partly by alterations in the body chemistry.
3 Depression and irritability; emotional problems such as these may be caused by the decrease in the production of hormones experienced by men as well as women.
4 Skin wrinkling; wrinkles are usually most noticeable around the eyes, and are caused by the loss of elasticity in the skin tissues.
5 Eyesight; a gradual deterioration is common in middle age.
6 Hearing; this too sometimes becomes less sensitive during middle age.
7 Bones; the structure of the bones alters in middle age and they become more porous and brittle, and therefore more likely to break.
8 Muscles; the muscles tend to become slack and lose some of their strength. The slackness can lead to changes in the physique such as "middle-age spread," when the muscles are no longer capable of maintaining a trim shape.
9 Lungs; decreased activity and decreased lung capacity often lead to breathlessness and rapid tiring after exertion.
10 Urinary tract; this area tends to lose its elasticity and therefore makes the middle-aged person increasingly liable to inflammation and infection of the urinary tract. In addition the pelvic floor muscles may weaken, causing incontinence.
11 Fat deposits; even in lean people, fat deposits tend to occur in middle age around the shoulder blades, waist, hips and thighs in particular.

Physical changes
The middle-aged person may become very sensitive about the changes experienced in his or her appearance. Wrinkles inevitably form, the hair begins to gray, the contours of the figure change, and the skin starts to lose some of its elasticity. The best way to deal with these changes is to change with them. Don't try to dress younger than you are, as this will look incongruous and make you a figure of fun. Instead, buy clothes that play up your best points and play down your weaknesses; alter your hairstyle if necessary to suit your new facial contours, and keep your body fit with regular exercise and a balanced diet.

Psychological changes
An individual's self-image can change dramatically during middle age. A man with teenage children may feel that his position as head of the house is no longer important, or he may feel outstripped in his job by younger, more ambitious men. A woman may feel unfeminine after the menopause now that her childbearing years are over. However middle age is the time when you and others can benefit from the maturity and experience that you have developed during earlier adulthood, and it is also an ideal time to take up new opportunities for travel, interests or education.

Social changes
Many Western societies place a great emphasis on youth, and much of the advertising, merchandise and entertainment is aimed specifically at young people. It is easy for the middle-aged person to feel that his needs and wishes are not catered for, or indeed that his position in society is scarcely acknowledged. A little searching, though, will reveal areas where maturity and experience are of paramount importance, such as in further education, advisory services, pastoral work and the local community. Specialized knowledge in any discipline will always be valuable to new students.

Family changes
It is often difficult for young parents to encourage independence in their children, and it is sometimes equally hard for middle-aged parents to see their children become physically, sexually and intellectually mature and both emotionally and financially independent. Parents who have made their children their whole life are dismayed when they leave home, and a great deal of maturity and understanding is necessary on both sides to establish successfully a new parent-child relationship. Once this is done, parents and their grown-up children can come to look on one another as assets rather than encumbrances.

Menopause
The menopause, which marks the end of a woman's reproductive life, may begin as early as 40 or as late as 55. The illustration shows the parts of the body most affected by the changes at this time.

1 Emotional and nervous disturbances, often taking the form of irritability or depression; these result from hormonal changes in the body.
2 Headaches; these often occur during the menopause.
3 Insomnia; this is also a result of changes in the woman's hormone balance.
4 Fatigue; many women become easily tired during the menopause.
5 Hot flashes; these occur when blood is unexpectedly diverted to the face and neck.
6 Sweating; profuse sweating often accompanies hot flashes, especially at night.
7 Increase in susceptibility to heart disease; this occurs as a result of the drop in the level of the female hormones, which give premenopausal women a considerable measure of protection.
8 Metabolic changes; these are often the cause of a sudden gain in weight after the menopause.
9 The ova first of all deteriorate, which accounts for the high risk of congenital abnormalities in babies born to older mothers, and eventually ovulation ceases altogether and the woman is no longer fertile.
10 Menstruation becomes irregular and finally ceases as the uterus no longer needs to prepare for possible pregnancy.
11 The vaginal and pelvic muscles lose their elasticity because of decreased production of the hormone estrogen.
12 The internal and external genitals shrink.
13 The vaginal lubrication decreases considerably, which may make intercourse uncomfortable.

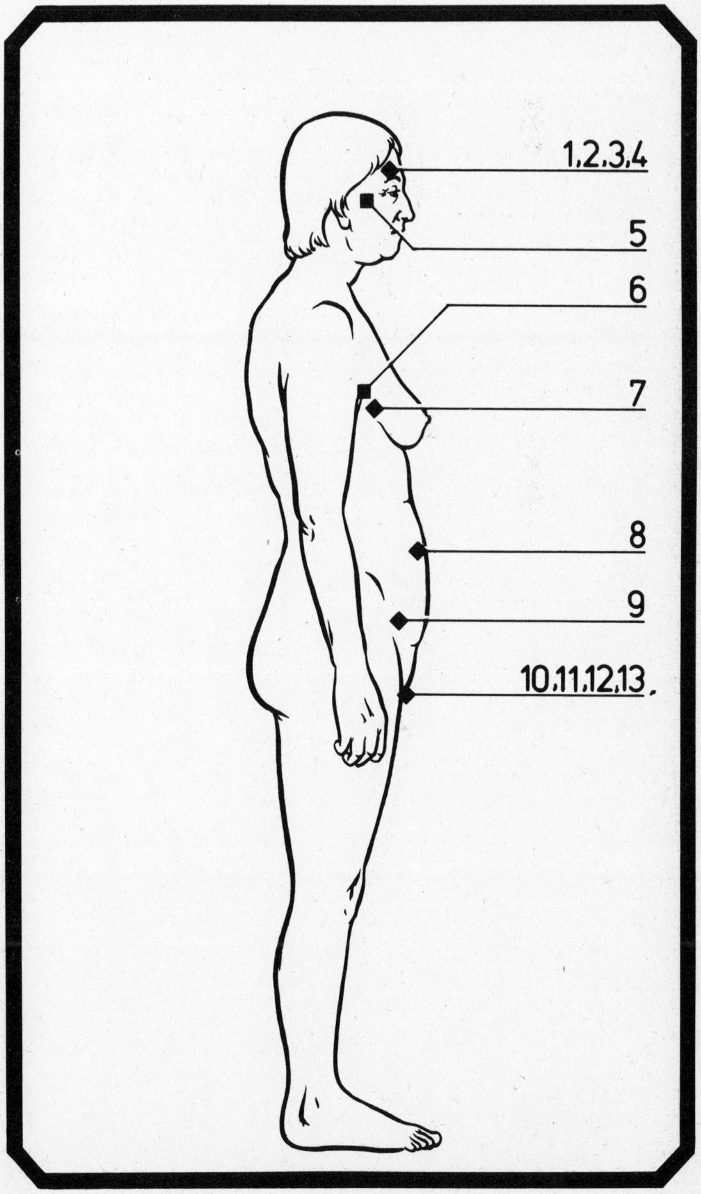

Middle age 2

During middle age, joints may swell and work less easily, and muscles have a tendency to sag and lose their elasticity. These processes lead to a feeling of general unfitness, with shortness of breath, lack of exertion, and weight gain, which can easily form a vicious circle. This state of unfitness is usually unnecessary, and can often be remedied by the application of deliberate countermeasures such as loss of any excess weight and regular repetition of simple exercises such as the ones on these pages. These measures won't halt the process of aging, but they will slow down its effects and produce a feeling of greater wellbeing combined with confidence in your improved appearance.

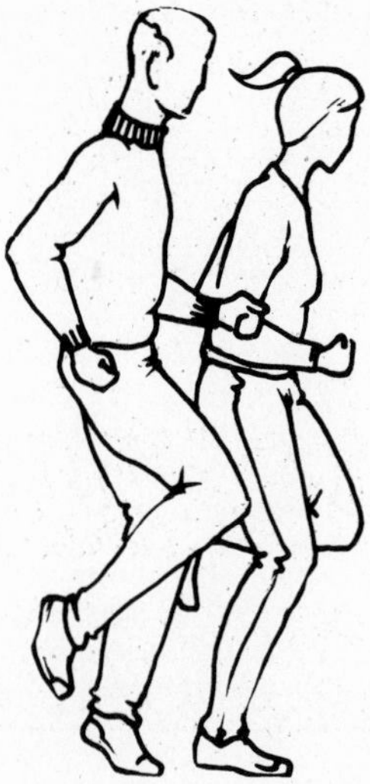

Starting to exercise
No elaborate apparatus is needed to start to get your body into good shape; all these exercises are designed to be easily done at home and ideally fitted into your daily routine. If you are very unfit, or have not indulged in any strenuous exercise for several years, ask your doctor to give you a full physical examination to ascertain that you are in good health and that you can begin your exercise program. Check your maximum pulse rating from the chart on p.81, and make sure that you do not exceed it; stop at intervals during your exercise session if you find yourself becoming over-tired.

Sports and activities
The types of sport suitable for you in middle age will depend very much on your physique, health and fitness. If you have been unused to strenuous activity, middle age is not the time to begin a highly competitive or demanding sport, but if you are in good physical shape most sports and exercise activities can be continued during middle age. From age 40 or so it is wise to give up competitive sports that are very strenuous, such as rowing, canoeing or weight-lifting, but these activities can be continued non-competitively and are all good forms of exercise. Activities such as gymnastics, soccer, tennis and sprinting may be continued into middle age if you are in good health, and golf, hiking, skating, jogging, cycling, archery and bowling can be continued indefinitely. Sports in which very careful and accurate judgement is necessary, such as parachuting, hang-gliding, motor racing, trampolining or motor-cycle racing may be affected by the gradual deterioration in sight and reaction times experienced in middle age, and should be discontinued as soon as any impairment of judgement is noticed.

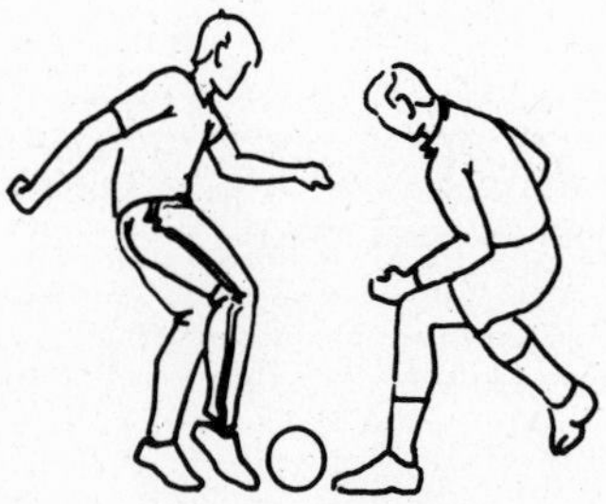

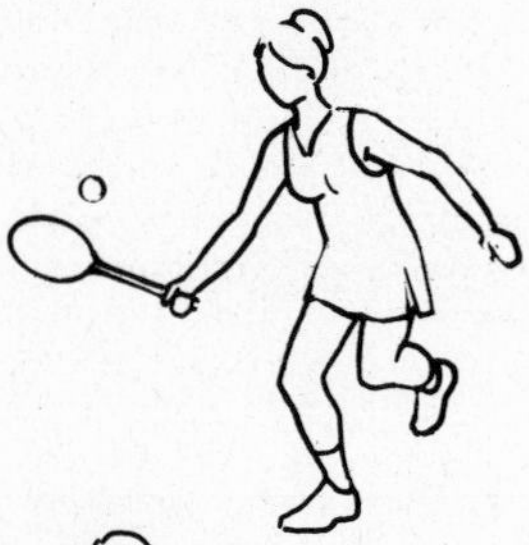

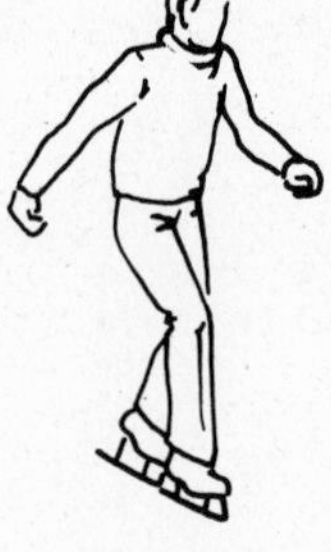

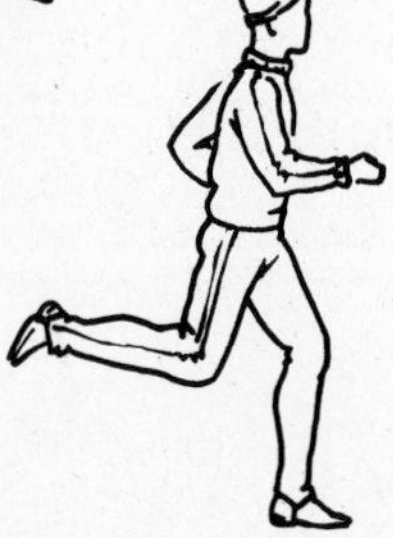

Warming-up exercises
Choose a time for exercise when you will have time to cool off and relax afterward, and start each exercise session with these exercises or similar ones. This kind of exercise gets the blood circulating faster, and eases the heart and other muscles slowly into their greater exertions as you move on to more strenuous exercises. Begin your program with one or two repetitions of each exercise, building up slowly by one or two repetitions each day to a maximum of 25 or 30.

1 Stand on one spot with your arms stretched out to your sides, and twist your body from side to side as far as you can, allowing your arms to swing loosely.

2 Stand with your feet flat on the floor and your arms hanging down, and bend your knees to a squatting position while your feet remain flat. Rise up slowly and repeat several times.

3 Hold the back of a chair as shown and swing your outside leg loosely forward and back from the hip. Turn round and repeat with the other leg.

4 Stand straight and raise one leg, bending the knee and hugging it as close to your body as possible. Repeat several times with each leg.

5 Stand in front of a low stool and step up and down from it several times.

6 Stretch your arms as high above your head as possible, inhaling deeply as you do so.

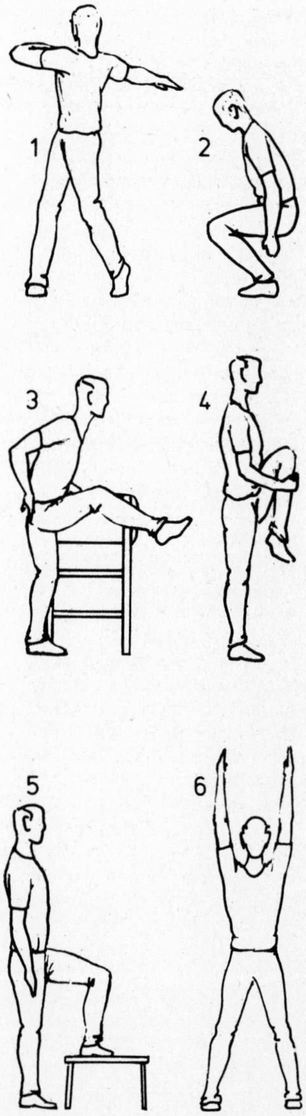

Death in middle age
The diagrams show the breakdown of deaths occurring in middle-aged men (**A**) and women (**B**) by cause of death. These statistics show that nearly half of all male deaths are caused by circulatory diseases, and this underlines the importance to the middle-aged man of avoiding as many of the contributory factors as possible (see pp. 80–89). Only half as many women die from circulatory problems. However, cancer causes twice as many deaths in women as in men, and these figures emphasize the need for middle-aged women to note any pre-cancerous changes in breasts or reproductive organs (see pp. 164–169).

Causes of death
a Circulatory diseases.
b Cancer.
c Respiratory diseases.
d Diseases of the digestion and metabolism.
e Other medical problems.
f Accidents.

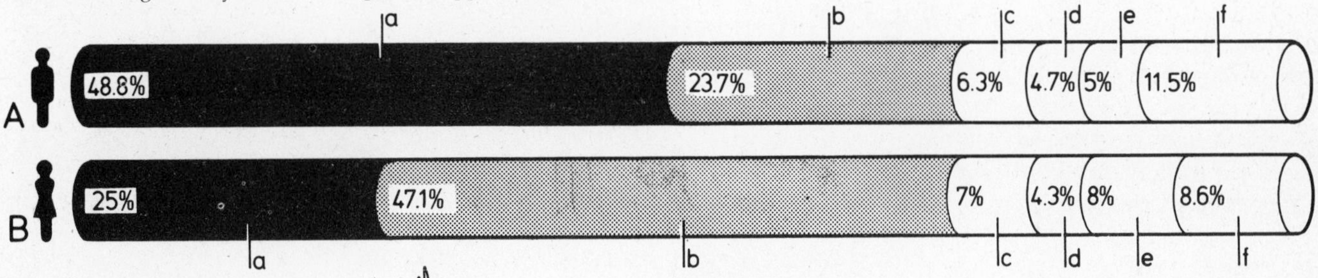

Waist, arm and trunk exercises
7 Sit firmly on a chair with your arms out to your sides, then bend to one side and touch the floor with one hand. Repeat to the other side.
8 Stand with your legs apart and your body bent forward; swing one arm to the side, and with the other hand touch the opposite foot. Repeat to the other side.
9 Stand with your feet astride and one arm bent over your head. Bend your trunk to the side, then repeat with the other arm and to the other side.
10 Lie flat on your back with your arms by your sides and your feet slightly apart. Raise your head and shoulders until you can see your ankles; lower them slowly, then repeat.
11 Lie face down with your arms stretched out to the sides, palms down. Raise your head and shoulders as high as possible, bringing your arms back in line with your shoulders. Relax, and repeat.
12 Stand with your feet astride and your hands stretched out above your head; move your arms in large circles, first forward and then backward.
13 Move your arms and legs vigorously as though jumping rope.

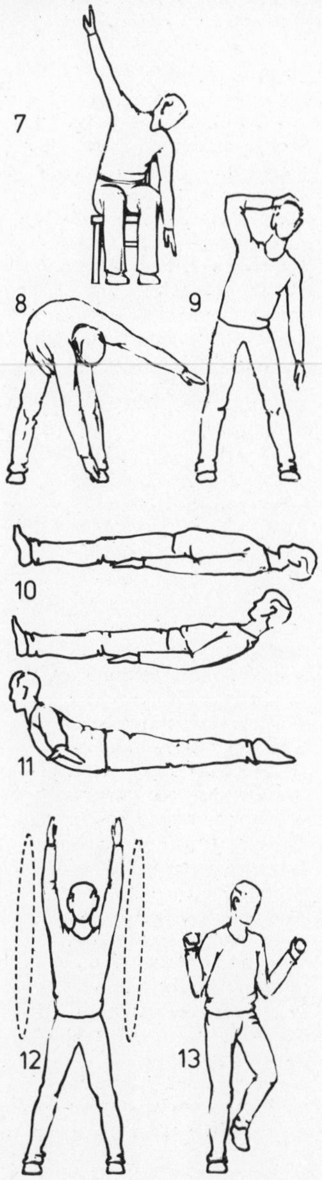

Leg and hip exercises
14 Stand behind a chair, holding its back with both hands. Bend your knees, keeping your feet flat, until you are squatting, then straighten up slowly.
15 Balance on your hands and feet as shown, with your knees bent and your back parallel with the floor. Kick each leg in turn as high in the air as you can, keeping your toes pointed.
16 Stand behind a chair and hold its back with both hands. Swing one leg sideways several times, and then repeat with the other leg.
17 With your arms above your head and your trunk upright, lunge forward first onto your right leg and then onto your left. Repeat several times.
18 Lie on your back with your arms down by your sides. Raise one leg vertically, then lower it to the ground slowly. Repeat with the other leg.
19 Lie face down with your hands under your chin, then lift one leg as high in the air as you can. Lower it slowly, and repeat with the other leg.
20 Lie on your back with your arms stretched out to the sides. Swing one leg over the other as far as you can, then return to the starting position and repeat with the other leg.

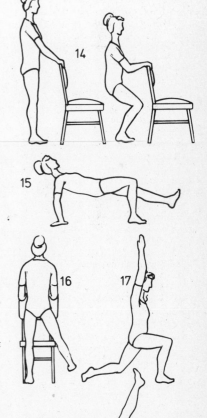

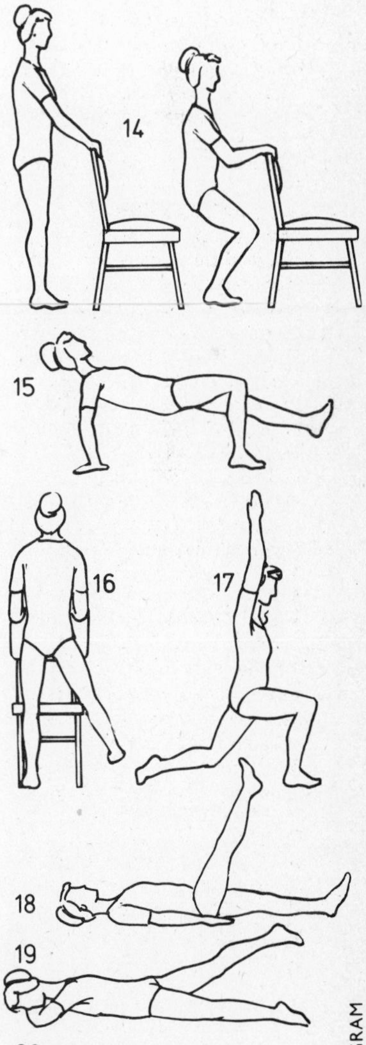

Growing older 1

As the human body grows older it becomes gradually less efficient and requires more attention to keep it in good health. Parts of the body such as the joints, the muscles or the digestive system, which may have functioned previously with very little specific care, may begin to cause problems in old age, and many of the body's functions slow down or deteriorate. In contrast the intellect, provided its functioning is not impaired by any physical disorder, may improve during old age; the comprehension of words is greater in old people, and crystallized intelligence – the kind that bases judgments on experience – is greatly increased. Here we look at some of the ways in which the older person can help to minimize some of the adverse effects of aging.

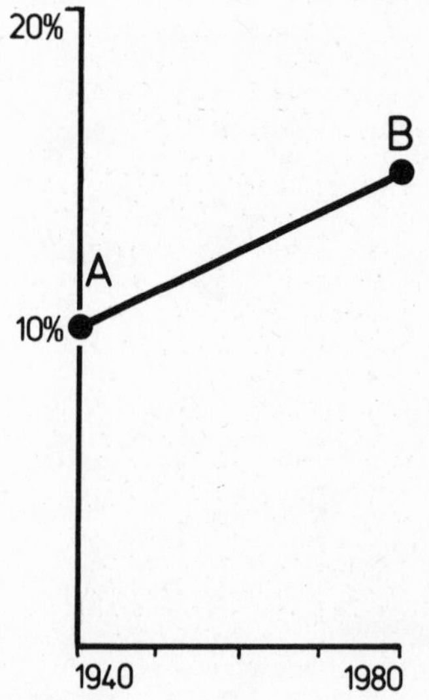

Ratios in the population
With increased medical knowledge and skill, many more people now survive middle age and live into an active old age. In 1940, only 10% of the population of the United States was over the age of 60 (**A**); by 1980, over 15% of the population was over the age of 60 (**B**), with every indication that this trend is increasing. These figures underline the importance of ensuring that elderly people continue as valuable and valued members of society, by helping to ensure that they remain healthy and happy.

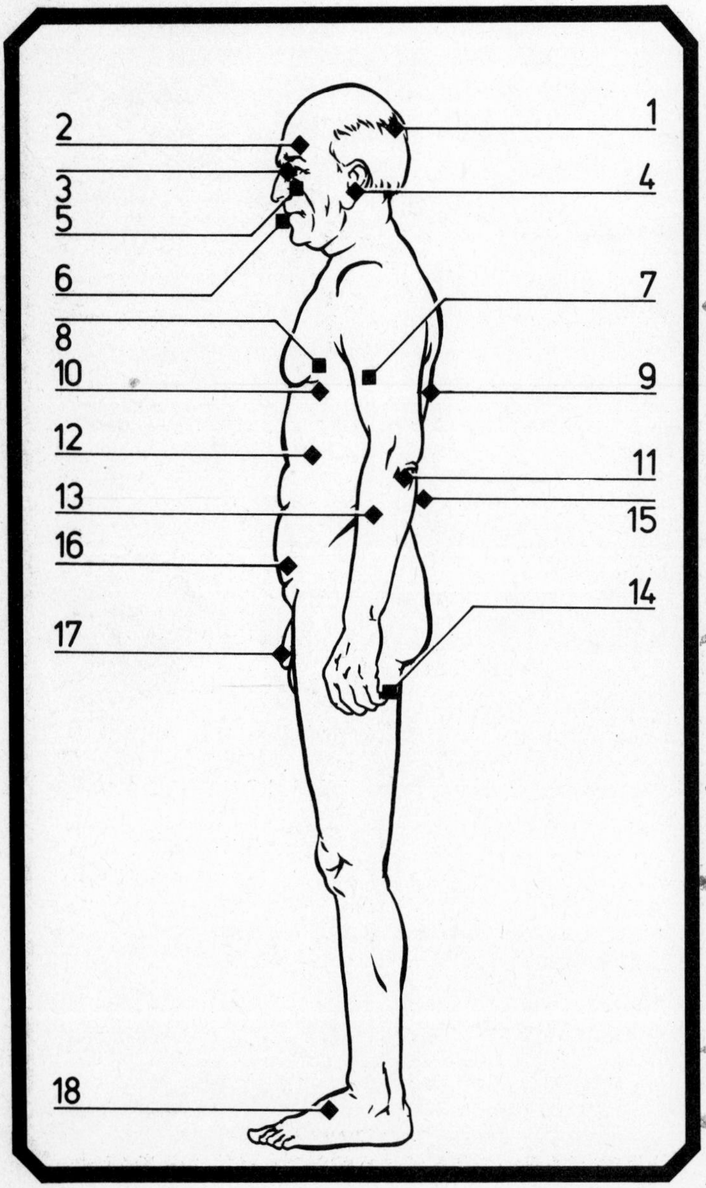

Changes in old age
The illustration plots the locations of some of the physical changes that take place during old age.

1 Hair; many older men have lost a great deal of their hair, and in other men and most older women the hair is thinner than in middle age. Graying is often total in elderly people.
2 Sleep; this is more shallow during old age. Old people may readily fall asleep during the day.
3 Eyes; the eyesight often deteriorates gradually, and the lens and cornea become less transparent.
4 Hearing; older people find that their hearing is less efficient.
5 Face; the facial muscles tend to lose their elasticity and the facial expression may change.
6 Appetite; the acuity of the sense of taste deteriorates, and food may taste less appetizing.
7 Muscles; the muscles begin to sag and folds of skin appear around the jowls, upper arms, etc.
8 Respiration; the efficiency of the lungs lessens.
9 Spine; the intervertebral disks compress as the body ages, often causing a slight decrease in height.
10 Chest; the muscles of the chest wall sag and cause drooping breasts in women and less efficient respiration in both sexes.
11 Skin; the skin loses moisturizers, causing a loss of elasticity.
12 Age spots; these are small brown areas of pigment that may form in the skin during old age.
13 Bones; as the body grows older, the bones become rarified and more brittle.
14 Touch; the sense of touch deteriorates slightly as the nerves just under the skin lose some of their sensitivity.
15 Kidneys: the kidneys take longer to process waste materials into urine.
16 Bladder; the bladder capacity often lessens during old age, and may cause a more frequent need to urinate.
17 Genitals; older men take longer to gain an erection during sexual stimulation, but can maintain it for much longer without feeling the urgent need to ejaculate.
18 The feet often swell, and muscles weaken causing fallen arches.

Illness
During old age, physical problems caused by the declining efficiency of the body's systems are compounded by such circumstances as decreased mobility, the absence of caring relatives, or depleted finances that make adequate nutrition difficult, and illness is frequently the result. If the older person is very isolated, relatives and neighbors may not realize that he or she is ill for days or even weeks, which will increase the serious effects of the illness, and many old people have to be hospitalized because there is no suitable person to nurse them at home.

Loneliness
Isolation is a situation that many older people have to contend with. A spouse may die after several decades of marriage, leaving the partner living alone for the first time in many years; in other situations, for instance that of a bachelor or spinster, a life of independence may give way to a life of loneliness when friends die or the person concerned becomes housebound. Physical difficulties prevent many old people from leaving their houses to visit relatives or to join in social activities, and their interests may be necessarily curtailed by failing sight or hearing.

Family
Family relationships are often strained by some of the changes and problems associated with aging. If an elderly relative is ill or otherwise needs support, this can create feelings of resentment in the younger members of the family and embarrassment in the older person concerned. Elderly people may wish to keep their independence at all costs, even at risk to their health, which may worry relatives, or they may become unnecessarily demanding on their families. Siblings may argue about the responsibility of caring for the father or mother, whether this involves nursing, visiting or financial support.

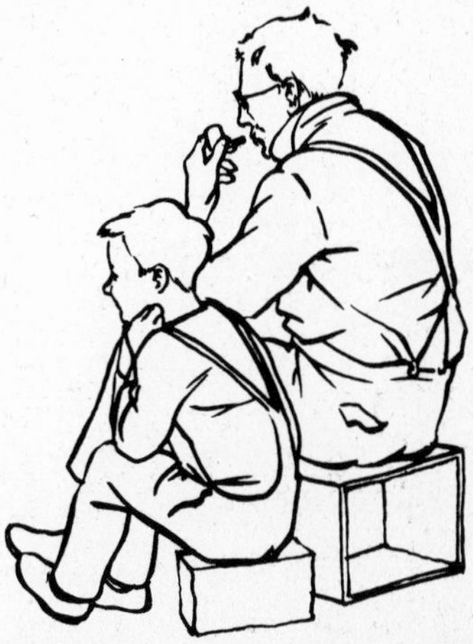

Problems in old age
The illustration here shows the sites of some of the problems that may occur commonly in old age.
1 Coordination; difficulties in coordination and mental confusion may well occur as a result of a decrease in the amount of oxygen reaching the brain. This situation arises because of decreased lung efficiency in oxygenating the blood.
2 Eye problems; glaucoma, detached retina and cataracts are eye problems that affect many people as they grow older. Regular visits to an ophthalmologist will ensure early detection of the problems.
3 Social isolation; this can occur as a result of hearing difficulties.
4 Teeth and gums; tooth decay and gingivitis are common in old people when they lose mobility and their personal hygiene routines deteriorate.
5 Malnutrition; this may occur because of the decreased acuity of the sense of taste, which may make foods less than tempting.
6 Excess weight may be a result of decreased activity, too much carbohydrate and fat in the diet, a change in metabolism, or a combination of these factors.
7 Hypertension; high blood pressure, or hypertension, is a condition that increases in frequency among older people.
8 Pneumonia; decreased activity in old age means that infections have a tendency to spread to the lungs, where they may cause pneumonia.
9 Hypothermia; in this condition the body receives insufficient warmth. This may be caused by inadequate heating or clothing, aggravated by changes in the skin's responses to temperature that occur in old age.
10 Clumsiness; this can occur as coordination, balance and the sense of touch deteriorate in old age.
11 Stiff joints; the connective tissue of the joints and muscles becomes less elastic in old age, and joints may become stiff and painful.
12 Kidney problems; changes in the functioning of the kidneys and bladder tend to increase the incidence of kidney problems.
13 Incontinence; this may be a result of lessened bladder capacity combined with a slackness of the pelvic floor muscles.
14 Genitals; changes in this area include atrophy of the internal and external genitals and a decrease in the vaginal lubricating fluids.
15 Broken bones; older people are very likely to suffer broken bones after falls and other accidents because of their increased skeletal frailty.
16 Arthritis and rheumatism; pain and swelling of the joints or their membranes is very common in old age, particularly in the hip and knee joints.

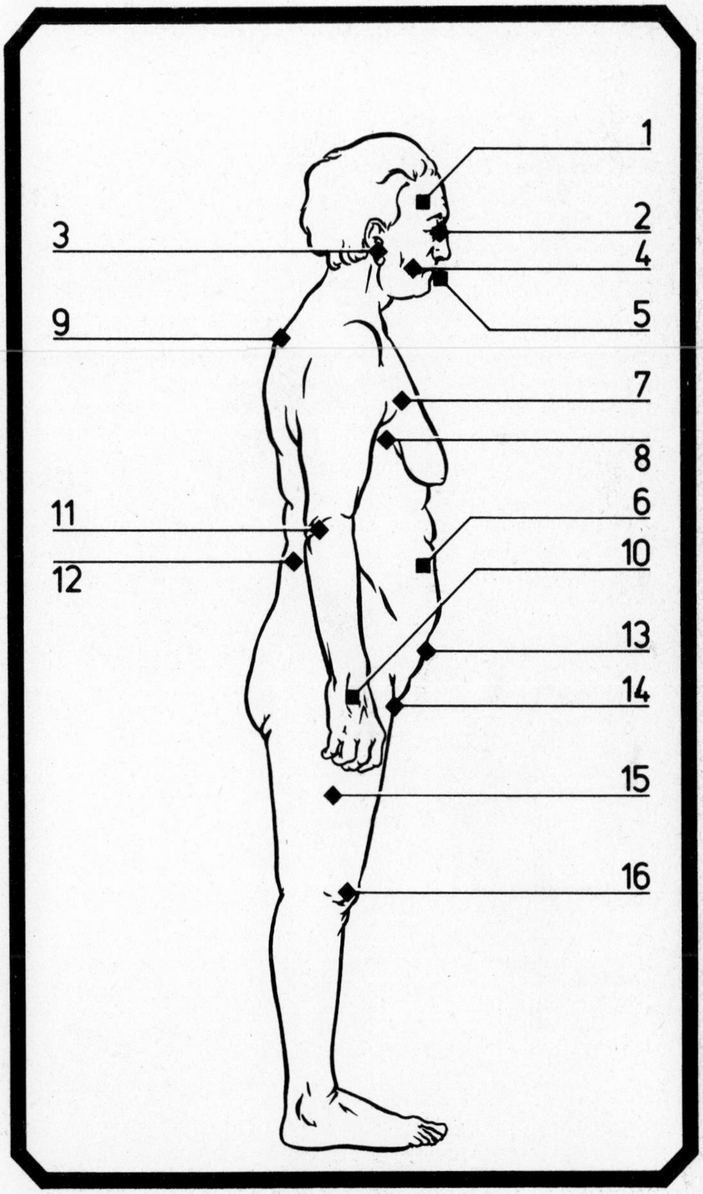

Growing older 2

Exercise and recreation play as important a part in the life of the elderly as they do in the young and the middle-aged. The stiffness and swelling of joints and connective tissue associated with aging worsen rapidly if the limbs concerned are immobilized, but improve if they are exercised gently and regularly. In addition, physical and social recreation help to prevent the boredom and ennui that may develop in later life, especially after retirement from a demanding career or when housebound after a life of outdoor activity. On these pages we look at recreation and exercise for the over-sixties; the simplest of these exercises can be done even by people who are bedridden, and will help to keep as many muscles and joints as possible well-conditioned and flexible.

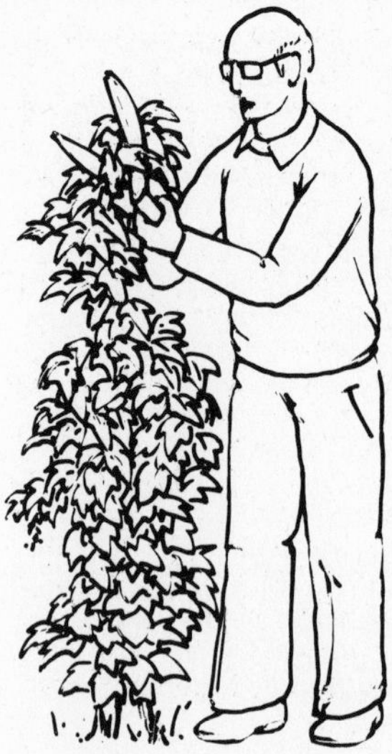

Hobbies and pastimes
Of all the phases in a person's life, retirement offers perhaps the best opportunity for indulging an old hobby or taking up a new one. If you find that your interests are being curtailed by decreased mobility, develop new ones that can be followed more easily in your home, such as painting, weaving, cooking, creative writing, carving, gardening or listening to new kinds of music. Reading is a hobby that can introduce you to many new areas of interest.

Sports and activities
If you are fit and well, and if you have regularly taken part in sporting activities in the years leading up to old age, there is no reason why you should not continue gentle sports during your older years. Because of the increased frailty of the skeleton in old age, sports that include a risk of falling should be avoided, and sports that place a great strain on the heart and respiratory system should also be slowly phased out by this time. Archery and bowling are excellent recreations and will also help to maintain your coordination skills. Hiking and gentle hill walking provide good heart and lung exercise for elderly people, and golf gives the opportunity for walking in pleasant surroundings. Swimming provides good exercise, and can be varied in intensity to suit your own level of fitness; and gardening is another healthy outdoor activity. Painting and sketching out-of-doors can be an effective way of getting fresh air, and the same is true of outdoor photography.

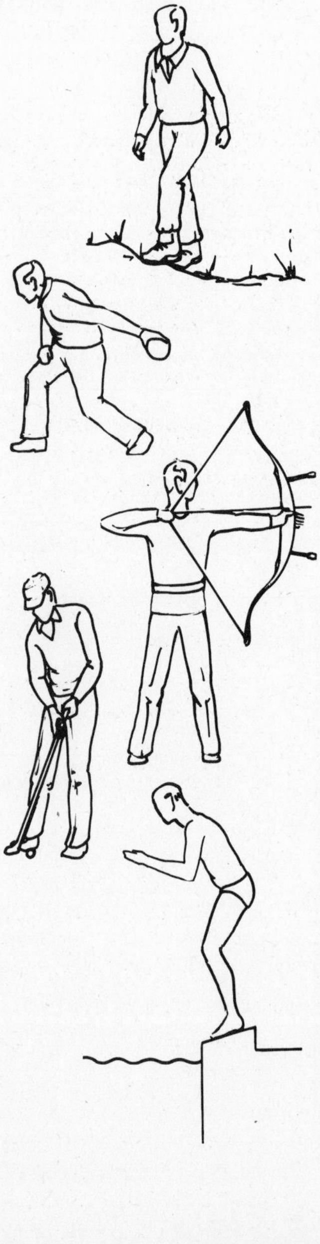

Feet and leg exercises
These exercises will help to improve your circulation, increase your mobility, and maintain the health of your legs and feet. Gradually increase the number of times that you repeat each exercise per day, starting with one or two repetitions and reaching a maximum of 15 or 20.
1 Stand upright with your arms down by your sides. Bend your knees as far as you can while keeping your feet flat on the floor; straighten up and repeat.
2 Stand with your back straight and your arms by your sides, and raise first one knee and then the other as high as possible.
3 Stand upright with your weight balanced on your toes and your heels raised off the ground. Rock slowly back onto your heels and raise your toes off the ground, and then return to the starting position.
4 Stand upright with your weight balanced on your toes and your heels raised off the ground. Bend your knees slightly while still balancing on your toes.
5 Sit on a chair with your feet extended in front of you. Rest your feet on the heels, and turn your feet alternately inward and outward.
6 Lie on one side with your head resting on one hand; raise your upper leg a few inches. Turn over, and repeat with the other leg.

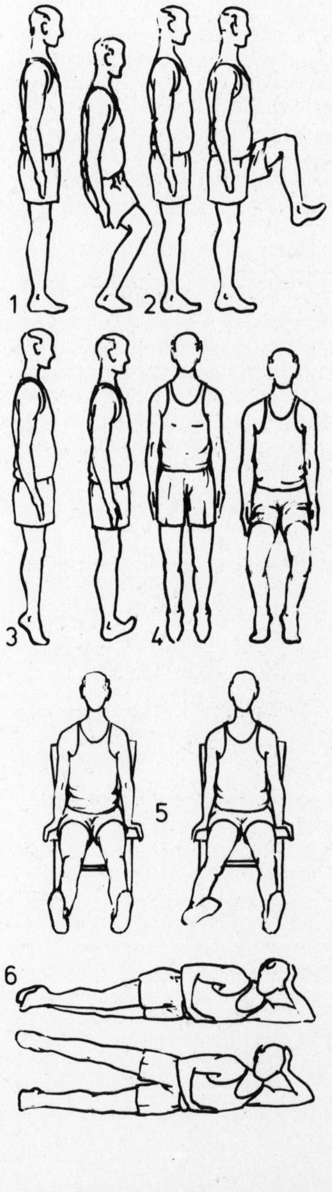

Hygiene
Through both forgetfulness and a decrease in physical ability, it is easy for an elderly person to allow his or her hygiene routines to lapse. Stiffness or trembling in the hands may make it hard for the elderly person to wash adequately or to handle a toothbrush, and infections may set in that will then be hard to control. Care of the feet is very important for elderly people, as problems there can lead to immobility, wasting of muscles and stiffness of the joints in the rest of the body. If personal hygiene is well maintained, many health problems will be avoided.

Diet
A nutritious diet is essential for the wellbeing of elderly people, as it is for younger people, but reduced finances and limited mobility may often lead old people to live off snacks and cheap foodstuffs. Protein foods such as meat, fish and eggs are quite expensive and may require a good deal of effort for preparation and cooking, and so are often skimped on by elderly people. Fresh vegetables, also, are harder to prepare than canned or frozen ones, and are often omitted, so that the elderly person may be deficient in vitamins. Malnutrition may cause a totally needless deterioration in health.

Sleep
The periods of deep sleep experienced during the night become less frequent during old age, and so the sleep of the elderly may become less refreshing. Although the total sleep requirement diminishes in old age, bedridden or housebound old people may tend to cat-nap during the day, which frequently leads to insomnia at night; this readily becomes a vicious circle. It is best to try to sleep only at night unless the person is ill or excessively tired. The bed should be warm, comfortable and fairly soft, so that stiff or painful joints are cushioned.

Sex
The nature of sexual relationships changes as the partners grow older because of the physical changes associated with the aging process. Many older people see these changes as indications that their sex lives are coming to an end, but this is far from true; if care is taken to understand and accept the changes, a healthy sex life can be continued well into old age. Men take longer to achieve an erection but are often able to prolong intercourse; women may experience a decrease in vaginal lubrication, and a slackness of the vaginal muscles. For both sexes the intensity of orgasm diminishes slightly.

Hand and arm exercises
For exercises **7** to **19**, begin with one or two repetitions per day and work up slowly to a maximum of 10 or 15 per day.
7 Hold your arms out in front of you with the palms of your hands flat and the fingers extended. Clench your fists tightly, then extend your fingers again.
8 Alternatively raise and lower your hands so that the muscles of the forearm are exercised.
9 Clench your hands and raise your elbows to the side so that your hands are on your chest. Push first one arm and then the other out to the front.
10 Stand with your arms bent at the elbows and your fingers resting on your shoulders. Extend your arms upward and outward, and then return them to the starting position.
11 Sit with your arms stretched out to the sides. Raise one arm while lowering the other, and then alternate.
12 Stretch your arms out to the front and down as low as possible, and then lift them as high as possible over your head.
13 Hold your arms out to the sides, and swing them slowly in large circles, first forward and then backward.

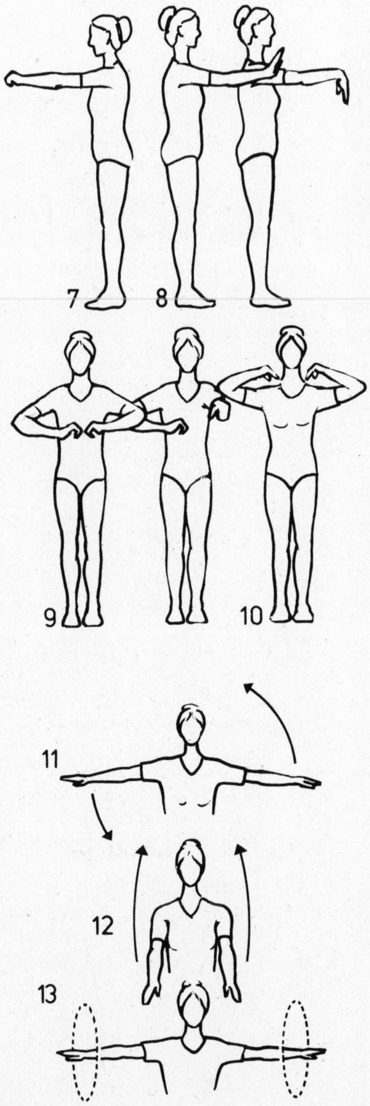

Trunk exercises
14 Stand upright with your arms by your sides. Raise first one shoulder and then the other.
15 Stand upright wth your feet apart and your arms by your sides. Bend forward and try to touch one foot with the opposite hand, then repeat with the other hand to the other foot.
16 Stand with your feet apart and your hands clasped behind your head. Turn your head and trunk first to one side and then to the other.
17 Stand against a wall with your back straight and resting on the wall. Bend your knees and slowly slide down the wall until you are as near a sitting position as possible, then slowly return to the starting position.
18 Lie on the floor with your knees bent up and your arms out to the sides. Swing your knees over to one side to touch the floor, and then to the other side.
19 Lie flat on your back with your arms stretched out above your head. Raise one leg and the opposite arm, hold in that position for a few seconds, then lower and repeat with the other arm and leg.

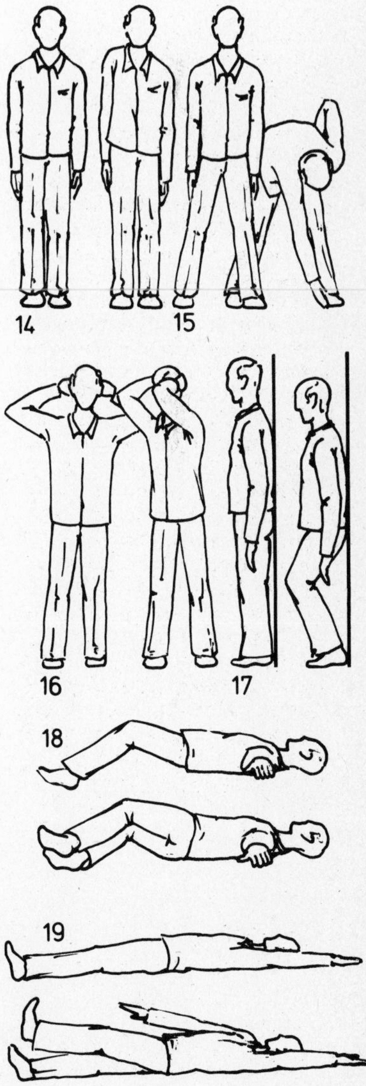

CHAPTER 4

In this chapter we look at some of the problems that men and women face in their everyday lives in the contemporary world. Some of these have been present for centuries, but in some way each of the problems has been altered or increased by recent changes in lifestyle. Tobacco, alcohol and drugs are now more widely distributed than ever before. Pollution and changes in dietary habits have increased the incidence of many cancers. Urban living, and competitive and demanding jobs, take their toll of greater stress on individuals. With the latest developments in contraceptive technology many couples are confused over which is the best method for them, but greater openness about sex and sexuality has made more people aware that sexual problems can be diagnosed and treated.

PROBLEMS OF CONTEMPORARY LIVING

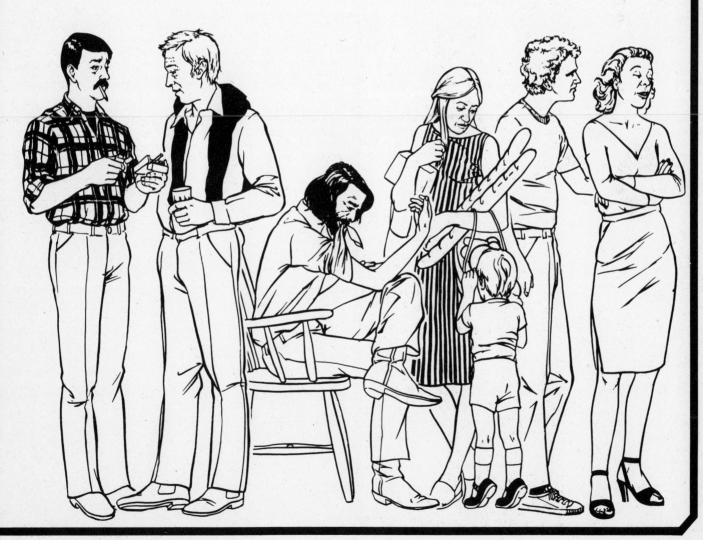

Stress 1

Biologically, the origin of stress lies in survival. All animals that live by hunting and are likely to be hunted need to be able to react either by fighting to overpower their prey or by taking flight. The body prepares itself for these responses by releasing large quantities of hormones into the blood. The 20th century has produced its own stressful stimuli attacking mainly the mind, the senses and the emotions; the body undergoes the same physiological processes even though the source of the stress and the main response is psychological. An individual's ability to cope with different levels of stress will play a large part in determining his state of mental health. Here we look at some of the causes and effects of stress.

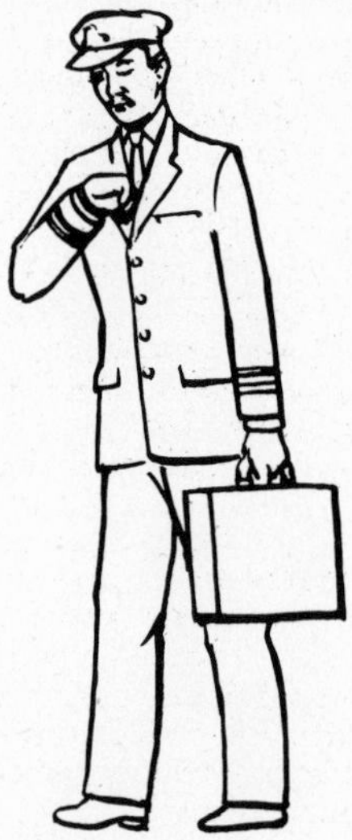

The need for stress
The human body and mind are built to thrive on a certain amount of stress. Many people find high levels of stress pleasurable when they provide challenges that have to be overcome physically or mentally. Such people include those taking part in highly competitive or dangerous sports, and those who thrive on careers such as journalism or air traffic control that put them under constant pressure.

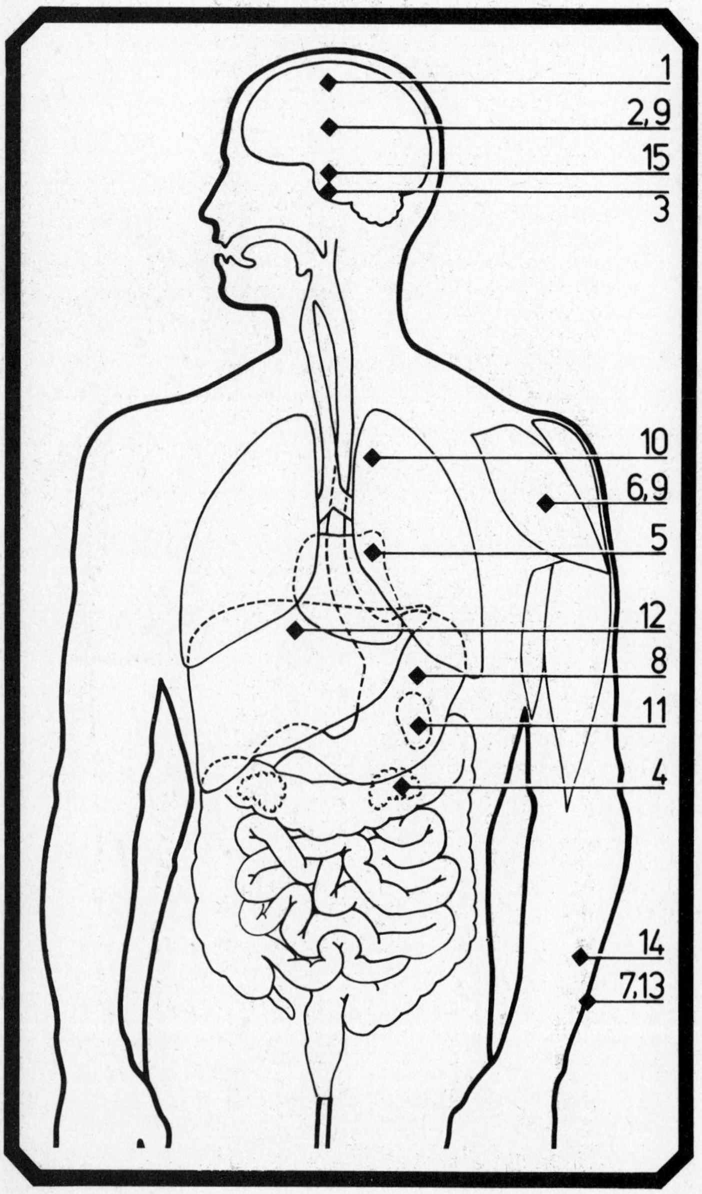

Physical effects of stress
The diagram shows the parts of the body affected when under stress. The body's instinctive reaction is either to fight or take flight.

1 The cerebral cortex receives and analyzes the incoming source of stress via the senses and interprets its meaning.
2 The brain then instructs the alarm center in the lower brain and brain stem to prepare the parts of the body which may need to take action.
3 The pituitary gland, which is attached to the hypothalamus at the bottom of the brain, releases a hormone (ACTH) which will be carried in the bloodstream.
4 The hormone is carried to the adrenal glands which sit just above the kidneys. The glands release two hormones, adrenaline and noradrenaline, and cortisones. These substances will adjust the body functions so that the source of stress can be tackled.
5 The heart speeds up, pumping blood around the body more quickly. The rate can go up from 70 beats per minute to 120 or 130.
6 More oxygen is delivered to the muscles.
7 Blood vessels constrict at the skin.
8 Blood vessels constrict at the stomach.
9 More blood is diverted to the muscles and brain as a result of actions **7** and **8**.
10 Breathing increases in speed, and air passages in the lungs dilate to bring in more oxygen.
11 The spleen contracts, releasing more red cells into the blood to carry more oxygen.
12 The liver releases supplies of sugar while fat or cholesterol is released into the blood from deposits in the body, skin and gut. Stress can increase the blood sugar level to the point where it overflows into the urine causing temporary diabetes.
13 The skin begins sweating ready to shed excess heat.
14 The body's repair system is also on the alert. There is an increase in fibrinogen and platelets, which clot the blood and stop bleeding, and white blood cells called lymphocytes which help repair body tissues.
15 The hormones released in the body through stress may reduce the hormones which control the sex drive and so reduce it.

Stress and young people
A child's development is often the key to psychological problems in later life. Frustration is part of growing up but it can lead to either aggression or withdrawal. Children from broken homes or with overprotective parents may be particularly vulnerable. The situation may get worse during adolescence – a time of intense emotions – when even a well-adjusted child has to come to terms with his or her own sexuality and demonstrate success with members of the opposite sex. Pressure of exams, bullying at school, family favoritism or the death of a parent may be additional sources of stress.

Stress and adults
Adult life calls for social adaptation in achieving economic independence, in forming new emotional ties, and possibly in preparing to marry and raise a family. For most people it is an exciting and challenging time, but it can also be a time of stress. Finding a new job and new home and making new friends can be frightening, and the reality of marriage and children may not match up to expectations. Postnatal depression is one problem women may suffer. Adults may experience marriage or relationship difficulties, problems with adolescent children, or job and money worries.

Stress and middle age
Middle age may bring on what is commonly called the "mid-life crisis," a time when some people feel that their hopes of achieving the ambitions of their youth have permanently disappeared. Most people are well settled into their jobs, marriages and lifestyles by this stage of life, and may begin to feel trapped. Men may suffer from overwork, lack of promotion, or promotion above their capabilities. Women may be approaching or experiencing the menopause, or they may be unduly distressed by their children leaving home. Divorce, separation and extramarital affairs can be other sources of stress.

Stress and the elderly
Depression, often brought on by the loss of a loved one, is the most common psychological disorder affecting the elderly. But it may go untreated since poor concentration, indecisiveness and poor memory may be the results of depression or of natural aging. Enforced retirement may bring on anxiety or a feeling of hopelessness and lack of confidence. Poor mobility, travel costs and fewer visits from friends and relatives may cause a sense of isolation, perhaps aggravated by deteriorations in eyesight and hearing. Anxiety about death, illness, housing and money are additional sources of stress.

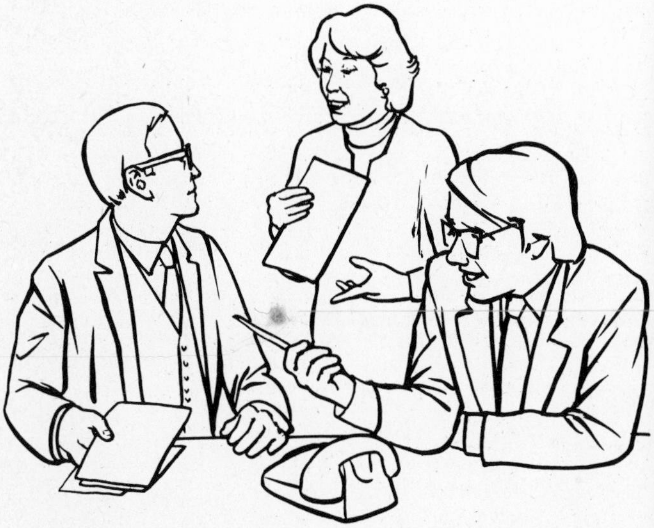

Stress and the environment
The pace, pollution, noise and congestion of urban civilization are a major source of stress in the 1980s. Being caught up in a traffic jam when you have to keep an appointment, or fighting your way through crowds, creates frustration. Living in a high-rise or a ghetto may instill a feeling of isolation and despair. The noise and smell of traffic and the rubbish that accumulates in city streets can irritate and numb the senses. The situation seems particularly stressful in the city because often a person can see no way out of the lifestyle, and so the natural instinct to take flight and escape is frustrated. The stress caused by this kind of environment may arouse anger and aggression; it is rarely socially acceptable to let out this aggression, and so the problem is bottled up and the stress is increased. But while noise and crowds produce stress, the opposite end of the scale may also have the same effect. Complete isolation and quiet may be unendurable to some people.

Types at risk
Most people suffer stress at some time in their lives, but the following groups are particularly vulnerable.

- Racial, religious or ethnic minorities.
- Homosexuals or other sexual minorities.
- New mothers or mothers with several small children.
- Bereaved, divorced or separated people.
- Middle-aged women during the menopause, particularly if their children have left home.
- People living in bad housing conditions.
- People living alone in a big city with no friends, particularly those who are always on the move from one hotel or boarding-house to another.
- People who are unemployed or retired; they may suffer from boredom or a lack of self-esteem.
- Adolescents, particularly those from broken homes, those with overprotective parents, or those studying hard for exams.
- Men and women with stressful careers, such as doctors, nurses, journalists, airline pilots, business executives, athletes etc.

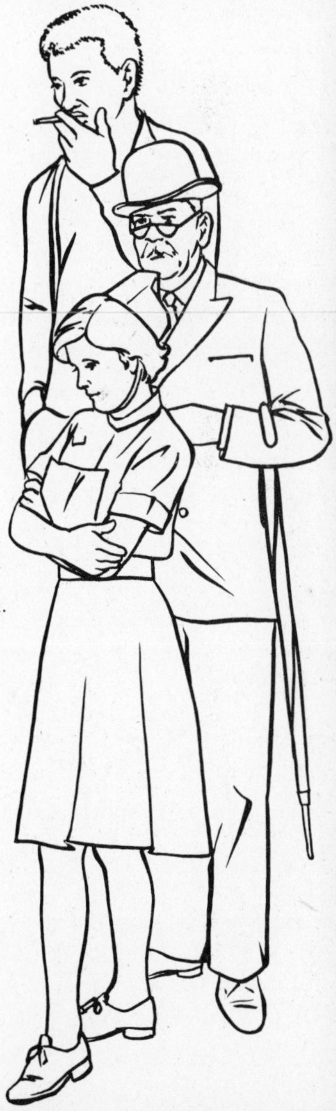

Stress 2

About 15% of the US population suffers a significant psychiatric or psychological disorder at some time in their lives, according to a recent study. More people are being treated both in and out of hospitals than in previous decades, although the stays in hospitals tend to be shorter. We outline some of the types of treatment available. But rather than pointing to an increase in mental illness the pattern may suggest that more people are willing to seek treatment and to admit to themselves that they might have a problem. The stigma once attached to psychiatric illness is gradually decreasing. But the onset of mental disturbance can be so gradual that you may be unaware that anything is wrong; here we describe what can go wrong, what to look for, and how to help yourself before you need professional treatment.

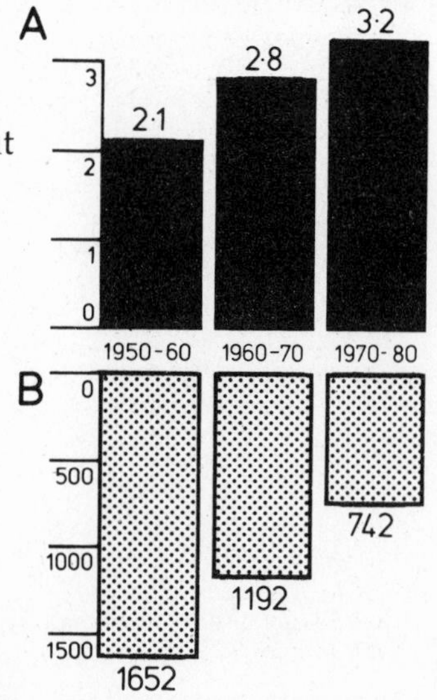

Incidence
The diagram shows the increase in the number of admissions of psychiatric patients in the USA since the 1950s. Although this in itself does not point to an increase in the amount of mental illness it does suggest that more cases are being recognized and being referred for specialized treatment. The diagram also shows how the number of days spent in hospitals by psychiatric patients has been considerably reduced in the same period, suggesting a belief that short-term treatment is more beneficial and reduces the risk of institutionalization.
A Admissions per 1000 population
B Days in hospital per 1000 population

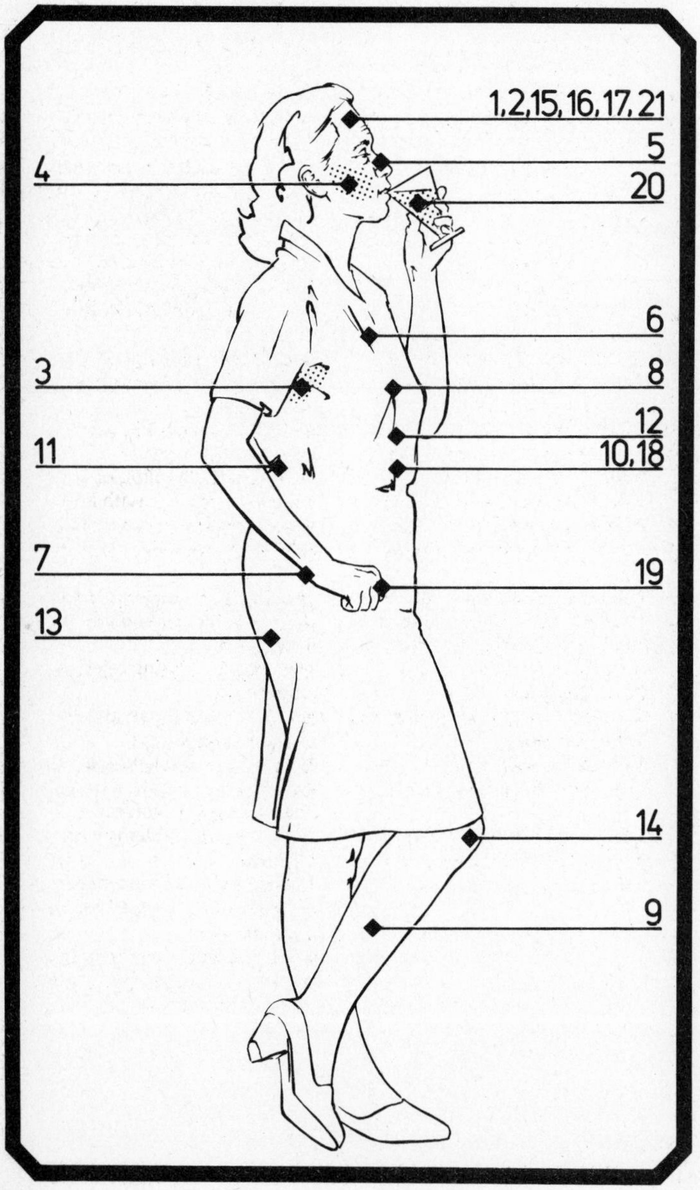

Complications of stress
Stress may contribute to the following physical disorders and can also aggravate many preexisting physical complaints.
1 Headaches.
2 Exhaustion.
3 Excessive sweating.
4 Facial flushing.
5 Nasal catarrh.
6 Asthma attacks.
7 High blood pressure or fast pulse.
8 Heart disease or heart attacks.
9 Skin diseases.
10 Stomach problems such as indigestion and ulcers.
11 Vague pains in the back and limbs.
12 Diabetes.
13 Diarrhea.
14 Rheumatism and arthritis.

Excessive stress may also result in the following psychological disorders.
15 Depression; this may be mild or severe. A minority of severely depressed people may suffer from manic depression, extreme cycles of agitated, euphoric behavior alternating with deep depression.
16 Postnatal depression may last for days, weeks, months or even years. It may be caused by such factors as hormone changes, breastfeeding problems, separation from the baby or lack of confidence.
17 Schizophrenia is often brought on by stress within the family. Symptoms may include deterioration of personality, illogical thought, the hearing of imaginary voices, and delusions of persecution (paranoia).
18 Anorexia nervosa is self-starvation usually indulged in by insecure or overpressurized adolescent girls (see p. 28).
19 Prolonged aggressive behavior may be brought on by stress.
20 Overdependence on drink or drugs is frequently used to escape from stress.
21 Neuroses such as panic attacks and palpitations, phobias (extreme, illogical fears), hypochondria, hysteria, amnesia and obsessive rituals may develop in a person anxious to escape from stressful reality.

Psychotherapy
Psychotherapy aims to help someone find the cause and solution to his problem through individual or group discussion with a doctor or therapist. By talking with the patient and tracing his troubles back to his earliest remembered life experiences the psychotherapist tries to help him understand his emotions and reactions to events. He may give advice or reassurance – "supportive therapy"–or remain non-committal, encouraging the patient to look closer at himself – "analytic therapy." Hypnosis or drugs may be used with either.

Drugs
Many drugs for treating the symptoms of psychiatric problems have been developed in the last few decades. Antidepressants relieve depression, tranquilizers help the patient who suffers from anxiety attacks, sedatives can reduce nervous tension, and hypnotics can induce sleep. Unfortunately some of the drugs allay the symptoms rather than treating the root problems, so they are really only a stop-gap measure in full treatment. Some of them also produce unpleasant side-effects, such as drowsiness, dry mouth, blurred vision, rashes, constipation, weight increase, a drop in blood pressure, or addiction.

ECT
Electro-convulsive therapy (ECT) involves the passage of an electric current through the brain, under anesthetic. It is not known how or why ECT works but its effect on chronic, severe depression can be dramatic. On some people its immediate effects wear off and further treatment is necessary; on others it has little or no effect. Still others complain of loss of memory after the treatment, which makes it a controversial method. A course of ECT usually involves 6 treatments spread over 2–3 weeks. Like drugs, ECT tends to treat the symptoms rather than the causes of the problem.

Hospitalization
Psychiatric hospitals or psychiatric units in general hospitals provide treatment for patients with psychiatric problems when there is a need for close medical supervision of drugs, therapy or ECT. Most people are in the hospital for only a short period. They may have to return if their illness recurs, but by being sent home each time they are less likely to lose touch with the outside world – one of the main reasons why psychiatric hospitals were frightening to so many in the past. Few patients are hospitalized against their will now; most are there because they want to receive help.

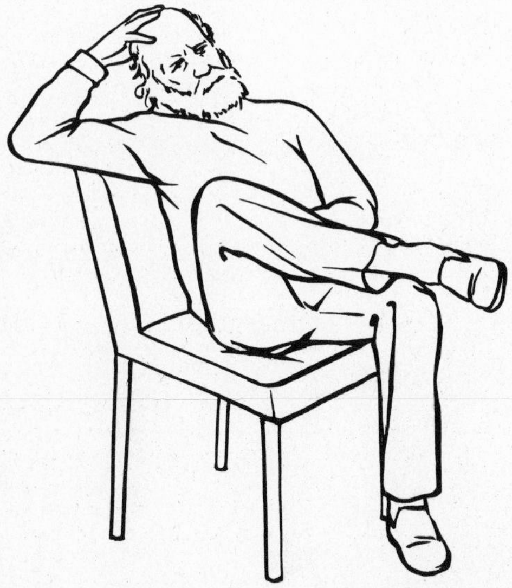

Self-help
Some psychiatric problems will need specialist help, but the following suggestions may help to prevent or alleviate some of the harmful effects of too much stress. Ensure that you are in good physical health. This will involve eating a balanced, nutritious diet, getting enough sleep and exercise, and making sure that you take time off regularly to relax. Try to talk out any problems that are bothering you with your family or friends; this will often reduce the mental strain associated with coping alone. Try every practical measure to reduce stress wherever you see it in your life.

If a restrictive home situation is depressing you, join a club, do voluntary work or take up a new interest. If you are overtired, work out ways in which you can delegate some of your tasks. If you are prone to anxiety attacks, prepare yourself thoroughly for interviews, public occasions, conferences and journeys so that as many of the arrangements as possible are made before the event.

Physical warning signs
The following signs may be symptoms of a stress problem.
- Excessive weight for your age and height.
- High blood pressure.
- Lack of appetite.
- A desire to eat as soon as a problem arises.
- Frequent heartburn.
- Chronic diarrhea.
- Constipation.
- Inability to sleep – either waking up early or not being able to drop off at night.
- Constant fatigue.
- Headaches.
- A need to take aspirin or some other medication every day.
- Muscle spasms.
- A feeling of fullness although you have not had anything to eat.
- Shortness of breath although you have not had any exercise.
- Fainting attacks, possibly preceded by nausea.
- Inability to cry.
- A tendency to burst into tears at the least thing.
- Problems with sex – impotence, frigidity or fear of intercourse.
- Excess nervous energy that prevents you from sitting still and relaxing.

Mental and emotional warning signs
The following signs may be symptoms of a stress problem if they are constantly present.
- Out-of-character personality changes, such as unpunctuality, untidiness, obsessions, drinking too much, driving too fast etc.
- A reversal of personality from placidity to aggressiveness or from being extroverted to introverted.
- A constant feeling of unease.
- Irritability with family or colleagues.
- Boredom with life, or excessive lethargy.
- A recurrent feeling of not being able to cope with life.
- Overanxiety about money.
- Morbid fears of disease and death.
- A sense of suppressed anger.
- An inability to find anything humorous.
- A feeling of being rejected by your family.
- A sense of despair at being an unsuccessful parent.
- Dread of the weekends.
- Reluctance to take a holiday.
- A feeling that you cannot discuss your problems with anybody.
- An inability to concentrate, or to finish one job before you start another.
- Inexplicable terror of heights, open spaces, certain people etc.

Stress 3

Relaxation techniques aim to combat stress by bringing the "fight or flight" response of the body under control. Eastern methods, although they are not widely recognized by the Western medical profession, are often beneficial as they are not merely physical exercises but aim to integrate the mind and body. Hatha yoga, the physical side of yoga, is a series of postures or poses; some are illustrated here. Correct breathing and slow, graceful progress toward the more advanced poses are essential. Chinese exercises, originally based upon the movements of animals, put the emphasis on continuous movement sequences designed to allow the body energies to flow freely, instead of being halted by holding the breath or maintaining a set position.

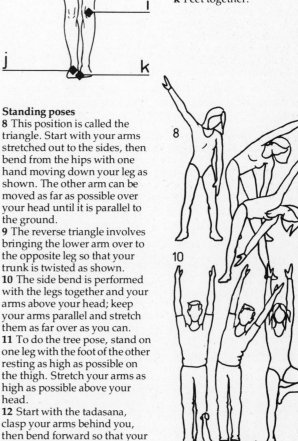

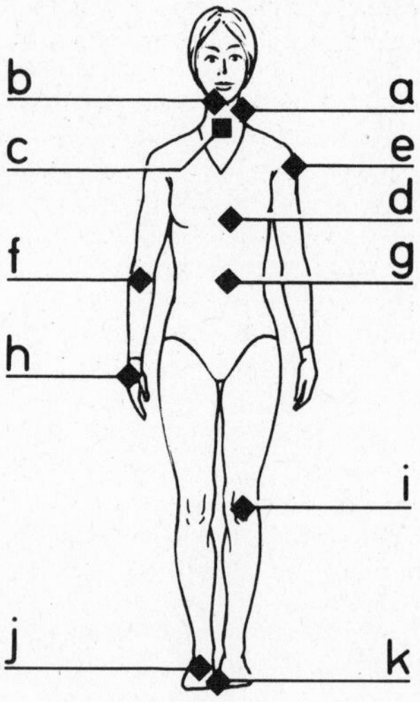

Tadasana
This is the basic standing pose used in yoga. Its characteristics are:
a Back and neck pulled up.
b Chin slightly tucked in.
c Throat relaxed.
d Chest open.
e Shoulders back.
f Arms hanging loose.
g Stomach pulled in.
h Hands loose.
i Knees pulled up.
j Weight evenly on heels and toes.
k Feet together.

Relaxing and recuperative poses
1 This posture, the corpse, is one of deep relaxation. Lie flat on your back with your arms at your sides, palms up, and your feet together. Allow your arms and feet to go limp; your feet will fall apart gently. Raise your chin, close your eyes, and take deep relaxed breaths.
2 This relaxation pose is preceded by the tadasana. Allow your body to fall forward as far as it will go, until your hands touch the floor.
3 This is one of many poses preceded by the corpse. Raise your legs together as high as you can; hold the back of your knees if this helps.
4 Following on from pose **3**, bring your legs right over your body, supporting your back with your hands.
5 For this position, the plow, raise your trunk as in **4** but without supporting it with your hands, and take your legs right over to touch the floor.
6 Starting from the tadasana, clasp your hands behind your back and then raise them as shown.
7 A number of relaxing poses can be carried out in the lotus position. You can turn your head with the chin raised and then lowered to your chest, or you can roll your head from left to right.

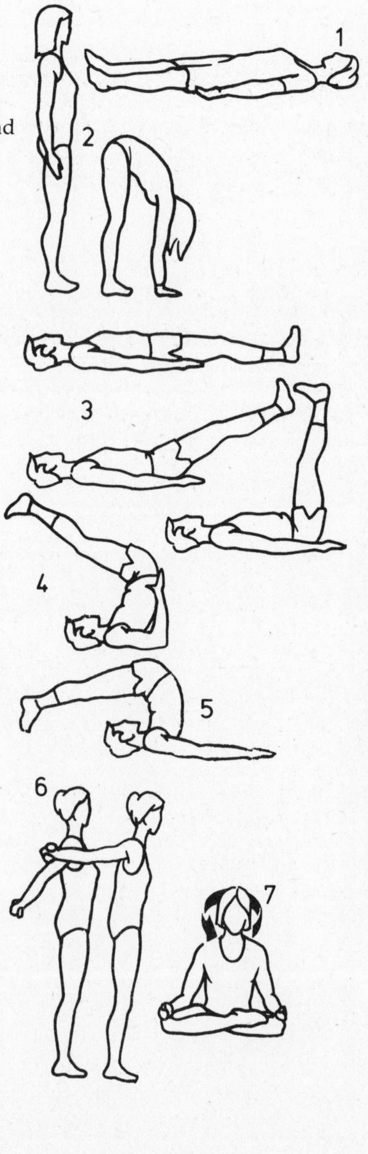

Standing poses
8 This position is called the triangle. Start with your arms stretched out to the sides, then bend from the hips with one hand moving down your leg as shown. The other arm can be moved as far as possible over your head until it is parallel to the ground.
9 The reverse triangle involves bringing the lower arm over to the opposite leg so that your trunk is twisted as shown.
10 The side bend is performed with the legs together and your arms above your head; keep your arms parallel and stretch them as far over as you can.
11 To do the tree pose, stand on one leg with the foot of the other resting as high as possible on the thigh. Stretch your arms as high as possible above your head.
12 Start with the tadasana, clasp your arms behind you, then bend forward so that your trunk is perpendicular to your legs.
13 Lunge forward on one leg so that your front leg is bent and your back leg straight. Two alternate positions for the arms are shown.
14 Form an equilateral triangle by stretching your arms forward and your legs back as shown.

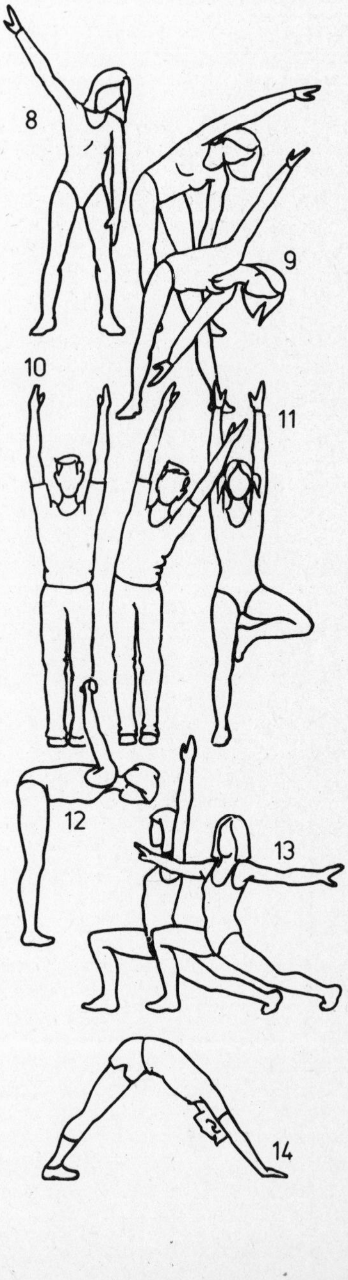

Breathing exercises
The type of breathing that is most helpful in yoga involves exhaling deeply to empty the lungs and then expanding the chest as you inhale deeply. Your stomach muscles should be pulled in and your nostrils should be relaxed; you should be aware of your chest and stomach movements.

a To practice deep breathing, kneel with your knees together and your feet apart; keep your back straight and hold your hands loosely with the palms upward.

b To practice full lung breathing adopt the lotus position or sit cross-legged. Breathe in slowly to fill first the lower, then the middle, then the upper parts of the lungs. Swallow, press your tongue against the roof of your mouth, and hold your breath. Exhale steadily.

c For alternate nostril breathing adopt a sitting or kneeling pose. Place the first and second fingers of your right hand on your forehead with the thumb beside your right nostril and your third and fourth fingers beside the left nostril. Breathe in slowly through the right nostril, closing the other with your fingers, then breathe out slowly through your left nostril, closing the other with your thumb. Repeat with the other hand.

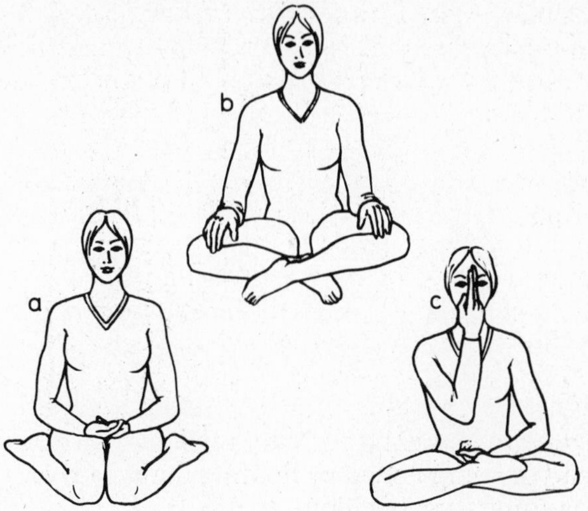

Sitting poses
15 Sit with your legs stretched out to the front, and lean forward to grasp your toes. With practice you will be able to pull your head down onto your knees.
16 This is the classic lotus position. Place your right foot on your left thigh and then your left foot on your right thigh.
17 Sit between or on your feet as shown, then raise your arms above your head. Breathing out, lower your arms, place your hands on the soles of your feet, and bend your trunk forward as shown. Then sit up, breathing in.
18 Balancing on your bottom, raise your legs and hold them up with your hands as shown.
19 This position requires a good deal of suppleness; sit with your legs wide apart and stretch your arms so that you can grasp your feet.
20 Sit with your knees flat and the soles of your feet touching; clasp your feet with your hands.
21 Sit with one leg straight across your body while the other leg is brought up to the body and held by the hands.

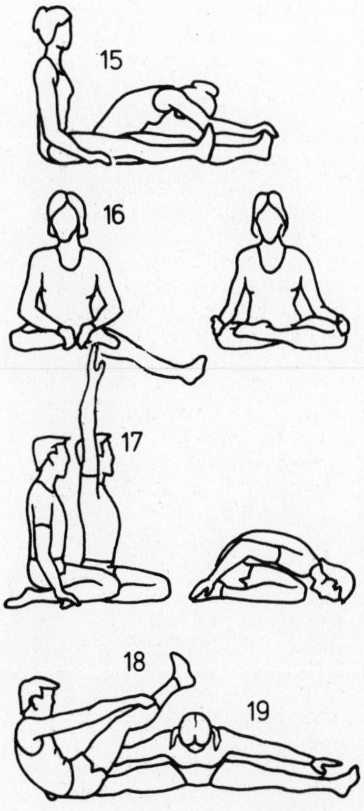

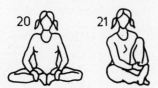

Lying poses
22 Lie face down with your hands under your shoulders. Push down with your hands and straighten your arms so that your trunk is raised, then look up.
23 Lie face down with your legs bent at the knees; clasp your ankles, and then raise your head and your knees simultaneously. This pose requires a great deal of flexibility.
24 Two forms of the locust pose are shown here. Lie face down with your arms at your sides and lift either one leg or both legs a few inches off the ground.
25 This is a still more difficult version of the locust pose. While raising both legs off the ground, pull your arms back as far as possible.
26 Two variations of the side raise pose are shown here. Lie on one side with your head supported on one hand and the other placed flat in front of you as shown. Lift either one leg or both legs a few inches off the ground.
27 Lie on one side with your head resting on one hand; lift your upper leg as high as possible and hold it there with your other hand.

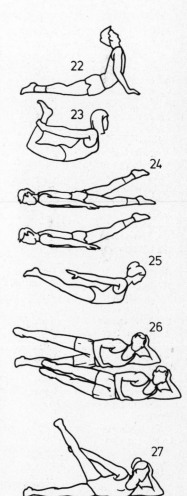

Smoking 1

During this century the smoking of cigarettes, cigars and pipes has almost totally replaced tobacco chewing and snuff-taking as ways of using tobacco, and since the invention of the cigarette-making machine the consumption of cigarettes has soared. Over the last thirty years, medical research has proved that smoking constitutes a grave health risk, with more and more diseases proving to be associated with or aggravated by smoking. Women who smoke while pregnant can cause damage to their babies, and in recent years smoking has been recognized as a major air pollutant. Here we look at some of the risks associated with smoking, and examine some ways of lessening those risks.

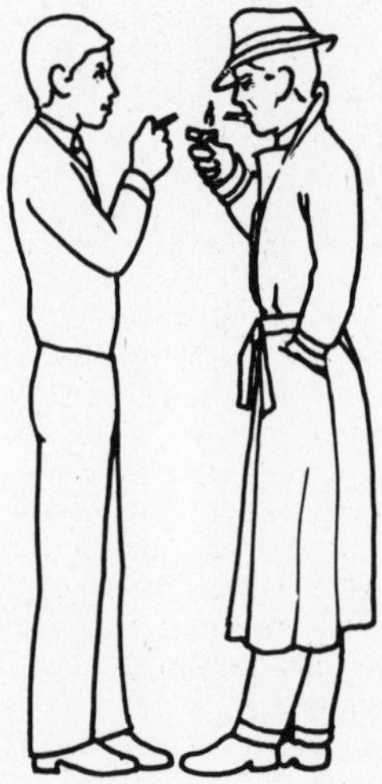

Reasons for smoking
People generally smoke for a mixture of psychological and physical reasons. Some receive physical pleasure from smoking, while others smoke to relieve boredom or stress or to receive a "boost" when they need to work harder. Some smokers are physically addicted to nicotine and their bodies crave it; others are pyschologically dependent and restless in its absence. Many people smoke for sociability or conformity to their peer groups, or for an appearance of sophistication. Smoking depresses the appetite and may unwisely be used as a weight reducing aid.

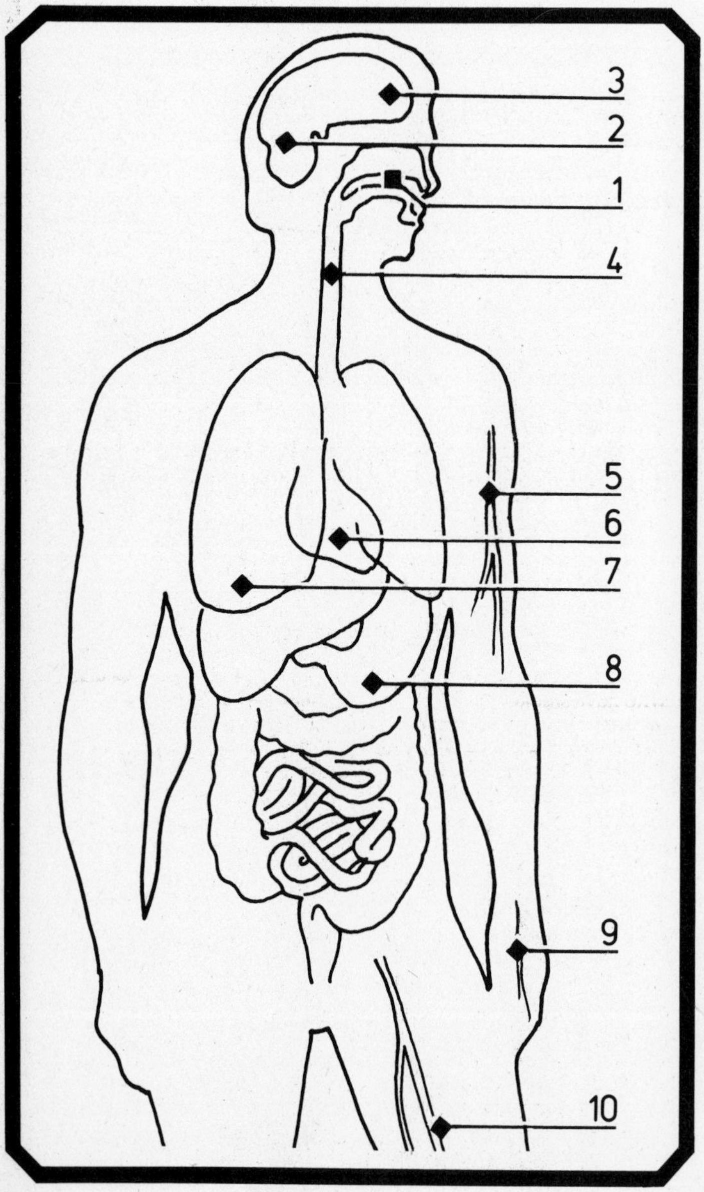

Immediate effects of smoking
This diagram illustrates some of the parts of the body affected when a pipe, cigar or cigarette is smoked. These effects wear off gradually when the smoking stops, but if smoking is frequent or continuous the affected parts of the body have no time to revert to their normal states.

1 Nicotine is absorbed through the lining of the mouth (as well as through the lungs) and enters the bloodstream.

2 The nicotine releases a small quantity of catecholamines, which subdue the transmission of nerve signals and so reduce feelings of fatigue.

3 The toxins carbon monoxide and cyanide in the smoke may cause a headache. Carbon monoxide is only absorbed through the lungs, and its presence in the bloodstream indicates that the smoker inhales the smoke into the lungs.

4 Nicotine acts on the nerves, and paralyzes the cilia of the airways. Cilia are the tiny hair-like projections responsible for removing the mucus that traps harmful particles; when they are put out of action the mucus, and the particles, remain in the airways. Nicotine also inhibits the alveolar phagocytes, which are normally responsible for engulfing and destroying the bacteria and viruses in inhaled air; one cigarette puts them out of action for 15 minutes.

5 The blood pressure rises because of the constriction of the blood vessels caused by the nicotine absorbed fom the smoke.

6 The heart rate increases because of the action of the chemicals, and so the reserve energy of the heart is decreased, rendering the person less capable of physical exertion or strain.

7 The lungs fill with a mixture of air and tobacco smoke, which deposits minute amounts of tar on the insides of the lungs.

8 Hunger is abated because of the action of the nicotine on the autonomic nervous system, the part of the nervous system that governs the actions of the involuntary muscles including those in the digestive system. Slight nausea may be experienced if the stomach is empty, but this soon passes.

9 The blood vessels to the hands and feet are constricted; this leads to poor general circulation.

10 Certain chemicals, as yet unidentified, contribute to the raising of the serum cholesterol level in the bloodstream.

Smoking in this century
Tobacco has been smoked in pipes by American Indians for centuries, but the cigar and cigarette were not introduced until the nineteenth century. The sudden boom in cigarette smoking in this century has a variety of causes, perhaps mainly the ability of new machinery to produce them quickly and cheaply. Many people took up smoking during the two World Wars, and as it slowly became socially acceptable for women to smoke the potential market for cigarettes doubled. Pipe and cigar smokers are very much in the minority among the smokers of today.

Smoking in the United States
The diagram *right* shows the male (**A**) and female (**B**) populations of the United States over 20 years of age, divided into groups according to their smoking habits. The first group consists of those who have never smoked (**1**), the second of those who formerly smoked but have now given up (**2**), and the third of those who are currently smokers (**3**) based on 1979 figures. Over 50% of women over 20 have never smoked, compared with roughly 40% of men, but few women who have started smoking have given up – 14% of the total adult female population compared with 24% of men.

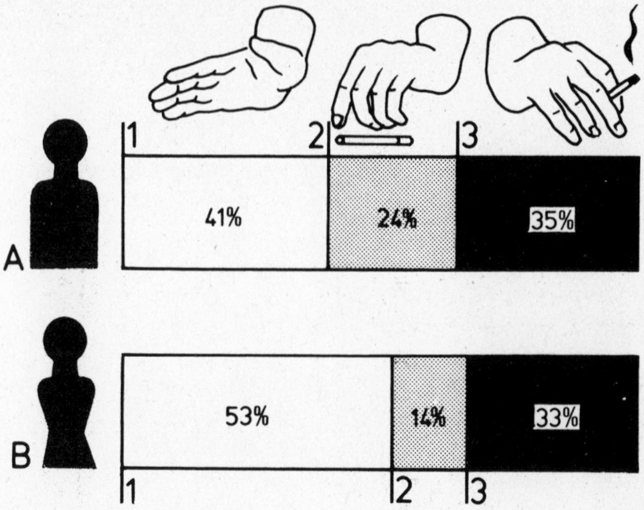

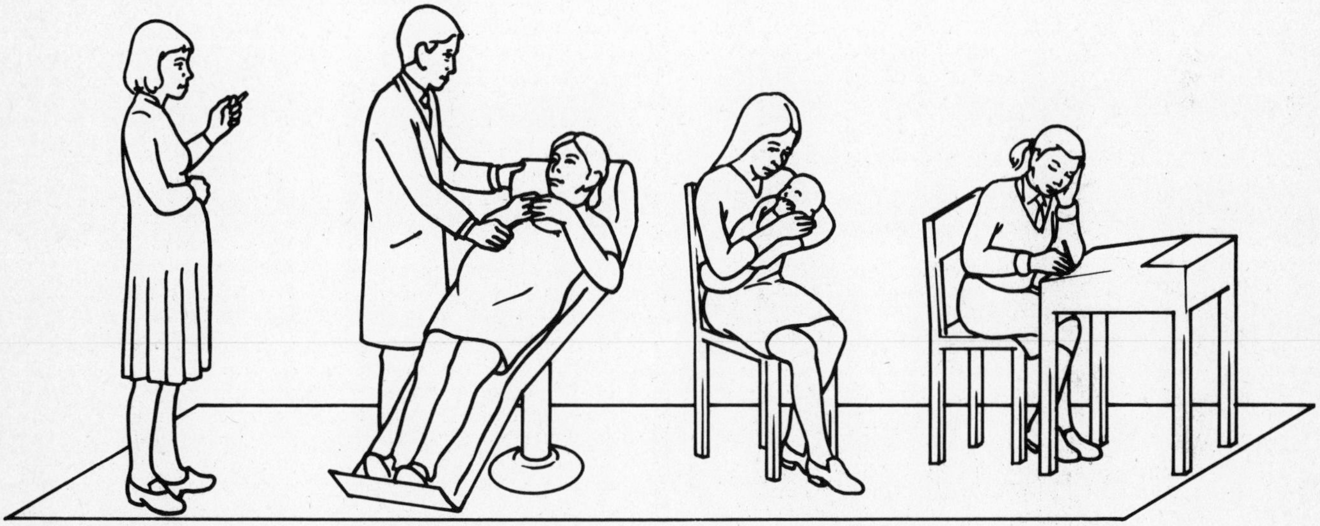

Smoking during pregnancy
The effects of tobacco smoke on the body can have far-reaching consequences for a woman who is pregnant. The decreased efficiency of the circulation while the mother is smoking means that less blood reaches the fetus; there is also a deficiency in the amount of oxygen reaching the fetus, since the carbon monoxide in the smoke combines with hemaglobin and blocks oxygen transport. Both of these circumstances are likely to affect the fetus adversely and slow down its growth and development.

Effects on the fetus
The likelihood of a pregnant woman miscarrying her baby is doubled if she smokes. Fetal malformation, congenital heart disease and breathing difficulties are more likely among the babies of mothers who smoked through pregnancy, and the premature separation of the placenta from the uterus is also more common. The likelihood of stillbirth is doubled. However, most ill effects seem to be associated with mothers who continue to smoke beyond the fourth month of pregnancy, so a pregnant woman who has not stopped smoking by the fourth month must accept that her continued smoking constitutes a grave risk to the life and wellbeing of her unborn child.

Effects noticeable at birth
Research has shown that full-term babies born to mothers who have smoked through pregnancy have a lower birthweight and are smaller and less robust than full-term babies born to non-smoking mothers. Because of difficulties with the placenta, premature births among smoking mothers are common, which lead to still lower birthweights. The chances of the baby dying within the first few months after birth are double those of the babies of non-smokers. Mothers who have stopped smoking before the fifth month of pregnancy count as non-smoking mothers as far as these statistics are concerned.

Effects later in life
A survey of 17,000 children in the UK whose progress was followed from birth suggests that smoking through pregnancy may lead to an educational disadvantage for your child later in life. Among these children at age 11, those whose mothers had smoked through pregnancy tended to be several months behind the average in educational progress, and also slightly shorter than the children of non-smokers. The more cigarettes the mothers had smoked per day during pregnancy, the more marked these effects were.

Smoking 2

Smoking-related causes of death
When tobacco smoke is taken into the mouth, various chemicals are absorbed into the bloodstream through the mouth lining. These include nicotine, toxins (poisons) and carcinogens (cancer-inducing substances). The nicotine and toxins alter the blood vessels and heartbeat, increasing the likelihood of circulatory and heart disease. If the smoke is inhaled deeply, tar collects in the lungs and the cells lining the airways are destroyed, causing respiratory diseases.

Mortality before age 65
The diagram *right* illustrates the chances of dying before age 65 of male adult non-smokers (**A**) and male adults smoking 24 or more cigarettes per day (**B**). 18% of the non-smokers are likely to die before age 65, while 40% of the heavy smokers will not reach that age. For smokers of 1–23 cigarettes per day, the chances of death before age 65 will be between 18% and 40%; for smokers of considerably more than 24 per day, the chances of death will be considerably higher. For women the corresponding percentages are slightly lower, mainly because women tend to inhale less, and also to start smoking later in life.

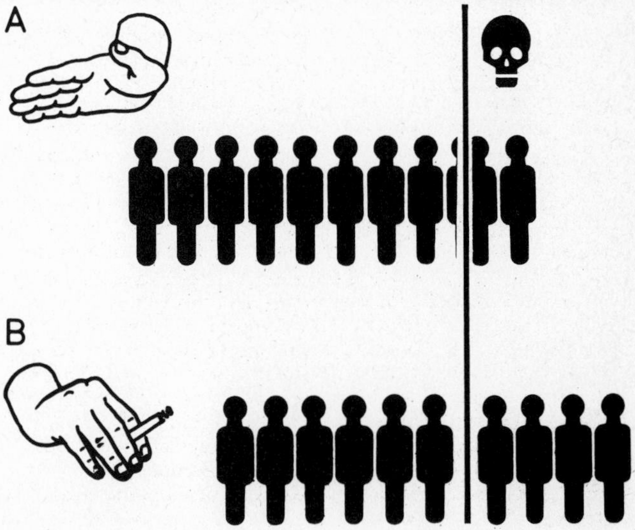

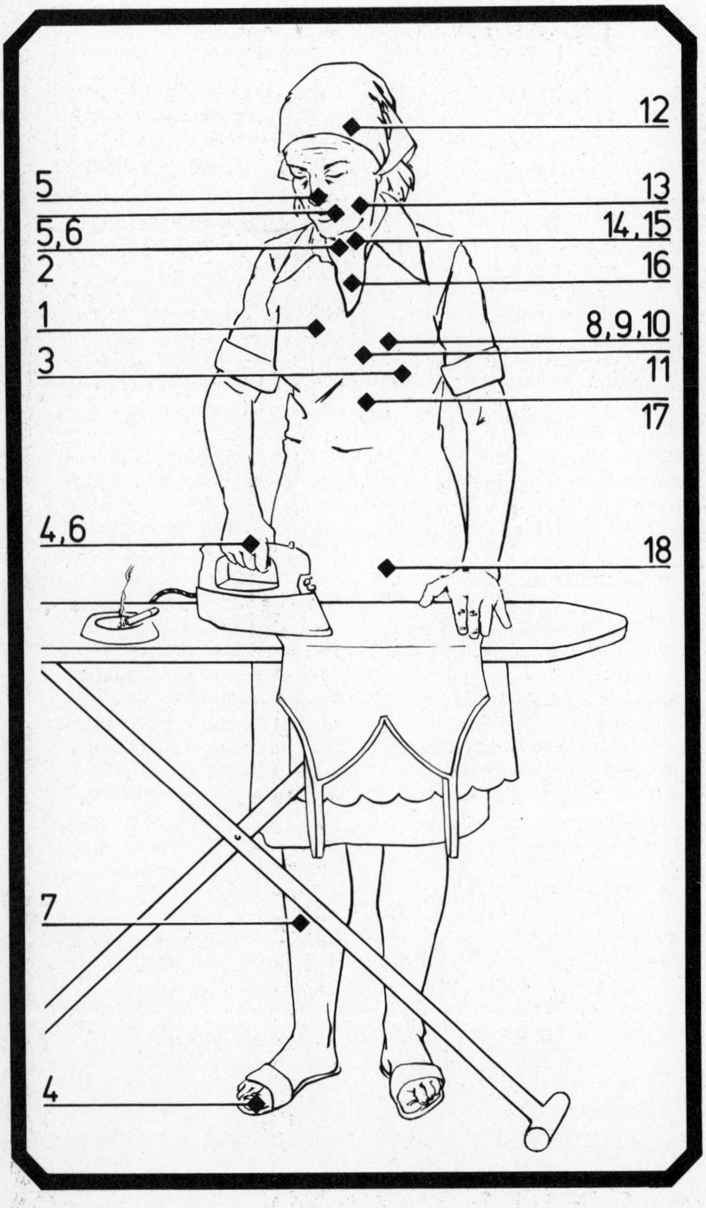

Unpleasant or disabling results of long-term smoking
Any or all of these symptoms may appear in long-term smokers.
1 Decreased lung efficiency caused by modification of the lung tissue; this makes exertion unpleasant or even dangerous.
2 Persistent cough, caused by the hypersecretion of mucus in response to the irritant constituents of the tobacco smoke. The mucus is at first clear, but later becomes purulent if infection occurs.
3 Permanently depressed appetite caused by the effect of nicotine on the autonomic nerve supply. This often leads to poor or inadequate nutrition among heavy smokers.
4 Severe circulatory problems in the hands and feet; people with peripheral vascular disease continue to smoke at their peril and often have to have limbs amputated.
5 Decreased senses of taste and smell caused by prolonged contact with tobacco smoke.
6 Discolored teeth and fingers from nicotine staining.
7 Varicose veins caused by decreased blood supply to the legs.

Potentially fatal results of long-term smoking
Long-term smokers run an increased risk of dying from each of the following diseases; in heavy smokers the risks are approximately double those of non-smokers.
8 Lung cancer, or more correctly cancer of the bronchus; only rarely is the actual lung tissue the site of the tumor.
9 Chronic bronchitis.
10 Emphysema.
11 Coronary artery disease.
12 Stroke.
13 Cancer of the cheek.
14 Cancer of the pharynx.
15 Cancer of the larynx.
16 Cancer of the esophagus.
17 Gastric or duodenal ulcer; this applies chiefly to men.
18 Cancer of the bladder; this also applies mainly to men.

As well as their increased risks from the diseases listed above, smokers are far more likely than non-smokers to die if they contract some of the more common diseases such as pneumonia, influenza, kidney disease and diabetes. Children brought up in a house in which the parents smoke are more likely to get chronic bronchitis than the children of non-smoking parents.

Individual attitudes
The dangers of smoking are nowadays widely publicized, especially as more diseases are found to be caused or aggravated by smoking, and individual smokers are increasingly aware of the damage they are doing their own bodies. Many of those who become concerned give up smoking totally; many others cut down their consumption, or change to a brand of cigarette that is lower in tar. Some people establish a no-smoking rule in their house, especially if a pregnant woman or a baby is part of the household, and it is becoming once again the rule to ask permission to smoke rather than taking it for granted.

Public attitudes
The results of recent research on the health and pollution dangers of smoking have led to public pressure for banning or reducing smoking in public areas. Smoking is forbidden in most food shops, especially where unwrapped food is sold, and in the kitchens of most restaurants. Many theaters and concert halls either ban smoking or have particular areas set aside for smokers, while public transport is usually divided into smoking and non-smoking areas. Various pressure groups are campaigning for still more stringent regulations, such as banning all smoking in hospitals or shopping areas.

Reasons for giving up
There are many reasons, covering a variety of considerations, for giving up smoking. Perhaps the most pressing reasons are medical; if you give up smoking, you reduce drastically your risks of developing many fatal or disabling diseases, especially those involving the lungs and circulation, and thus improve your life expectancy. You will feel fitter, be more able to exert yourself, and be more competent at sports. You will reduce the risk of harming your unborn child if you are pregnant, and children in your household will be less likely to develop respiratory diseases. Those around you who suffer from asthma or respiratory disorders will not have their conditions aggravated by your tobacco smoke, and you will also be reducing their risks of developing lung cancer.
Other factors are more social in emphasis. If you stop smoking your breath, clothes and hair will no longer smell of smoke, and your fingers and teeth will gradually lose their yellow tinge. The atmosphere in your home will not be clouded by tobacco smoke, and you will not be contributing to the pollution of the atmosphere. Your senses of smell and taste will improve considerably. In addition, you will save a great deal of money and earn a great deal of respect for your self-discipline.

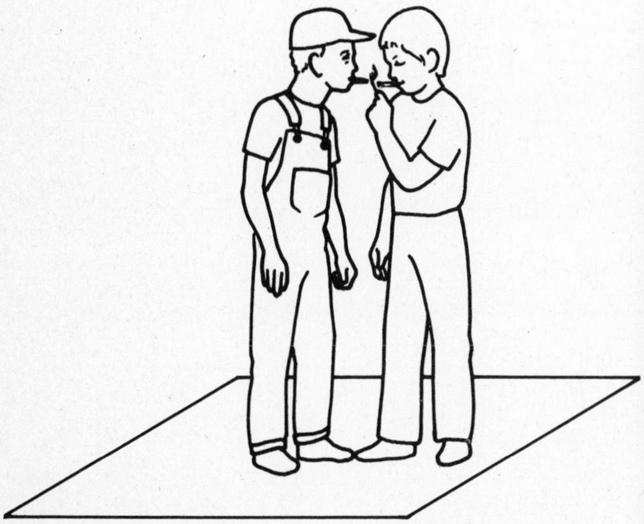

Why children smoke
Children who are brought up in families where they have the example of a parent or older sibling who smokes are very likely to start the habit themselves. Any person in authority who smokes, such as a teacher, doctor or minister, invites emulation from children who respect them. However, if you go too far in your condemnation of smoking, this may lead to rebellion on your child's part. Very often, smoking is associated by children with maturity, sophistication and sexual attractiveness — an image that is reinforced by advertising — and this is perhaps the main reason for juvenile smoking.

Discouraging children from smoking
Setting an example of non-smoking is one of the best ways of discouraging children from smoking; if they respect you, they will tend to follow your example. Children are unlikely to be greatly influenced by the threat of diseases that occur later in life, but if they are taught about the immediate effects of smoking on the lungs and circulation this may prove more effective. Environment-conscious children may well be concerned about the polluting effect of tobacco smoke on the atmosphere. Never offer a child a cigarette, and do not allow others to do so.

How to cut down
- Even if you find it impossible to give up smoking, there are various ways in which you can decrease the amounts of nicotine and tar to which your body is exposed.
- Smoke fewer cigarettes, cigars or pipes.
- Cut out first of all the "least vital" smokes, or set a time of day before which you cannot smoke and keep making it later.
- Change your daily routine so that situations where you smoked out of habit will no longer exist.
- Don't do anything else while you are smoking, such as reading, talking or working; this will help you think about why you are smoking each cigarette.
- Take fewer puffs per cigarette.
- Never leave a cigarette, cigar or pipe in your mouth for more than one puff.
- Leave the last third of any cigarette or cigar, as this is where the most tar collects.
- Change to filter tips if you smoke untipped at present.
- Change to a brand that is lower in tar than your present one.
- Use one of the special cigarette holders that help to filter out the tar.
- Aim to continue to cut down the number of smokes you have per day, setting yourself a fresh target each week.

How to give up
- If you plan to give up totally, it is probably better to do so all at once rather than to cut down slowly. Your body will get over its craving for nicotine more quickly, and it will be easier for you to refuse cigarettes if you can say you have given up.
- Think about the many reasons you have for giving up.
- Set a particular day for giving up, and smoke your last cigarette ceremoniously the night before; give away any spare cigarettes and your lighters etc.
- Tell as many people as possible, at home, at work and in your social life, so that it is hard to go back on your word.
- Change your routine so that you don't become bored.
- Save up your tobacco money for a particular luxury.
- If possible, give up with someone else for moral support.
- Join an anti-smoking clinic.
- Travel in non-smoking train cars and sit in non-smoking areas of theaters.
- Keep reminding yourself of the health benefits of giving up.
- If you smoked to relieve tension, learn other relaxation techniques.
- Chew gum if you need to have something in your mouth.
- Use nicotine tablets or gum for a few months if you find that your body cannot be instantly weaned away from nicotine.

Alcohol 1

Alcohol is an intoxicating drug known since ancient times. It has anesthetic properties and acts as a tranquilizer and a depressant; it induces mood changes not by acting as a stimulant, as many people think, but by depressing the part of the brain that controls impulsive behavior, judgment and memory. Alcohol in small quantities can be used effectively to ease tensions and overcome shyness, but heavy drinking can lead to alcoholism, fatal diseases and serious social problems such as traffic offenses, violence and marital strain. Here we look at the nature and effects of alcohol and suggest ways of preventing abuse and its serious consequences.

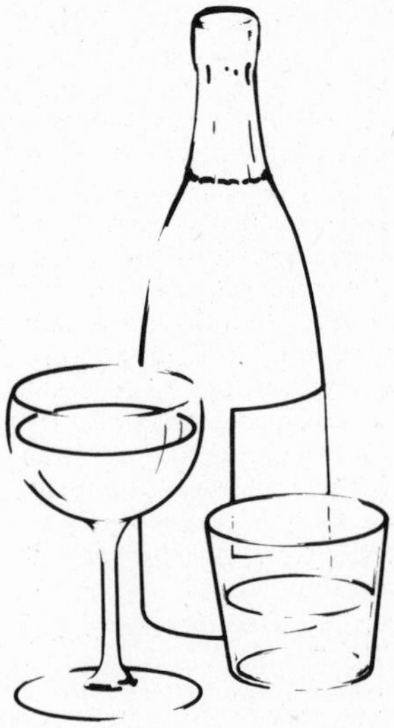

Contents of alcoholic drinks
Alcohol is prepared from a number of natural products including fruit, cereals and grain. Whiskeys are made from grain — usually barley, maize or rye — plus water and yeast. Wines are fermented grape juice; fermentation may be brought about by yeasts present in the "bloom" on the grapes, or specially cultured yeasts may be added to the juice. Some wines have sugar or sulfur dioxide added to them. Beer is brewed from malted barley, hops, sugar and yeast.
Most of the alcohol in drinks is ethanol, but other alcohols – known as congeners – are present in small quantities and may cause toxic symptoms.

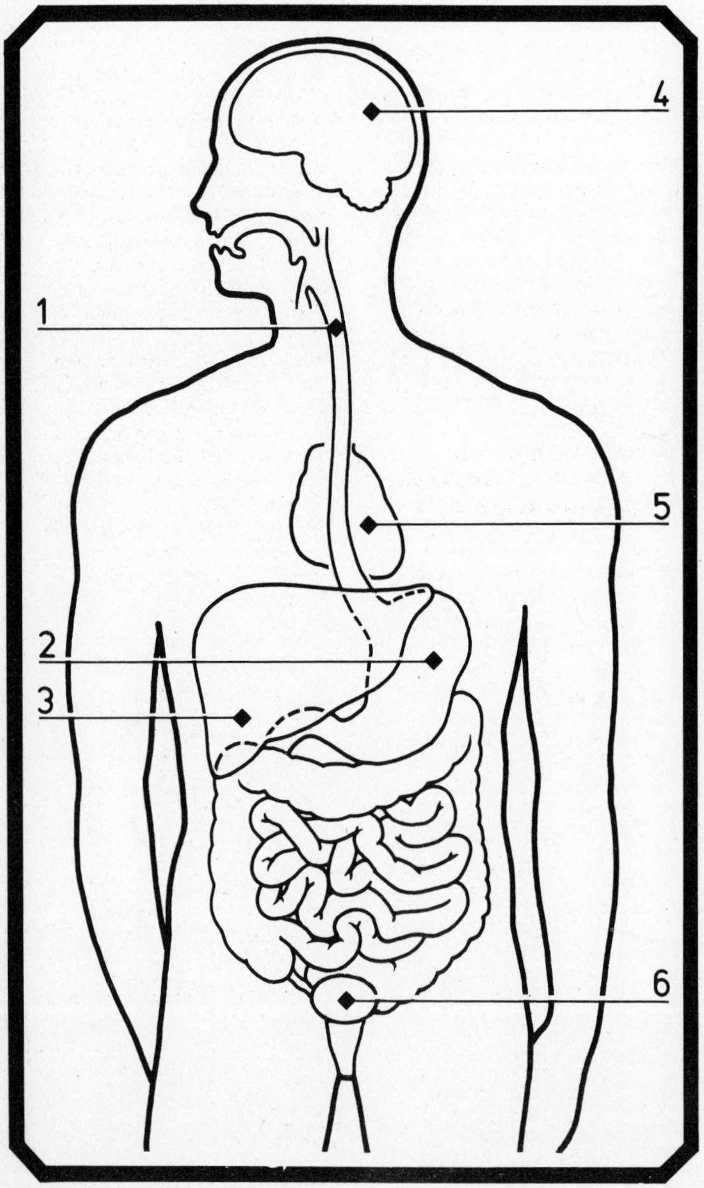

Immediate effects of alcohol
The diagram illustrates some of the parts of the body affected when a person drinks alcohol. These effects wear off gradually, but there could be lasting complications with continuous, heavy use of alcohol.

1 As alcohol passes through the mouth, throat and gullet it irritates the mucous membranes lining these passages and increases the secretion of saliva. Alcohol can be smelled on the breath.

2 Alcohol also irritates the lining of the stomach. Heavy drinking causes the stomach lining to become thickened and overactive; this leads to gastritis, with its symptoms of indigestion, retching and loss of appetite. Gastritis is often at its worst the morning after an evening's drinking; it may be impossible to eat or drink until midday or after.

3 Alcohol is absorbed from the stomach and intestines into the bloodstream, which carries it to the brain and other organs. In the liver alcohol is acted on by the enzyme alcohol dehydrogenase (ADH), which gradually metabolizes the alcohol and reduces the amount in the body.

4 The brain is the part of the body where alcohol exercises its main effects. Overt behavior is affected; this includes the retardation of such responses as perception, reaction time, the performance of motor tasks and skills, and the processes of learning, remembering, thinking, reasoning and problem-solving. Effects on emotional behavior produce such reactions as fear, anxiety, tension, hostility, goodwill and euphoria; these reactions vary with individuals and with the same person on different drinking occasions.

5 Alcohol often affects the cardiovascular system by increasing the heart rate and blood pressure, and dilating the blood vessels near the skin.

6 Alcohol removes body water by increasing the rate of urine formation; the urine contains considerable quantities of alcohol that have not been oxidized.

Spirits
Spirits are the strongest forms of alcoholic drink. They are manufactured by distilling brewed or fermented products so that liquids containing from 35-50% alcohol are recovered. The spirits in common use, such as gin, whiskey, vodka, rum, brandy and tequila, contain about 40% alcohol; a 1oz measure of spirits contains roughly 15mg of alcohol. Liqueurs, which are sweetened spirits with added flavorings, often contain still higher percentages of alcohol.

Wines
Wines are made by fermenting the juice of grapes or other fruits. Table wines, usually served with meals, have a natural alcohol content of roughly 9-12%. Other varieties such as sherry, port and muscatel are reinforced by the addition of distilled alcohol to bring their alcohol content up to as much as 18-22%; these drinks can be very intoxicating if several glasses are drunk in a short time. An average glass of wine (around 5oz) or an average measure of sherry (around 2½oz) contains roughly 15mg of alcohol.

Beers, ales, lagers, ciders
Beer and ale are derived from various cereals by brewing, and generally contain 3-6% alcohol; in strong ale, rough cider and barley wine this may rise to as much as 10%. Although many people consider that only spirits drinkers become alcoholics, the danger of alcoholism and cirrhosis of the liver is just as great for heavy beer and cider drinkers. Any man of average weight who drinks the equivalent of 4–5 pints of beer a day has a potential alcohol problem. Most beers contain around 30–35mg of alcohol per pint.

Alcohol in foodstuffs
Drinks that contain around 1% or less alcohol are sometimes treated in law as if they were nonalcoholic. The same is true for liqueur chocolates in which the amount of alcohol is similarly very small. Intoxication is impossible with these items as the sheer volume of food or drink would cause vomiting before the intoxicating level could be reached. Alcohol is also commonly used in cooking: meat may be cooked in wine, beer or cider, and brandy or sweet alcoholic drinks such as sherry and liqueurs are often included in luxury desserts.

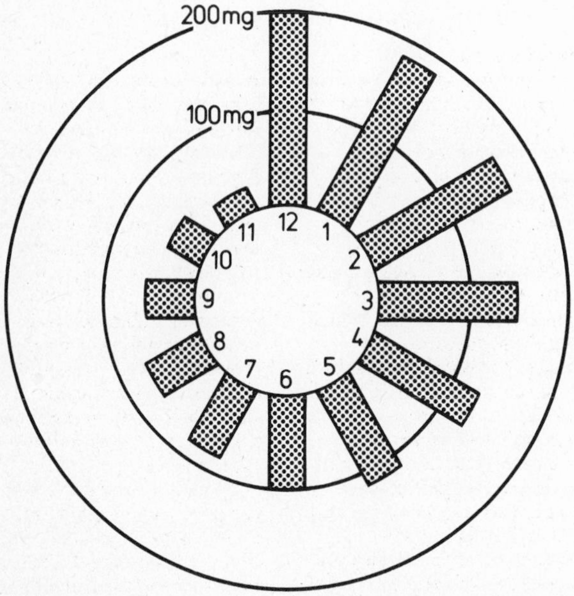

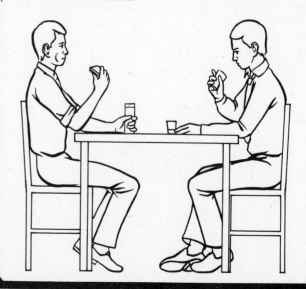

Blood alcohol level
An individual's blood alcohol level depends on a number of factors. Obviously the rate at which alcohol is consumed is important: the faster a person drinks, the faster he or she will become intoxicated. Other factors involve the rate of absorption. The alcohol in spirits is absorbed faster than that in beer or wine. Taking alcohol with a meal or on a full stomach reduces the rate of alcohol absorption, as do physical or mental exercise or a low body temperature. Also significant is a person's body weight: heavy people have lower blood alcohol levels than do lighter people after the same amount of drink in similar circumstances.

Reduction of blood alcohol level
More time is needed than most people realize to remove all alcohol from the bloodstream. The diagram *above* shows the effects of a heavy night's drinking on the bloodstream the following morning. If you go to bed at midnight with a blood alcohol level of 200mg your blood alcohol level would remain too high for you to drive legally in most places until about 7.30 next morning. Even up until midday you would be more likely than usual to have an accident as a result of your raised blood alcohol level.

Do
- Eat something or drink a glass of milk before drinking alcohol, or eat with your alcoholic drinks.
- Take care with unfamiliar drinks: they may be stronger than you think.
- Keep a careful count of the number of drinks you are having and don't exceed the number you know you can handle safely.
- Drink plenty of water before going to bed after an evening's drinking; this will help you to avoid a hangover.
- Respect alcohol and remember that it is potentially a dangerous and addictive drug.
- When in a large group, share costs of rounds as a way of avoiding the pressure on each person to contribute a round.

Don't
- Drink more than 90mg of alcohol in any one day, and don't drink this much habitually.
- Drink when you will be driving or using machinery.
- Drink when what you really need is rest, sleep or food.
- Drink if you are taking any form of medication that may react with alcohol.
- Drink alcohol to quench your thirst.
- Feel obliged to drink or feel embarrassed about ordering a nonalcoholic drink.
- Offer drinks to people who have obviously had enough.
- Force someone to have an alcoholic drink when they ask for a soft drink, or pretend that an alcoholic drink you have provided is nonalcoholic.

Alcohol 2

Problem drinking and alcoholism
The line between acceptable levels of alcohol intake and alcohol abuse is very difficult to define. Certainly, however, drinking has reached a problem level if it causes emotional, physical, social or financial problems, if it reduces the person's competence at work, if alcohol is taken instead of meals or specifically to produce oblivion, or if the person is physically or psychologically dependent on drink. Alcoholism is a condition in which a person with access to alcohol is unable to control the amount he drinks; problem drinking may be excessive, but the person remains in control of his own drinking habit.

Alcohol use in the USA
The diagrams *right* show the percentages of the population in three different age ranges who have ever used (**A**) or who currently use (**B**) alcohol. Over 50% of those in the 12–17 age range have at some time drunk alcohol, and over 30% of the people in that group are current users of alcohol, despite the fact that they are not old enough to purchase alcohol in most states. More people in the USA have tried alcohol, and more people are current users of alcohol, than any other drug (see p. 161).

1 Age 12–17
2 Age 18–25
3 Age 26+

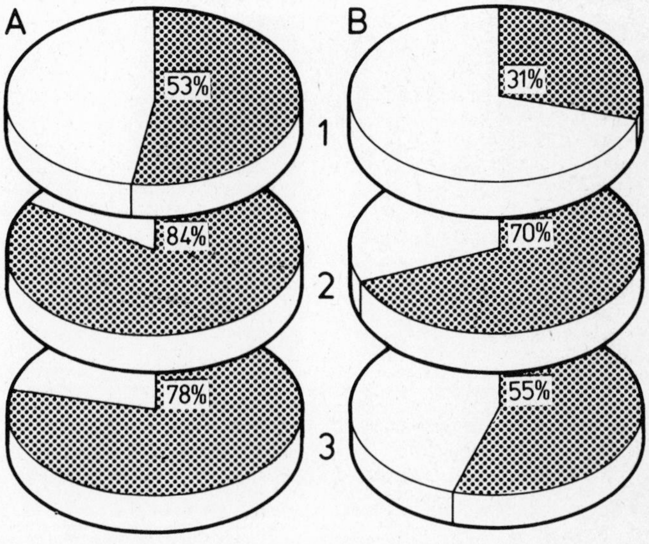

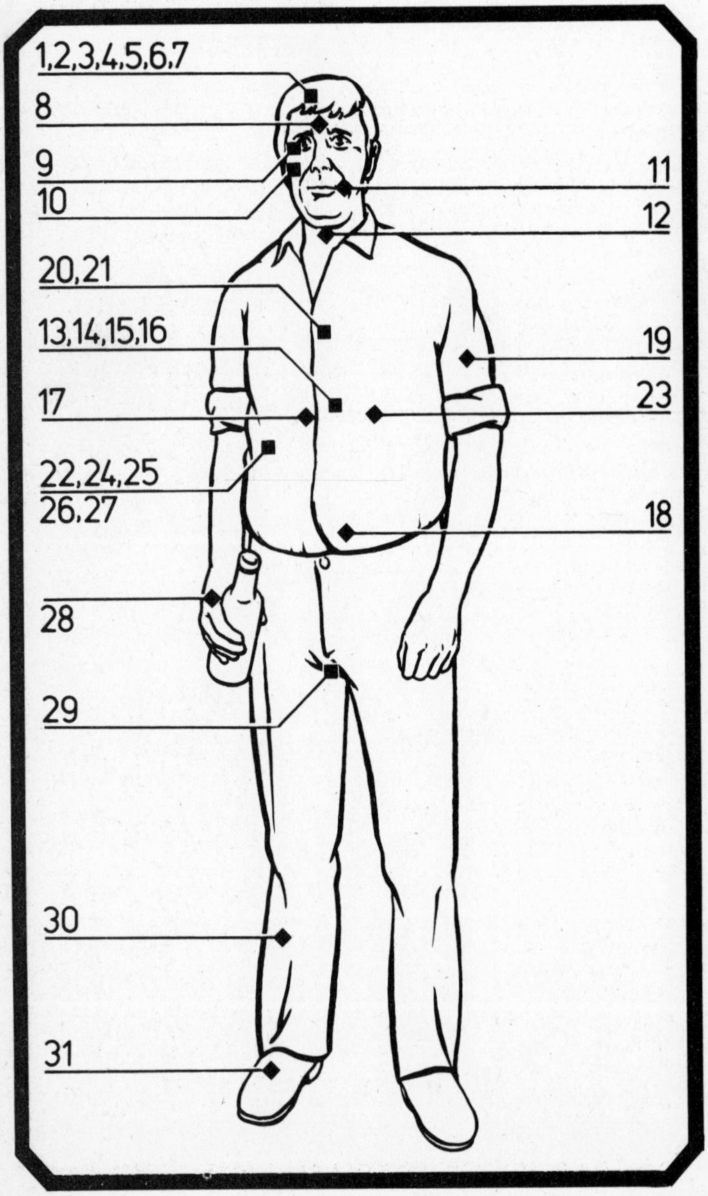

Effects of alcohol abuse
The following conditions may appear in a heavy drinker as direct or indirect results of excessive use of alcohol.
1 Alcoholism, a physical and psychological dependence on alcohol.
2 A frequent level of intoxication.
3 Persistent headaches.
4 Blackouts.
5 Epilepsy.
6 Brain damage or other injuries caused by falls when drunk.
7 Personality problems caused by dependency on alcohol.
8 Sweating, especially at night.
9 Anemia, caused by poor eating habits.
10 Facial flushing and enlargement of the blood vessels of the face.
11 Cancer of the mouth.
12 Cancer of the throat.
13 Permanent loss of appetite.
14 Vitamin deficiency or malnutrition.
15 Gastritis.
16 Gastric ulcer.
17 Duodenal ulcer.
18 Obesity, caused by the high calorie content of alcoholic drinks.
19 Hypertension or raised blood pressure.
20 Cardiac irregularities such as tachycardia and arrhythmia.
21 Cardiomyopathy, a disease of the heart muscle.
22 Gallstones.
23 Pancreatitis.
24 Fatty liver, an accumulation of fatty lipids in the cells.
25 Hepatitis.
26 Cirrhosis of the liver.
27 Primary liver cell cancer.
28 Delirium tremens (DTs), the physical shaking and mental distress that constitutes the withdrawal symptoms when alcohol is withheld from an alcoholic or someone who has recently had a heavy bout of drinking.
29 Impotence, caused by physical or psychological factors.
30 Varicose veins.
31 Gout.

An alcoholic or problem drinker is also likely to have a decreased capacity for work, to become violent, to commit traffic or sexual offenses, and to suffer from depression, loneliness, periodic self-disgust, and chronic lack of motivation.

Drink and finance
A tax on alcoholic drinks is a valuable source of revenue for many governments, but the economic cost of alcohol abuse is also considerable. Productivity is reduced through inefficiency, accidents or absenteeism; in addition, governments are obliged to spend more on health services and medical care, on research and public education, and on judicial proceedings following incidents resulting from intoxication. On a personal level, the family of an alcoholic often suffers financial hardship; the drinker may channel all the housekeeping money into drink, or his earning capacity may be seriously curtailed.

Drink and the family
Most people's first experiences of alcohol are in a family setting, and often the pattern of alcohol use (or abuse) will be repeated in future generations. The children of alcoholics tend to become alcoholics themselves, or to marry alcoholics, not so much because of an inherited tendency but because they have learned their attitude to drink from their parents. Marital stress or breakdown, sexual problems, violence, financial hardship, neglect and social alienation are problems that the family of an alcoholic often has to face; the alcoholic resents his family's hostility, and drowns his sorrows in yet more drink.

Drink and work
Drinking is an integral part of some occupations. Deals are often done over a drink in a bar, or in a restaurant over a meal complete with wine and liqueurs. Some jobs may require attendance at frequent parties and receptions. Senior executives and their wives, traveling salesmen and journalists are at particular risk. Other occupations, such as working in a bar or brewery, allow easy access to alcohol and carry a high risk of alcoholism, while people in the armed forces may be tempted to over-drink through loneliness or camaraderie. Alcoholics in all occupations have high records of accidents and absenteeism.

Drink and social life
Drinking is probably the most common social pastime in the Western world, and drink is often used as a "social lubricant" to help people to relax. Ironically, however, an addiction to alcohol that often starts with social drinking leads eventually to social alienation and rejection. The alcoholic is essentially a lonely person in his addiction, even when those around him are also drinking, and when drunk he invites laughter or contempt. Friends become reluctant to invite him to social gatherings because of his lack of self-control with drink, and this alienation may drive him once again to still more drinking.

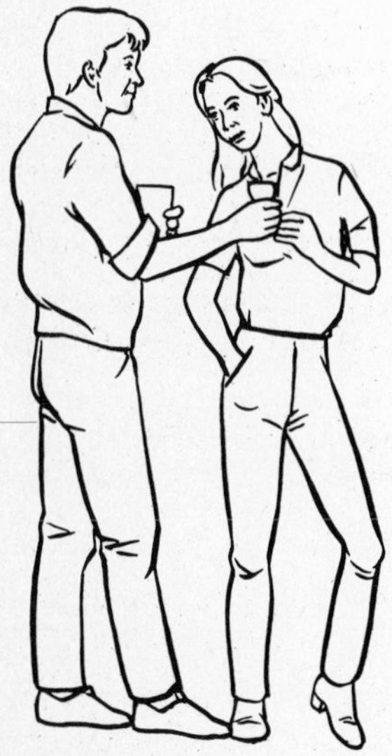

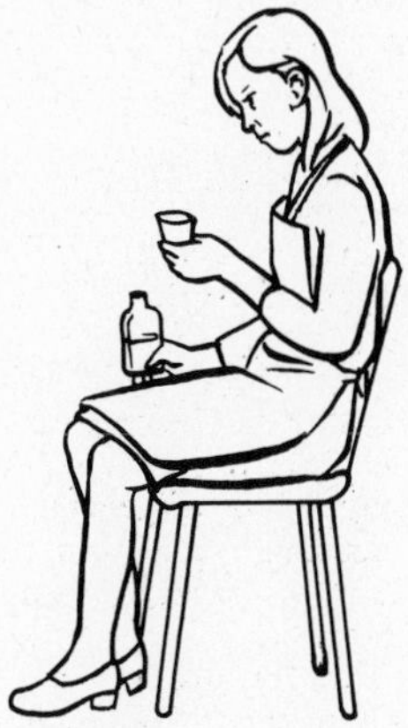

Danger times
Situations when alcohol abuse may begin to occur include the following. Young men in their teens or early 20s, seeking to prove their manhood, may spend too much time in bars and slip imperceptibly into a pattern of heavy drinking. Housewives who are alone a great deal or coping with a demanding family may turn to alcohol through boredom or frustration. Businessmen or career women under severe pressure may drink excessively to "unwind"; people facing a lonely old age, sudden unemployment or great emotional distress may turn to drink for comfort.

Attitudes to the alcoholic
The family of an alcoholic is often subjected to financial and emotional problems that tax their love and patience to the full. Happily, many societies now exist to help such families, and if you have an alcoholic in your family it will be invaluable to join one of these societies. Don't allow pride to prevent you from admitting that the problem exists; remember that the alcoholism is not your fault, and do not continue to cover up for the drinker's transgressions. It is possible for an alcoholic to build a new life, and he will need your help to relearn self-respect and self-control.

Danger signs
If you find yourself doing any of these things, examine your life carefully to see if you are in danger of alcohol abuse. If you are, or think you may be, seek the help of a doctor or an Alcoholics Anonymous group as soon as possible, for your own sake and your family's.

- Gulping drinks, or feeling that others drink too slowly.
- Looking for employment that offers opportunities for drinking.
- Finding yourself involved in frequent traffic offenses or car accidents.
- Having unexplained blackouts or periods of amnesia.
- Frequently expressing jealousy, aggression or resentment.
- Experiencing persistent depression.
- Taking a drink last thing at night, during the night, or first thing in the morning.
- Drinking in solitude.
- Drinking before attending a function.
- Experiencing persistent problems in your work or family that are related to your behavior.
- Inventing excuses for drinking.
- Giving up other activities in favor of drinking.
- Increasing your consumption of alcohol.
- Skipping meals in favor of drinking.
- Drinking for the relief of anger, insomnia, fatigue, depression or hunger.

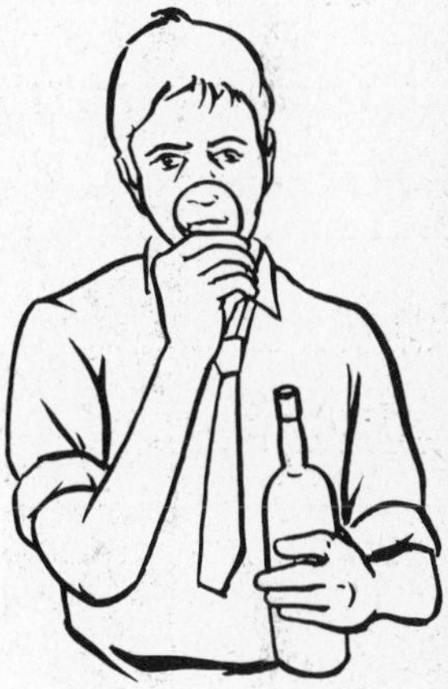

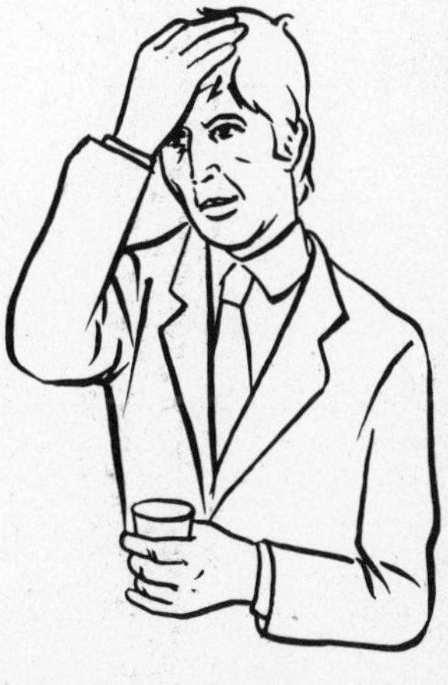

Drugs 1

Drugs are chemicals that act on the body to produce changes in the taker's physical or mental state. Drugs can be divided into three categories by availability. The first group comprises over-the-counter or nonprescription drugs. The second group consists of drugs recommended by a doctor and bought on his prescription, and the third group contains drugs that can only be obtained illegally. Drugs from all these groups, not only the third, can be over-used and cause health problems, and addiction can occur even with over-the-counter drugs. Here we look at the dangers of drug abuse and pinpoint situations that are likely to lead to over-use, showing you how to avoid those situations in your own life.

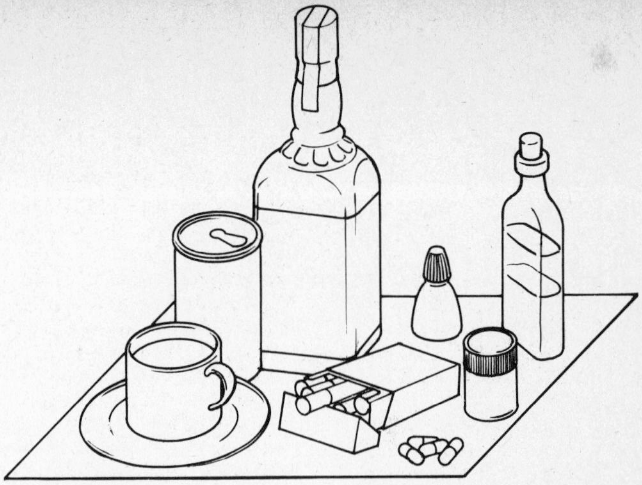

Everyday drugs
Drugs are contained in many preparations that are not always immediately associated with drug-taking. Alcohol and nicotine are drugs, and so is the caffeine in coffee, tea and cola. Additionally, most households also contain painkillers, laxatives, diarrhea medications, antacids, cough medicines and cold remedies, all of which are drugs. Even homeopathic medications are drugs; the difference is that they are naturally occurring materials rather them chemically manufactured ones.

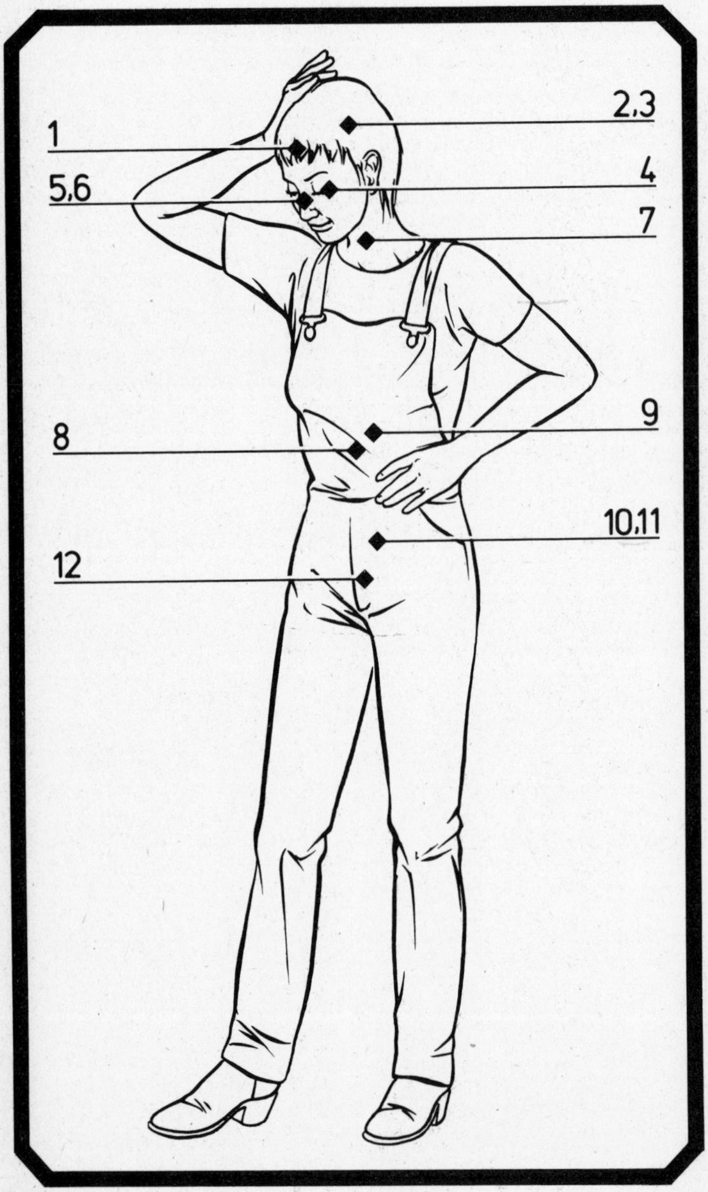

Use of over-the-counter drugs
Nonprescription or over-the-counter drugs are generally taken for the common conditions plotted on the diagram *left*. Over-use begins when the user takes the drugs daily as a "preventive" for those conditions, or takes the drug for its side-effects rather than to relieve pain or discomfort; physical dependence may soon follow.

1 Headache; this is perhaps the commonest reason for the use of nonprescription analgesics (painkillers) such as aspirin and acetaminophen.
2 Fatigue; overtiredness may well lead to the taking of stimulants, usually in the form of caffeine, or large doses of vitamins.
3 Insomnia; over-the-counter remedies usually contain antihistamines or analgesics.
4 Allergies; antihistamines are taken frequently to relieve troublesome symptoms.
5 Blocked nose; the decongestants taken for this condition constrict the blood vessels.
6 Cold; cold remedies contain analgesics, antihistamines, stimulants or decongestants, or a mixture of several.
7 Cough; many cough remedies – freely available in some countries but only with a prescription in the US – are based on codeine.
8 Overweight; appetite suppressants usually contain local anesthetics that numb the nerves of the mouth and stomach.
9 Indigestion; antacid remedies may contain salts of sodium, calcium, magnesium or aluminum.
10 Diarrhea; the drugs taken for this condition usually contain kaolin, aluminum or paregoric.
11 Constipation; laxatives are based on stimulants, salines, bulk-formers or lubricants.
12 Premenstrual discomfort; over-the-counter remedies often contain diuretics, analgesics and stimulants.

Prolonged use of drugs in this group, if they are taken regularly over several weeks or months, may lead, depending on the particular drug, to one or more of the following problems: digestive upsets, nausea and vomiting, kidney problems, constipation, loss of appetite, confusion (here used in its medical sense to describe a state of mental disorientation), headaches, and depletion of the necessary electrolytes, vitamins and fluid in the blood and body tissues. It is possible to become physically dependent on such drugs as laxatives and antihistamines as well as analgesics and anesthetic drugs; if the drug is stopped, withdrawal symptoms occur, but if the drug is continued it leads eventually to physical damage.

Fatigue and drug-taking
Overtiredness, lack of relaxation, and excessive working hours can lead to fatigue that sets in during the day. When this happens it can be tempting to take stimulants, which speed up the body's responses and make it more capable of activity and alertness. It is then difficult to slow the body down sufficiently to relax or to sleep properly, and when the effect of the drug wears off it can leave the body feeling even more drained than before. Even more stimulant is then required to wake it up the next time, and it is easy to fall into a pattern of increasing dependence.

Insomnia and drug-taking
Sleeplessness is usually the result of a body that is too tense or too active for sleep to come easily. This can be brought about by constant worry; by too much activity and insufficient relaxation during the day; by too much of a stimulant, such as caffeine, in the body; by eating a rich or heavy meal late at night; or by adverse sleeping conditions such as cold or discomfort. However, the drugs that are used to relax the body artificially do not produce a healthy sleep, and lead to depression as they wear off; the body then requires a stimulant, which makes sleep difficult the following night, and a vicious circle is created.

Headaches and drug-taking
Headaches can be caused by numerous different conditions, but perhaps the most common one is stress of some sort. The body becomes tense, which places strain on the muscles of the back and neck; lack of exercise aggravates the problem, and the pain is deferred to the head, causing a throbbing or stabbing pain. The easy way to relieve the symptoms is by taking an analgesic or painkiller, but when the effect of this wears off the headache will often return, as the root cause has not been dealt with. More analgesic is taken, and meanwhile stress is increased by the persistent headache.

Constipation and drug-taking
Constipation, like a headache, is generally a symptom rather than a complaint in itself. Laxatives may be taken that temporarily ease the problem, but the root cause, which is usually dietary, still remains. In addition, most laxatives work by irritating the colon, but over-use causes the muscles of the colon to weaken and eventually renders them incapable of functioning at all. The colon then becomes dependent on laxatives for its evacuation, and cannot work without them; if the laxatives are not taken, chronic and serious constipation results.

Contributory factors
The illustrations show some of the everyday situations that may contribute to stress, fatigue, insomnia and headaches. Avoidance of these, and similar, situations will lead to a healthier lifestyle and reduce the need for frequent consumption of everyday drugs.
1 Constant demands on your time can lead to stress.
2 Persistent worry and poor eating habits are contributory factors in insomia.
3 Working long hours without a break will cause tension and fatigue.
4 Reading or doing detailed work in a poor light may cause eye strain and headaches.

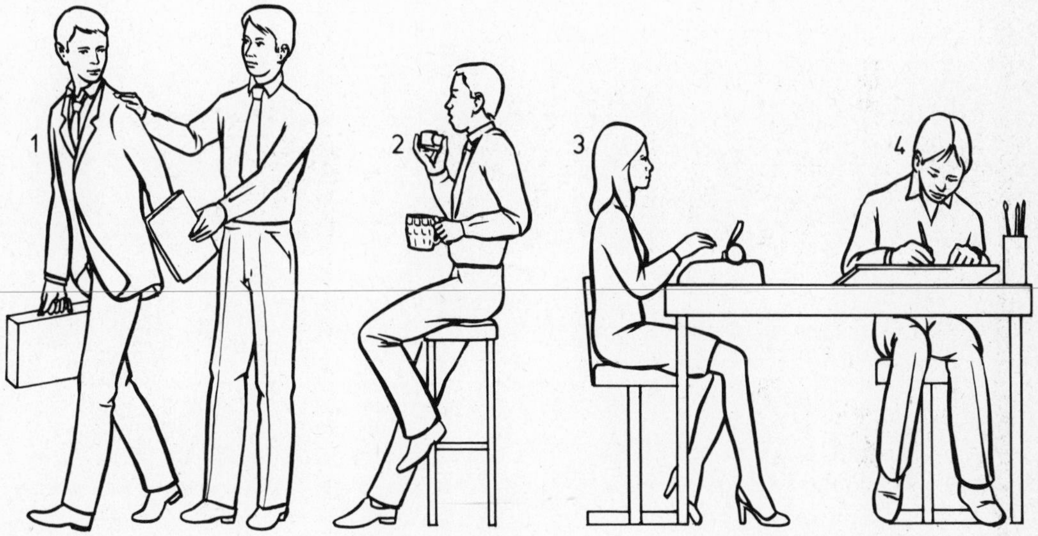

Avoiding fatigue
A busy life is the main enemy of the person prone to fatigue; even if you enjoy your occupation greatly you need a rest from the stresses and strains of long working hours. Make sure that you have some time completely alone every day so that you can relax from the demands of those around you; use this time to catch up on your sleep if necessary, or to pursue your own interests and hobbies. In this way, you will give both your body and your mind a rest and will not feel so fatigued. Do not take on more than you can easily cope with, and don't do things that other people could easily do for you.

Avoiding insomnia
Some of the factors that contribute to insomnia can be solved by minor changes in your sleeping habits. Your bedroom should be warm (not hot), and your bed and nightclothes should be comfortable. Discomfort of any sort is likely to keep you awake; you should not go to bed hungry or with a full bladder, and you should be relaxed. If worry tends to keep you awake, try to analyze the cause of the worry and either deal with the cause or learn to relax yourself so that you can leave the worry behind at night. If you cannot get to sleep, read or watch TV until you feel tired, or have a soothing warm drink.

Avoiding headaches
Since stress is one of the major causes of headaches, the avoidance of stress or at least the treatment of its symptoms plays a large part in headache therapy. Exercise not only removes you from stressful work situations but also relaxes the muscles of your back and neck that tend to stiffen and cause headaches; massage and warmth are also beneficial to these muscles. Avoid rooms that are stuffy, dry or smoky, or where strong chemicals are used; go out into the fresh air as often as possible. Cold compresses, rest, darkness and quiet are healthy treatments for headaches since they help to remove the causes.

Avoiding constipation
Since constipation nearly always reflects poor dietary habits, an improvement in the diet is far more effective than simply relieving the symptom by the use of a laxative. The usual cause of constipation is insufficient fiber in the diet. Fiber, or roughage, is found in whole grain breads and cereals and in fruit and vegetables, particularly if they are raw. These should be included as a natural part of the daily diet, and refined foods such as sugar and white flour should be avoided. If immediate relief is required, an enema is preferable to a chemical laxative so that the bowel does not become dependent on laxatives.

Drugs 2

Warning signs
Any drug can be dangerous if taken too often or in too large a dose, and so it is well worth examining your own use of common nonprescription drugs so that you become aware of any tendency to over-use them. Here we list some of the common warning signs.

- Finding that you need a cigarette, drink or pill to enable you to face the day.
- Using analgesics as preventives by taking them when you have no symptoms.
- Never leaving the house without a supply of drugs.
- Continuing to take a drug even against medical advice.
- Having a drink, cigarette, cup of tea or coffee, pill or dose of medicine at regular intervals throughout the day because you feel you cannot do without them.
- Having supplies of medication in several rooms of the house.
- Being unwilling to admit how frequently you take medication.
- Mixing several drugs to increase or heighten the effects of each.
- Taking a drug purely for its side-effects rather than to relieve symptoms.
- Feeling unable to sleep without a drink, cigarette or tablet to settle you.

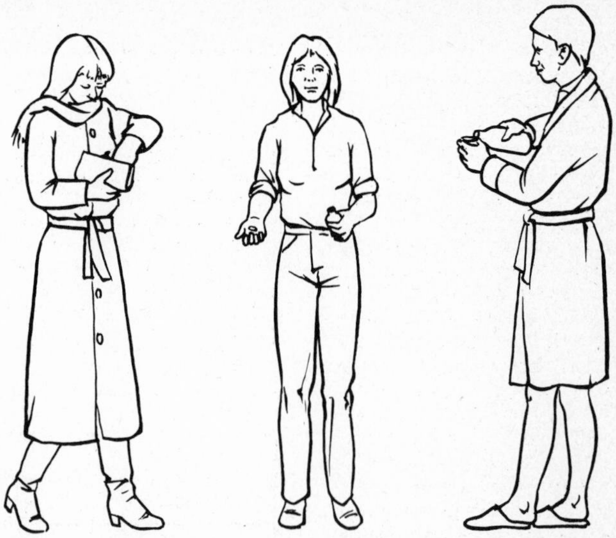

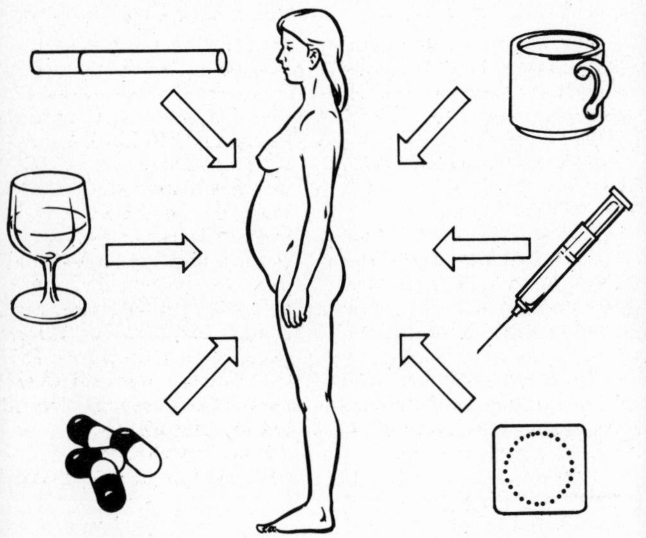

Pregnancy and drugs
There are many drugs that are capable of crossing the placenta and affecting the unborn child. These effects may be temporary, such as causing stimulation to the fetus, or they may be permanent, such as those that cause birth defects in the fetus. Some of the common prescription and nonprescription drugs that may affect the fetus include aspirin, sleeping pills, caffeine, antihistamines, thyroid drugs, tranquilizers, the antibiotics streptomycin and tetracycline, androgen hormones, the contraceptive pill, anticoagulants, alcohol, and tobacco. The fetus can also be affected by many of the illegal drugs, such as LSD and other psychedelics, cocaine, amphetamines, morphine and heroin. If the mother is addicted to hard drugs and has taken a dose within 24 hours before delivery, the baby may have to undergo withdrawal symptoms after birth or may require a complete blood transfusion. Some vaccines and general anesthetics may also affect the fetus. Always tell your doctor and dentist if you are pregnant or suspect that you might be; never take any drugs at all, even analgesics and cold remedies, during pregnancy without consulting your doctor and receiving his advice.

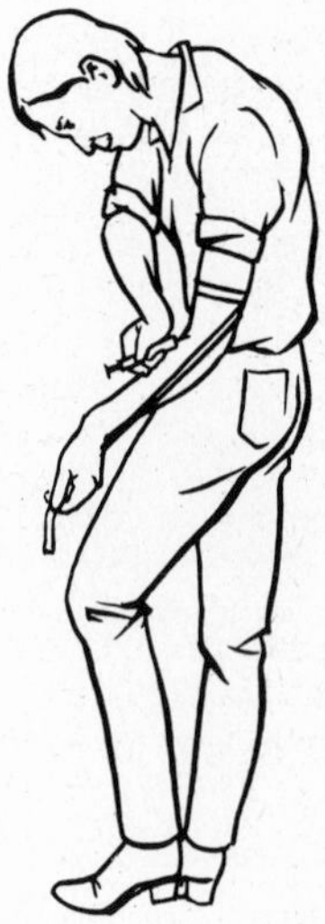

Drug users
There is no stereotype for the person who uses drugs for non-medical reasons. Some people find that they have unknowingly become dependent on a drug that they have been prescribed for medical reasons, for instance sleeping pills or appetite depressants, so that they begin to take the drug purely for its side-effects or to avoid withdrawal symptoms. Other people take drugs simply because they enjoy the sensations produced. Adolescents may experiment with drugs as part of their search for new experiences or in an attempt to conform to their peer group. People whose occupations necessitate erratic working hours, such as airline staff or those in the medical profession, may find that their metabolisms and sleeping patterns are disturbed; this may lead to overuse of drugs to combat these effects. People with problems such as severe shyness or a sense of inferiority may take drugs to give themselves false confidence, and drugs may also be used as a way of escaping from emotional, professional or financial worries.

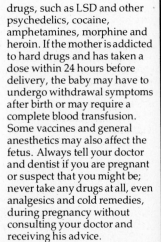

Drug use
The chart *right* shows the percentage of the US population in three different age groups who have ever used or who are currently using various drugs. The portion of the population who are at present in the 18–25 age range shows substantially higher figures for both past and present use of each type of drug than the other two age ranges, followed by the 12–17 age range. Considering that the third age group contains all those people from age 26 into old age, the figures suggest both that drugs have become more readily available in recent years, and that social disapprobation of their use has waned.

Drug	Age 12–17		Age 18–25		Age 26 or over	
	Ever used	Current user	Ever used	Current user	Ever used	Current user
Cannabis and/or hashish	28.2%	16.1%	60.1%	27.7%	15.4%	3.2%
Inhalants	9.0	0.7	11.2	x	1.8	x
Hallucinogens	4.6	1.6	19.8	2.0	2.6	x
Cocaine	4.0	1.0	19.1	3.7	2.6	x
Heroin	1.1	x	3.6	x	0.8	x
Other opiates	6.1	0.6	13.5	1.0	2.8	x
Stimulants*	5.2	1.3	21.2	2.5	4.7	0.6
Sedatives*	3.1	0.8	18.4	2.8	2.8	x
Tranquilizers*	3.8	0.7	13.4	2.4	2.6	x
*=prescription drugs	x=<0.5%					

Recreational drug use
Recreational drug use involves taking a drug (or drugs) for non-medical reasons— for example for its pleasant effects or as a social activity. Some drugs used recreationally are widely available, for instance many inhalants; others are legally available only on prescription. Many recreational drugs are illegal in most countries. Drugs may be taken to depress or stimulate nervous activity, or because they produce pleasurable physical or mental sensations; some drugs induce hallucinations or extraordinary sensations. Here we describe the main types of drugs and their effects.

Cannabis
Cannabis, or marihuana, is probably the most widely-used recreational drug. Cannabis is generally taken by smoking the chopped, dried leaves, but the leaves can also be eaten or made into an infusion. Cannabis resin (hashish) is a substance that is scraped off the leaves of the plants, and eaten, or mixed with tobacco and smoked. Cannabis produces a feeling of relaxation and cheerfulness, and tends to heighten sensory perception. Its physical effects include lowered blood pressure, reddening of the eyes, and increased pulse rate. It is not considered to be addictive.

Inhalants
Inhalants are drugs used by sniffing them in a concentrated form. Most of the commonly-used inhalants are everyday substances, including some glues, paints, cleaning fluids, and solvents such as nail polish remover. The inhalants usually produce dreamy feelings of wellbeing. Side-effects include headache, nausea, and in large doses blackout. Long-term use may lead to anemia, liver damage, and heart failure. There is also a danger of suffocation after blackout, as the inhalants are often sniffed from plastic bags or rags soaked in fluid. Inhalants are not addictive, but tolerance develops, requiring increasing doses to maintain the effects.

Hallucinogens
LSD is the most widely known of the hallucinogenic drugs; others are psilocybin, found in certain fungi, and mescaline, found in some cacti. Cannabis is a very mild hallucinogen. LSD can be sniffed or injected, but mainly it is taken orally. LSD tends to heighten the mental state of the user and so can produce mystical euphoria or terror and distress. Physical side-effects include increases in heart rate and blood pressure, and dilation of the pupils. The user feels little desire to eat or sleep. LSD is not considered to be physically addictive, although psychological addiction is certainly possible.

Stimulants
Stimulant drugs include nicotine (see pp.152–155), caffeine, amphetamines and cocaine. Stimulants subdue feelings of tiredness and increase feelings of wellbeing. Amphetamine (speed) can be sniffed, eaten, diluted and injected, or mixed with tobacco and smoked. In large doses amphetamine produces inability to sleep, confusion and irritability. Cocaine is usually sniffed; prolonged use damages the nasal membranes, and overdose may cause death. Stimulants are not physically addictive, but may produce psychological dependence.

Opiates
Opiate drugs are derived from the opium poppy, and include codeine, opium, morphine and heroin. The drugs have been extensively used as analgesics in the past, but use is limited today because of the dangers of addiction. The opiates produce feelings of drowsy euphoria and contentment. Side-effects may include nausea and vomiting. Long-term usage produces constipation, reductions in appetite and libido, and, in women, disturbed menstruation. The opiates are physically addictive, and withdrawal symptoms may range from minor physical disturbance to sweats, vomiting, cramps and personality instability.

Barbiturates
Barbiturate drugs depress the central nervous system, producing feelings of pleasant languor. They are frequently prescribed as sleeping pills in capsule form; when used recreationally the capsules may be taken orally, or diluted and injected. Barbiturates are highly addictive, and withdrawal symptoms are severe and potentially fatal. The fatal dose of barbiturates is fairly small, and accidental overdose, particularly when the drugs are taken with alcohol, is more common than with other drugs.

Tranquilizers
The two main types of tranquilizer prescribed in the Western world are Librium (chlordiazepoxide) and Valium (diazepam). Tranquilizers are used to relieve tension and anxiety, and produce feelings of relaxation. Side-effects include drowsiness and confusion, and reduced libido. Although tranquilizers are less potent than barbiturates, it is still possible to take an overdose, particularly if the drugs are combined with alcohol. Continued use of tranquilizers may lead to dependence.

Cancer 1

Cancer in humans is a group of over one hundred diseases that may arise in any of the body's tissues. If unchecked, cancer cells can spread throughout the body and destroy it, but in many cases the diseases need not be fatal if treated early. There has been steady progress in recent years in the understanding of the malignancies and of ways to cope with them. The reason why normal cells are transformed into cancer cells in certain people is not known, but some substances (carcinogens) which trigger off the disease have been identified. In the USA cancer deaths have risen from 6% of deaths in 1900 to 20% in 1969. Medical authorities believe that this figure could be dramatically reduced if people knew more about recognizing cancer symptoms.

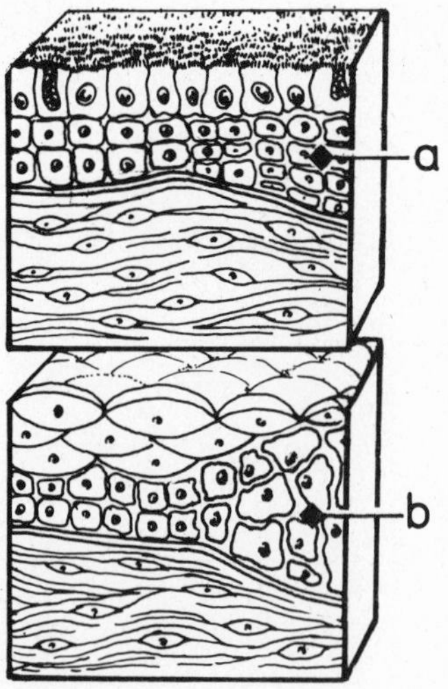

The nature of cancer
Cancer is a disturbance of normal cell growth. Under normal circumstances cell growth is controlled so that cells reproduce themselves only at a rate fast enough to replace cells that are dying (**a**). Where cancer cells are concerned, growth is unregulated. A single cell reproduces itself until there are a large number of cells which eventually give rise to a tumor (**b**), although not all tumors are malignant or cancerous. The growth is at the expense of the parent organ. Cancer cells can spread and invade surrounding tissue. They can break off and float via the bloodstream to other parts of the body and produce secondary growths.

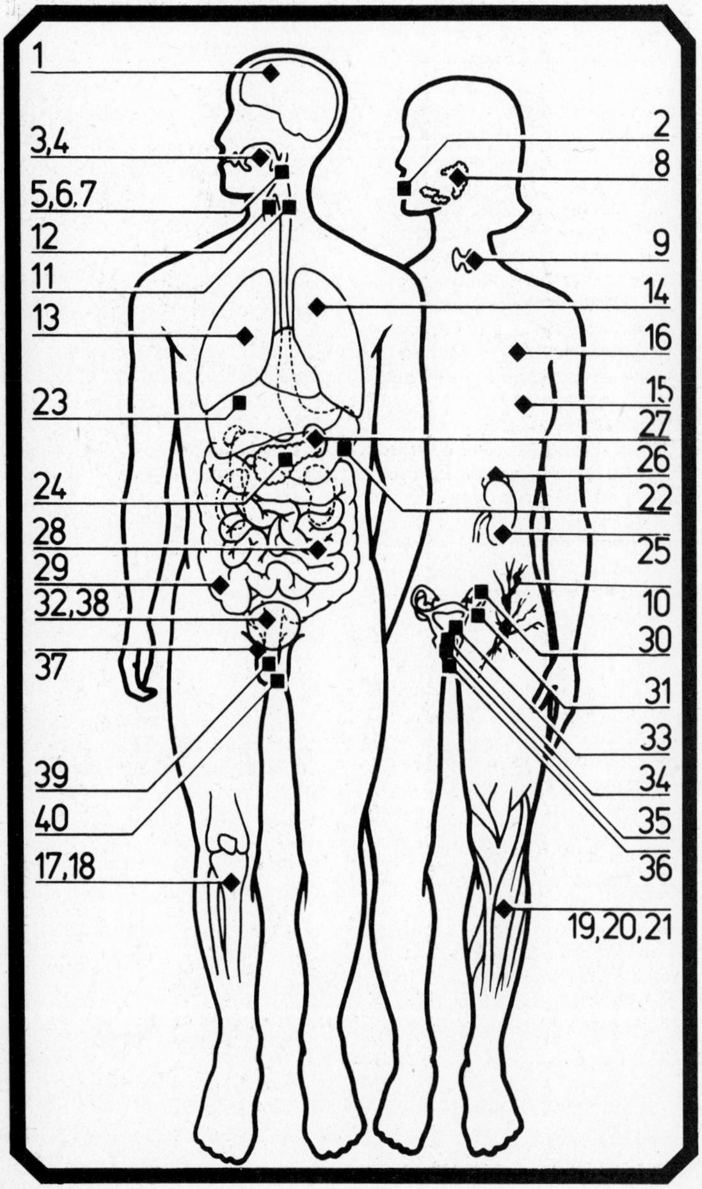

Sites of cancer
Cancer may arise in any of the body's tissues; we list the main sites.

1 Brain.
2 Lip.
3 Tongue.
4 Mouth.
5 Pharynx.
6 Throat.
7 Larynx.
8 Salivary glands.
9 Thyroid gland.
10 Lymph nodes.
11 Esophagus.
12 Trachea.
13 Bronchus.
14 Lung.
15 Breast.
16 Skin.
17 Bone marrow.
18 Blood.
19 Skeletal muscle.
20 Cartilage.
21 Nerve tissue.
22 Stomach.
23 Liver.
24 Pancreas.
25 Kidney.
26 Adrenal glands.
27 Spleen.
28 Small intestine.
29 Large intestine.
30 Ovaries.
31 Fallopian tubes.
32 Bladder.
33 Uterus.
34 Cervix.
35 Vagina.
36 Vulva.
37 Rectum and anus.
38 Prostate.
39 Penis.
40 Testes.

Deaths from cancer
In 1900 cancer was the seventh main cause of death in the USA. Today it is the second. Some people believe that this is because people are living longer and the likelihood of cancerous growths increases with age. But while there was little hope of a cure for patients at the turn of the century, now more than 35% of all cancer patients in the USA live at least 5 years after the illness is diagnosed and treated. The chart *right* shows the number of deaths from various cancers in the USA during 1979.

a Buccal cavity, pharynx and larynx.
b Esophagus.
c Lung, trachea and bronchus.
d Breast.
e Lymphatic and related tissue.
f Stomach.
g Leukemia.
h Intestine and rectum.
i Uterus and cervix.
j Skin.
k Prostate.
l Bone.

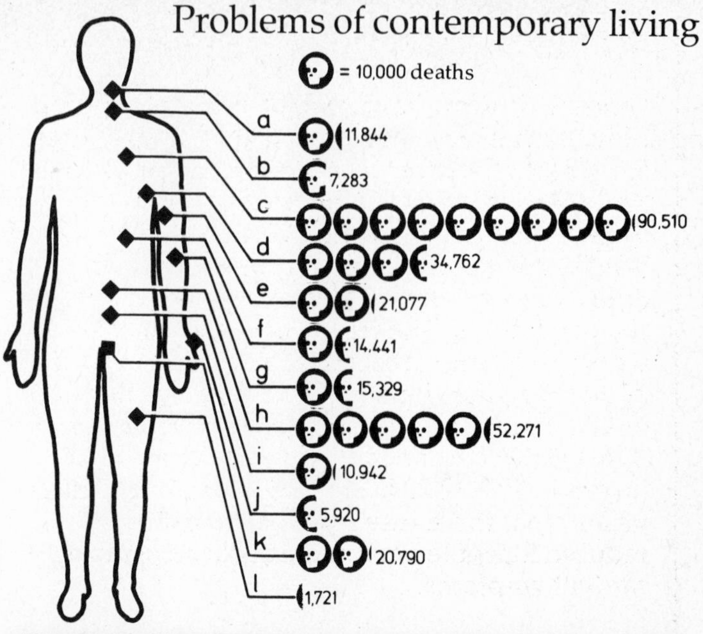

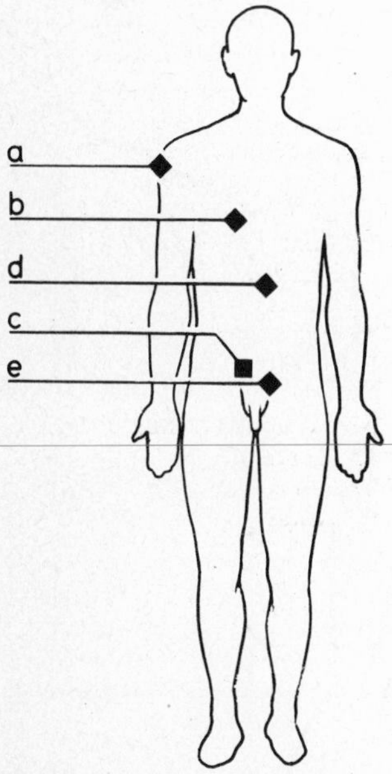

Most common sites in men
After 55, men have higher overall incidence of cancer than women. The most common cancer sites among men are the skin (**a**), lungs (**b**), colon (**c**) digestive system (**d**) and prostate (**e**). Lung cancer now kills 14 times as many men as it did in 1935. Men have more cancer than women in sites common to both sexes. This difference may be due to greater exposure of men to environmental cancer-producing agents or to greater genetic susceptibility.

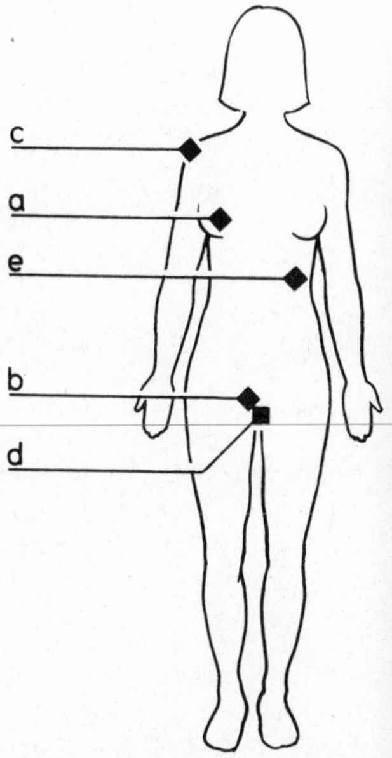

Most common sites in women
The incidence of all cancers in women exceeds that of men until the age of 55. The figure reflects the high incidence of cancers that attack the breast (**a**) and genital organs (**b**), which are the most common sites of cancer in women. Cancer of the breast most frequently strikes women between the ages of 40 and 60. It accounts for about 20% of all cancers in women and affects one in 18 women. Cancer of the cervix occurs in 1% of women usually between the ages of 45 and 50. The other most common sites in women are the skin (**c**), the rectum (**d**) and the other parts of the digestive system (**e**).

Known carcinogens
Several hundred chemicals are now known to possess carcinogenic (cancer-causing) properties. We list some of them.

- Tobacco smoke, which contains at least 16 carcinogens.
- Certain pesticides (now removed from the market).
- Hydrocarbons and other chemicals in the air from industrial waste, automobile exhaust and household waste.
- Some low-calorie sweeteners.
- Certain ingredients in some birth control pills.
- Aflatoxins – products of the food mold Aspergillus flavus.
- Ultraviolet rays of the sun.
- Ionizing radiation from X-ray, radium and other radioactive material encountered in industry and the general environment.

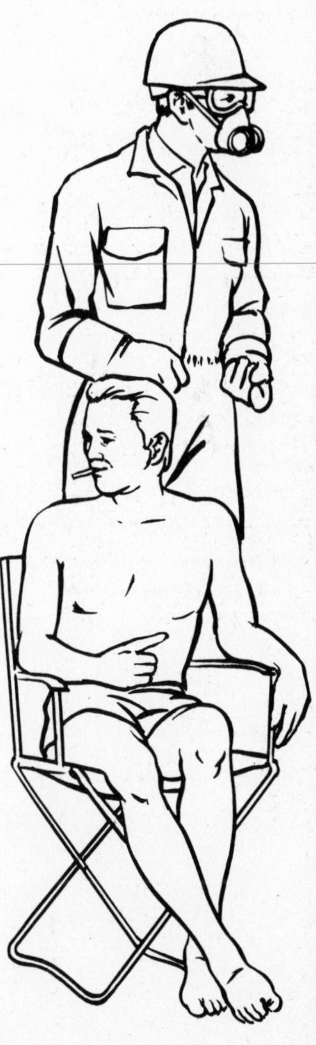

Workers in industries using the following chemicals are thought to be at risk from developing cancer.

- Coal tar and its derivatives – pitch, tar oils and creosote.
- Arsenic.
- Asbestos.
- Beta-naphthylamine used in the manufacture of synthetic dye.
- Chromates, iron oxide and dimethylnitrosamine used in drugs and rocket fuel.
- Petroleum.
- Benzene.

Cancer 2

Some cancers can be treated more successfully than others, often depending on the site. Cervical cancer can be detected in the early stages and cured, but lung cancer is usually diagnosed too late for successful treatment. Surgery and radiotherapy are the main forms of treatment, but both methods usually remove some normal tissue. Major advances have also been made in the restoration of structures altered by cancer and in the rehabilitation of patients who have undergone radical surgery. The use of drugs is becoming increasingly important although these are often used with other forms of treatment. Hormone therapy is also used in some cases. Here we examine the methods available and the types of cancer that might benefit from their use.

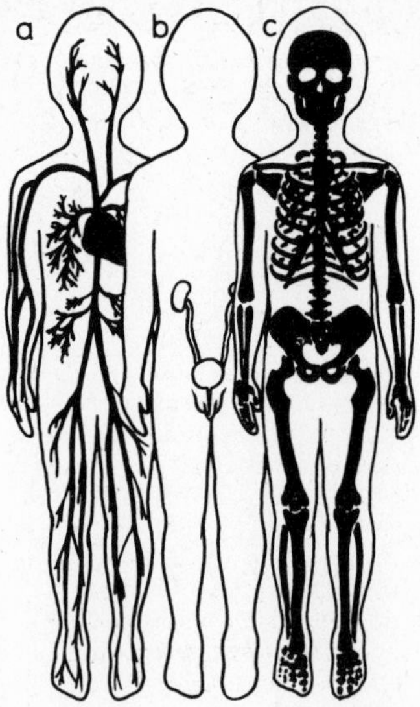

Cancer in children
The number of cases of cancer in children is small compared to those in adults and is generally confined to 3 types – leukemia (**a**), Wilm's tumor, a cancer of the kidney (**b**), and sarcomata, which often occur in the bones (**c**). Leukemia is the most common. It affects the bone marrow which produces blood corpuscles. The result is a shortage of red blood corpuscles and a large number of white corpuscles. Patients may become tired, pale and anemic, and they may be particularly prone to infection. Other symptoms include diarrhea, swollen feet and ankles, and hemorrhage.

Breast self-examination
The breasts should be examined once a month, after a period or on a particular date each month. You are looking for a change in the size, shape or color of the breast or nipple, puckering of the skin, lumps, alterations in outline, and any bleeding or unusual discharge from the nipple.

1 Sit naked in front of a mirror and observe your breasts first with arms at your sides and then raised.

2 Lie down on a bed or sit back in the bath. A pillow under the shoulder will help to spread the tissues.

3 Place your left hand under your head, keeping the elbow flat. With the flat of the fingers of your right hand, gently but firmly examine the top inner quarter of the breast working from the ribs and breastbone toward the nipple.

4 Examine the lower inner quarter of the breast, paying particular attention to the area around the nipple.

5 Examine the lower outer quarter, starting from the ribs below and at the side of the breast.

6 With your left arm at your side, examine the upper outer quarter.

7 Examine the armpit.

8 Repeat the procedure for the right breast.

If you discover anything unusual, see your doctor immediately.

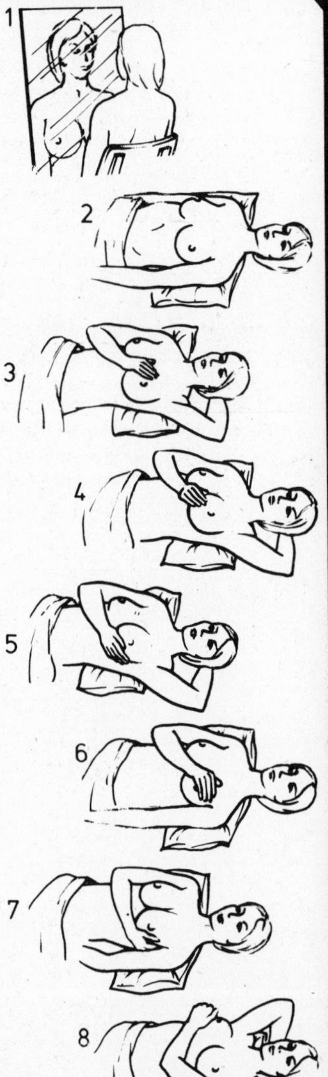

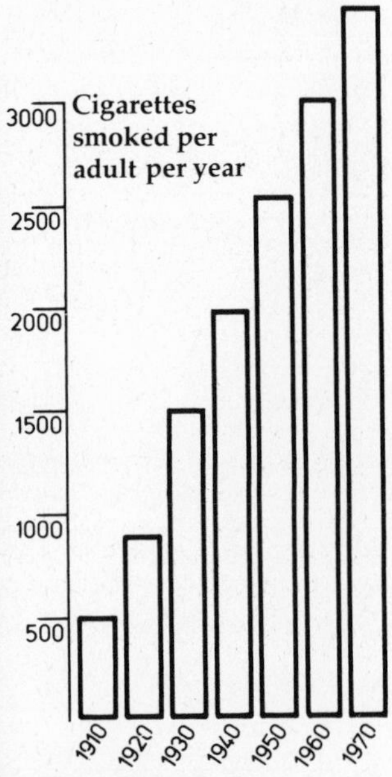

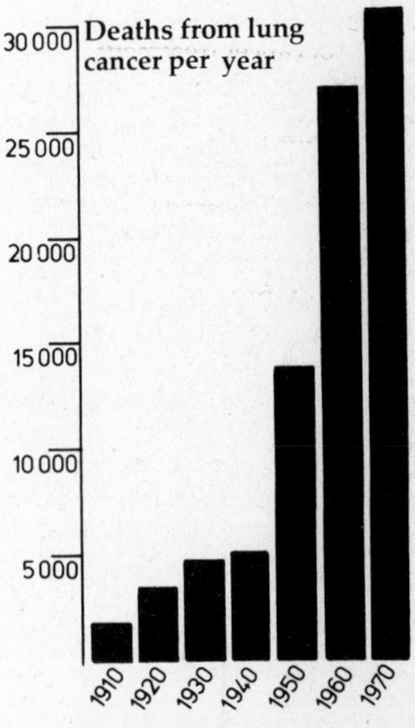

Lung cancer
Lung cancer is usually diagnosed too late for a cure. The average survival is 9 months but with successful surgical removal of the lung or lobe containing the tumor some patients live longer. The tumor begins in the walls of the bronchial passages or sometimes in the body of the lung, and usually produces no symptoms until it has become firmly entrenched in the lung tissue and even spread to other parts of the body. Sputum cytology may pick up early signs of the disease. Signs include a chronic persistent cough, blood in the sputum, severe pain in the chest, and a lingering chest infection. The chart *above* shows the results of a survey of lung cancer deaths and cigarette smoking in the United Kingdom; as the number of cigarettes smoked has increased, so has the number of deaths per year from lung cancer. In the USA, lung cancer at present is killing over 90,000 people per year. Over 95% of all lung cancer patients are smokers. The smoke paralyzes bronchial cilia, interfering with the natural cleaning mechanism, and the subsequent irritation to the tissues causes precancerous changes in the bronchial cells. The World Health Organization believes that lung cancer deaths would decrease by as much as 90% if cigarette smoking were abolished.

Mouth and throat cancer
Mouth and throat cancers have been linked to poor oral hygiene. There is also evidence that repeated trauma or irritation in the mouth, caused by jagged teeth or ill-fitting dentures, for example, may induce the disease. If a lump or ulcer is discovered in the mouth then its progress should be watched and if it has not healed in 10 days a doctor should be consulted. Persistent hoarseness or difficulty in swallowing should also be reported. Excessive alcohol consumption combined with smoking and poor nutrition are also related to cancer of the mouth and throat.

Stomach cancer
The sharp decline in stomach cancer during this century is thought to be linked with changes in techniques of food preservation. Those at risk from the disease include people with a family history of stomach cancer and people who eat a diet rich in smoked, pickled or salted food. Symptoms include persistent indigestion, difficulty in swallowing, loss of appetite, stomach pains, vomiting and the appearance of black, tarry stools, particularly in the middle-aged. Stomach cancer can be easily detected by a series of hospital tests and it is possible to live a normal life even after large parts of the stomach have been removed.

Liver cancer
Primary cell liver cancer is more frequent in persons with cirrhosis of the liver, a condition that is largely the result of consuming too much alcohol. Primary cell liver cancer is not common in Western countries. There is some evidence that liver cancer in Africans is connected with their poor diet which is almost bereft of the vitamins necessary for a healthy liver. Liver cancer is particularly common in sub-Saharan Africa where food molds and the protein antigen Australia are belived to be responsible carcinogens. The liver is a favorite site for the further growth of many types of cancer.

Cancer of the cervix
Cervical cancer is on the decline. It has been linked to general bad health, the smegma of uncircumcised males, and chronic vaginal and cervical infection. Routine screening (at least every 3 years) with a smear test will detect early signs. Affected tissue can be easily removed surgically, and the patient may still be able to have children. Advanced cases may require hysterectomy. Women who have had children or multiple sex partners, or those who have had intercourse at an early age are more at risk. Signs include bleeding after intercourse, bleeding between periods, heavy periods, or bleeding after the menopause.

Surgery
Surgery is the most common form of cancer treatment. Successful treatment requires the complete removal of all cancerous tissue to prevent recurrence, and the operation must be performed before the cancer has spread into organs and tissues that cannot safely be removed. Risks have been reduced by improvements in surgical techniques, anesthesiology, and preoperative and postoperative care, especially in the control of infection. Sites treated successfully include the larynx (**1**), lung (**6**), breast (**9**), stomach (**8**), ovaries (**13**), cervix (**14**), prostate (**15**), colon (**12**), and rectum (**16**).

Chemotherapy
Drugs are becoming more important in the treatment of cancers although the benefits must be weighed against the side effects. They are used with good results in the treatment of Hodgkin's disease (**7**), Burkitt's lymphoma (**18**), leukemia (**5**), and a rare tumor of the placenta in pregnant women, choriocarcinoma (**11**). Although complete remissions are rare using drugs alone patients with lung (**6**), colon (**12**), head and neck (**4**) or ovarian cancer (**13**) and those with malignant melanoma (**3**) may experience 20 to 70% remission rates with the use of one or more anticancer drugs.

Radiotherapy
The object of radiotherapy is to give a dose that will destroy the tumor without any great injury to any of the normal surrounding tissue. If the difference between the sensitivity of the two types of cells is large, as in the skin (**3**), treatment is easy and nearly always successful. Radiotherapy is also used to treat Hodgkin's disease (**7**), a generalized condition affecting the lymphoid tissue. Radiation is used as supportive therapy to surgery in some cancers including the stomach (**8**), the rectum (**16**), and the breast (**9**).

Hormone therapy
Hormone therapy is used mainly for tumors of endocrine glands such as the thyroid (**2**), pancreas (**10**), testes (**17**) and ovaries (**13**), and related organs. Cancers of the prostate (**15**) and breast (**9**) may respond well to hormone therapy. It is also useful in the treatment of metastases (secondary growths) originating from these areas, for instance it is used against disseminated breast cancer. The success of the treatment depends on whether the cancerous cells still have the specialized relationship with the hormone that the original tissue had.

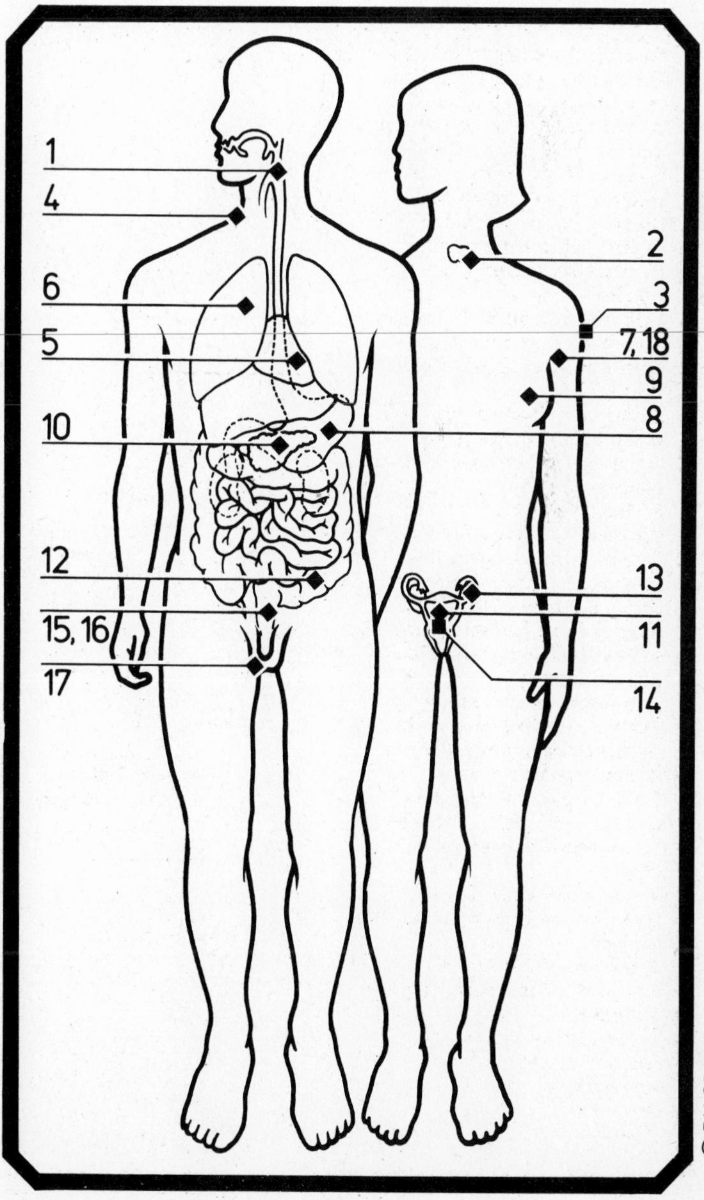

Cancer 3

Worldwide research is going on into the causes of cancer and ways to treat it. But existing knowledge has helped at least 1.5 million Americans who have been diagnosed and treated for cancer and are now apparently free from the disease five years later. Many cancer patients could be saved if known cancer detection methods and treatment were employed earlier; some form of effective therapy is available for virtually every cancer patient, but fears and fallacies surrounding cancer and ignorance about the disease may delay treatment and the chance of a cure. Here we list some of the signs to look for and some precautions that may help prevent cancer from developing.

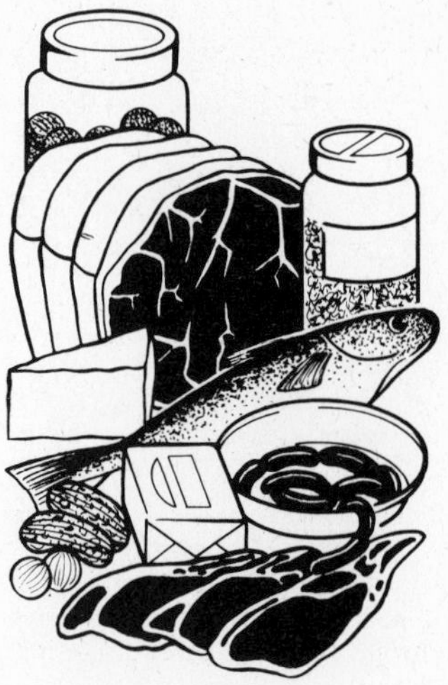

Diet
Cancers of the bowel, stomach and liver have been related to diet. The high-fiber diet of some countries in the developing world has been linked to a low incidence of large bowel cancer, but these high-fiber diets are also low in fats, animal proteins and sugar and rich in starch. Vitamin deficient diets in some parts of Africa have been linked to a high rate of liver cancer. A diet heavy in smoked, pickled or salted foods may put people at a higher risk of developing stomach cancer. It is generally the balance of the diet that is the important factor in prevention, rather than the presence or absence of any given foodstuff.

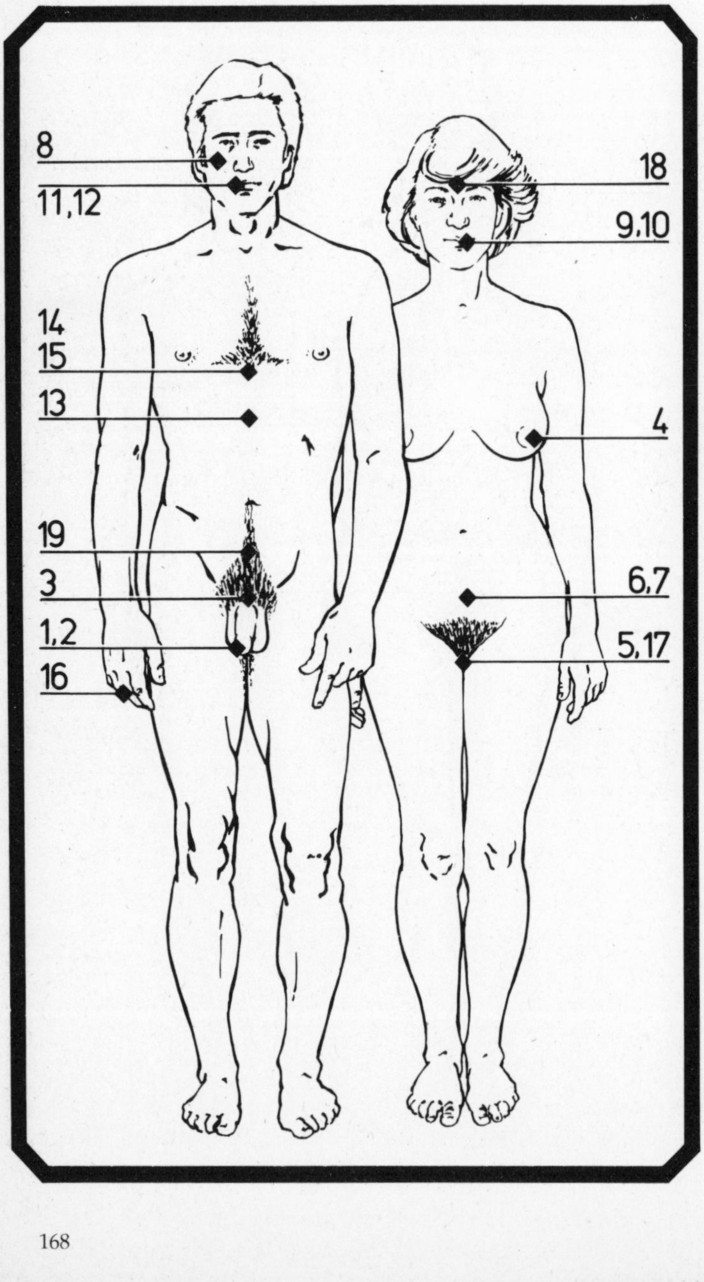

Self-help for men
1 Maintain good hygiene of the genital organs. Early circumcision helps prevent cancer of the penis, but so may scrupulous hygiene.
2 Examine the penis and testes regularly for any unusual sores, growths or other changes.
3 Have an annual examination of the prostate if you are over 60.

Self-help for women
4 Examine the breasts every month.
5 Examine the vulva regularly.
6 Have a cervical smear or "Pap" test every year, especially after the menopause.
7 Have a complete cancer-related check-up every year if you have never had children, never ovulated, had your first child after 30, began intercourse at an early age, have had multiple sex partners, are obese, or if you have ever had estrogen therapy or abnormal uterine bleeding.

Self-help for both sexes
8 Avoid over-exposure to the sun, particularly if you are fair-skinned.
9 Eat a well-balanced diet.
10 Avoid a diet heavy in smoked, pickled or salted foods.
11 Maintain good oral hygiene.
12 Have any jagged teeth repaired, as constant friction in the mouth can cause precancerous changes in the tissue.
13 Avoid excessive alcohol intake.
14 Don't smoke.
15 Have a chest X-ray at intervals recommended by your doctor if he feels this is a helpful inclusion in tests to screen you for cancer; at all other times keep X-rays to a minimum, as over-exposure can trigger off cancerous changes in cells.
16 Avoid prolonged contact with any known carcinogens.
17 Have a yearly rectal examination after the age of 45.
18 Be observant of changes in your body and its functions and report anything suspicious or persistent to your doctor.
19 Have a cancer-related check-up every 3 years between 20 and 40 and every year after 40, especially if there is a personal or family history of cancer, polyps in the colon or rectum, or ulcerative colitis.

Public education
Ill-founded fears and fallacies, and ignorance about cancer, leading to delay in diagnosis and treatment, are major reasons for death among cancer patients. Many cancers treated early enough are curable. More than 35% of all cancer patients live at least 5 years after the illness is treated, but the figure could be even better. Medical authorities estimate that 65% or more of patients with cancer could be saved with existing methods if they were aware of the danger signs, had an annual health examination, and did not allow fear to keep them from seeking a medical diagnosis.

Epidemiological research
Epidemiological research – the gathering of information about the pattern in which disease occurs – has been responsible for much of the evidence on carcinogenic agents, such as tobacco smoke. Comparisons of the number of cases of cancer in a group of workers or in people from different countries or regions have shown striking differences and suggested that cancer is strongly linked with the environment. As a result carcinogenic substances have been removed or measures have been taken to protect people from them. The research has also identified high-risk groups for health checks and screening programs.

Vaccines and drugs
Research is going on into the possibility that some cancers are caused by viruses and that it might be possible to develop a vaccine against them. Immunology, the study of the body's natural resistance to foreign organisms, is another area of research. Scientists believe that vaccines using cellular antigens, which stimulate antibody production, may suppress or destroy carcinogenic agents or the cancer cells induced by them. Anti-cancer drugs are also being developed. Some are naturally occurring, but most are synthesized in the laboratory.

Research into causes
Many scientists are now convinced that damage to the genetic chemicals in human cells, DNA and RNA, may be the key factor in the transformation of normal cells into cancer cells. Research is progressing on a rapid test to identify carcinogenic agents. It involves the use of human cells grown in flasks to determine in a day or two whether or not a suspected agent transforms normal cells. Conventional screening takes 2 to 3 years.

Warning signs in both sexes
The following symptoms do not necessarily indicate cancer, but they should be brought to the attention of your doctor.
1 Chronic indigestion or difficulty in swallowing.
2 Vomiting.
3 Loss of appetite.
4 Chronic, persistent cough or hoarseness.
5 Blood in the sputum.
6 Lingering chest infection.
7 Stomach pains.
8 Any new symptoms in a middle-aged person referable to the stomach.
9 A lump or thickening anywhere in the body.
10 A mole, wart or birthmark that begins to grow, bleed, change color or become tender.
11 The appearance of black, tarry stools (caused by blood lost in the stomach changing color during its passage through the bowel).
12 Any unexplained change in bladder or bowel habits.
13 The sudden appearance of constipation or diarrhea, or the alternation of the two.
14 Thin, pipe-like stools.
15 Pain in the bowel.
16 Blood, pus or a lot of mucus in the stools.
17 Unusual bleeding or discharge.
18 Any sore or ulcer that does not heal.

Warning signs in men
19 Feeling an urgency to get up in the night to urinate but then only being able to pass a small quantity.
20 Increased frequency of urination.
21 Difficulty or discomfort in passing urine.
22 Pain that appears to be located in the prostate.

Warning signs in women
23 Swelling in the armpit.
24 Alteration in the shape of the breast or the texture of its skin.
25 An unusual lump or dimple in the breast.
26 Blood-stained discharge from the nipple.
27 Heavy periods, or bleeding between periods.
28 Bleeding after intercourse.
29 Vaginal bleeding after the menopause.

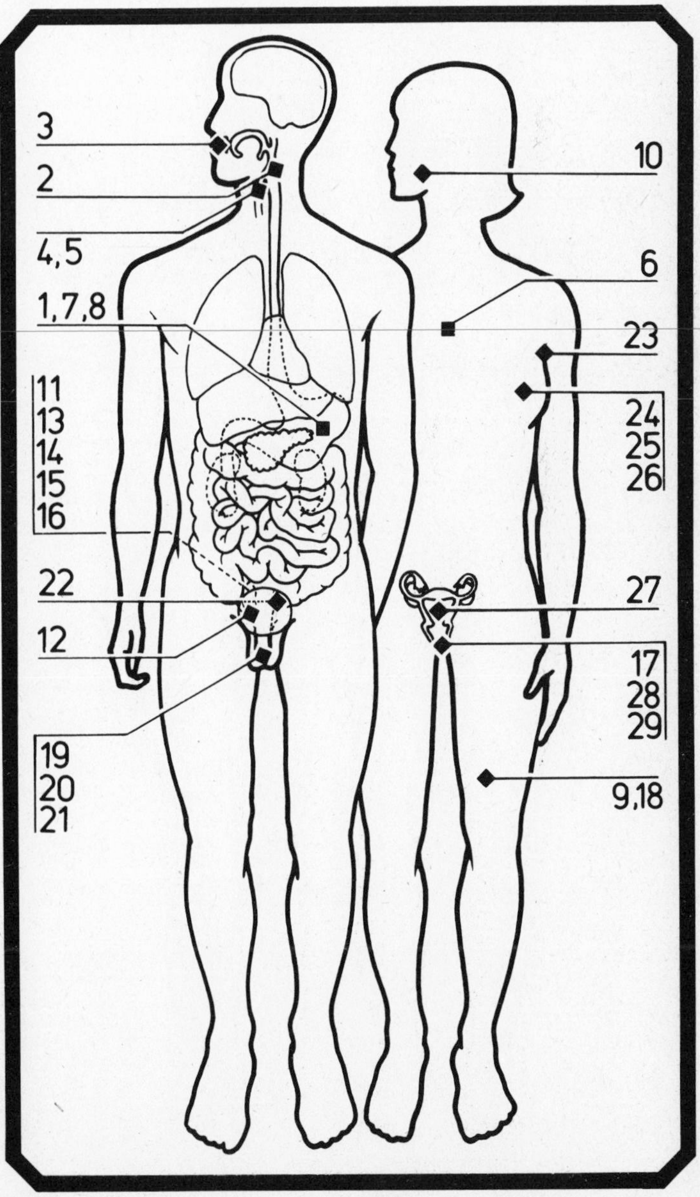

Contraception

Methods of birth control have been practiced for centuries, but still the search continues for the safest and most reliable form of contraception. In the USA about 80% of all couples use some kind of contraceptive. Many women choose the reliability of the contraceptive pill or the intrauterine device (IUD), but their side-effects and possible health risks have persuaded some to go back to using a diaphragm or other type of cap. The male forms of contraception, the condom and coitus interruptus, are still the most widely-practiced contraceptive methods in the West. The male pill has aroused much interest, but is still in the research stage, as are many other new methods and modifications and improvements of existing methods.

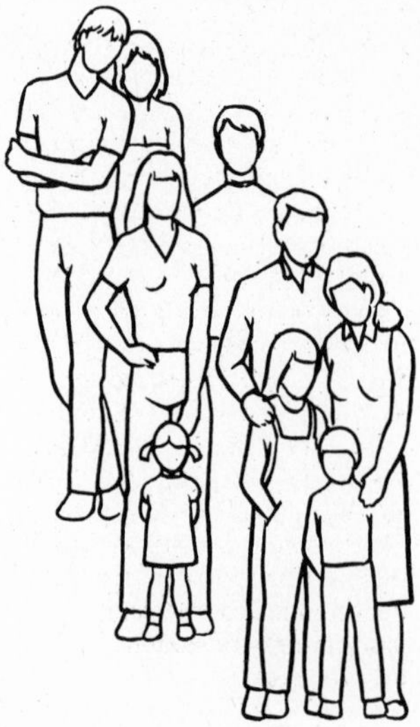

Choice of contraceptive
Choice of contraceptive will be influenced by individual needs. Teenagers or young adults at the start of sexual activity often use withdrawal or condoms. Once sexual activity is established many young women use the pill, but concern about the side-effects of pill hormones helps persuade others to choose one of the IUDs developed for women who have not had children. Between children some women continue using the pill or an IUD, others change to the slightly less effective diaphragm. Once the family is complete, some couples opt for sterilization of either the man or the woman.

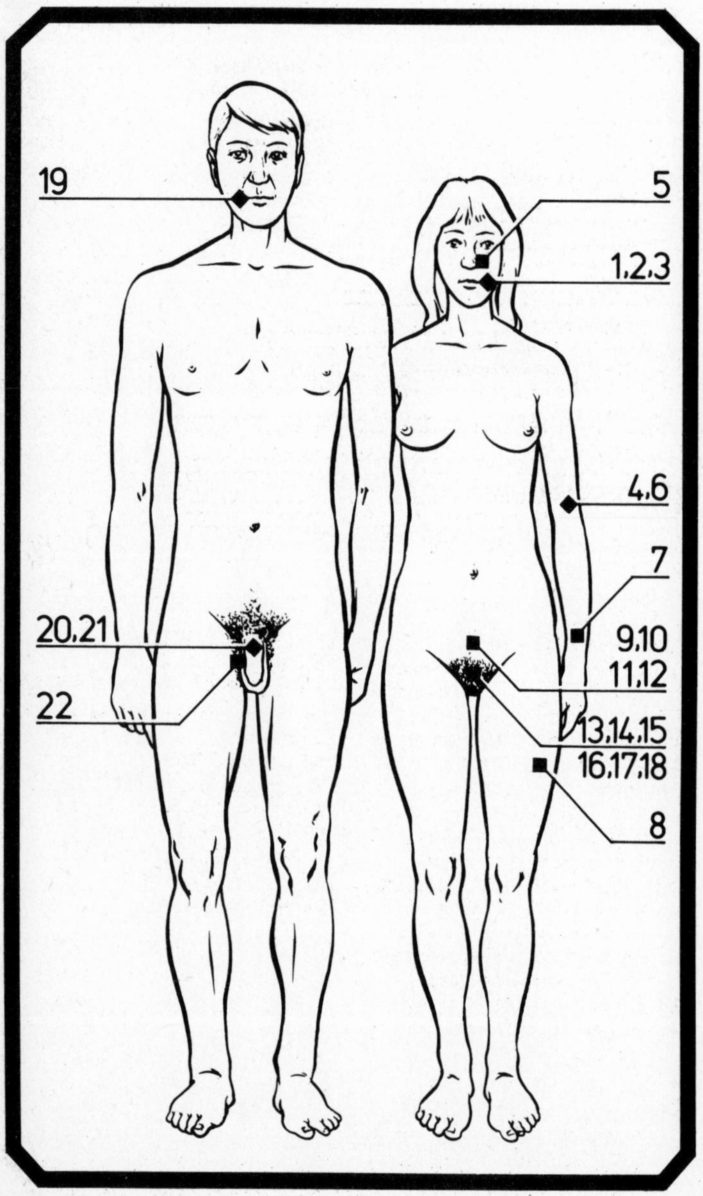

Contraceptive methods
The following methods have been developed; those marked with an asterisk are still at the research stage.
1 Oral contraceptives, or the birth control pill.
2 Temperature method of calculating fertile days; sometimes this is combined with observing cervical mucus and other body signs, and is then known as the sympto-thermal method.
3 Morning-after pill; available in some places as an emergency measure, this prevents implantation of the fertilized egg.
4 Injections of slow-releasing hormones.
5 Hormone nasal spray.*
6 Infertility vaccines.*
7 Contraceptive bracelet.*
8 Implantation of slow-releasing hormone capsules.*
9 Intrauterine device (IUD) to prevent the fertilized egg from establishing a pregnancy.
10 Progesterone-impregnated IUD.
11 Female sterilization.
12 Menstrual extraction, the removal of the uterus lining.
13 Vaginal sponge impregnated with spermicide.*
14 Intravaginal ring with slow-releasing progestogen.*
15 Cervical cap.
16 Vault cap.
17 Diaphragm.
18 Mucus and calendar methods of calculating fertile days.
19 Male pill.*
20 Condom.
21 Coitus interruptus or withdrawal.
22 Male sterilization.

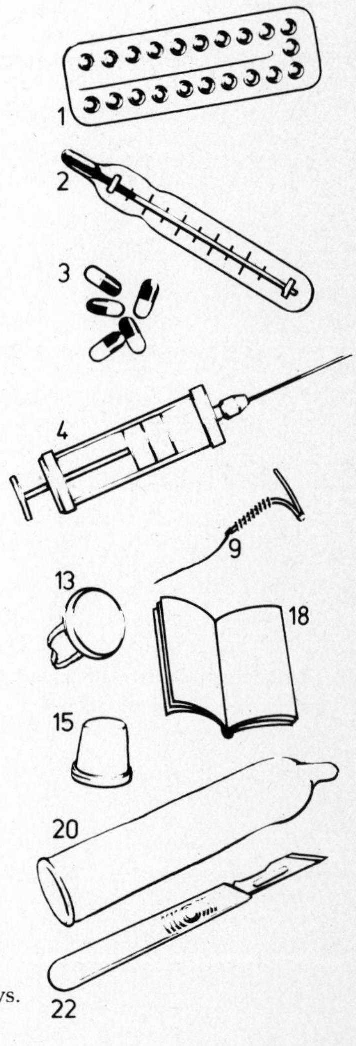

Natural or rhythm methods
All these methods – calendar, temperature, mucus, and sympto-thermal – are based on the recognition of changes in the woman's monthly cycle and involve having intercourse only during the infertile times of the month. The calendar method requires studying previous menstrual cycles to calculate the time of ovulation. The temperature method involves taking the temperature daily as this rises slightly after ovulation. The mucus method is based on the recognition of changes in cervical mucus around the time of ovulation. The sympto-thermal method combines various observations. All these methods are fairly unreliable.

Diaphragms and caps
Used together with spermicide, a diaphragm or other type of cap provides an effective barrier to sperm. It must be fitted by a trained person and requires regular checking. The cap must always be used with spermicide, which is smeared on before insertion, and should be left in position for at least six hours after intercourse. If intercourse is delayed or repeated more spermicide must be used. The method has no side-effects, and used properly it is extremely efficient, but some people find it messy and feel that it destroys the spontaneity of sexual intercourse.

Male methods
Coitus interruptus and condoms are the main male methods of contraception. In coitus interruptus, or withdrawal, the man takes his penis out of the woman's vagina before ejaculation; this method is very unreliable as some sperm may be released before ejaculation or the man may not be able to delay ejaculation.
A condom fits tightly over a man's erect penis so that when he ejaculates the sperm are trapped inside. Condoms are cheap, widely available, have no side-effects, give some protection against VD, and are reasonably efficient, but they may interrupt lovemaking and reduce sensitivity.

Sterilization
Female sterilization is achieved by cutting or blocking the Fallopian tubes, so preventing the eggs' normal journey from the ovaries to the uterus and their possible fertilization by sperm. Male sterilization or vasectomy is a minor operation that involves cutting and tying the vas deferens, the tubes that carry sperm from the testes to the penis. The man continues to ejaculate but the semen no longer carries sperm; these are reabsorbed by the body.
Sterilization is an extremely reliable method of birth control, but is rarely reversible; the couple must be sure they want no more children.

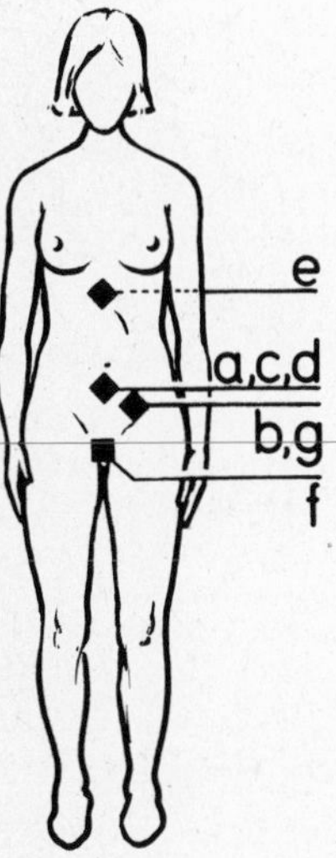

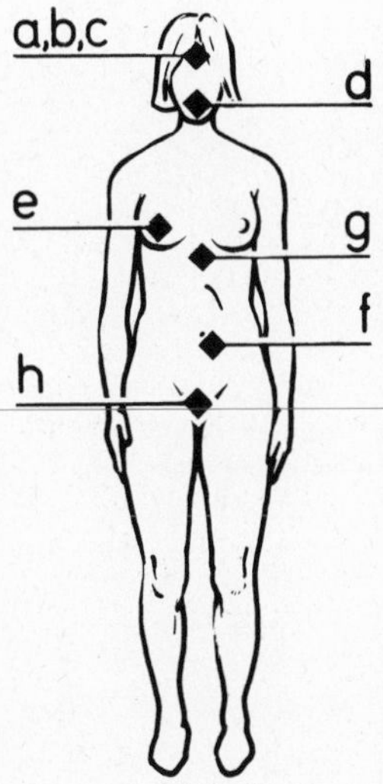

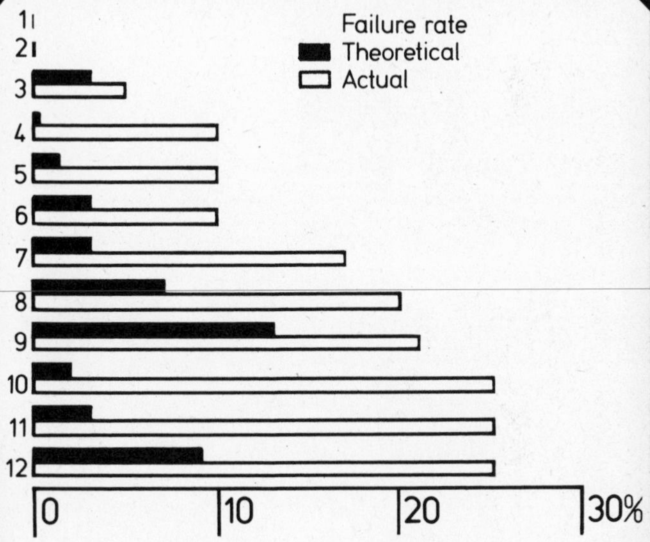

IUDs
Available intrauterine devices include several that can be used by women who have not had children. IUDs are nearly as efficient as the pill, are very convenient and do not interfere with lovemaking.
Complications, most of them uncommon, include: (**a**) perforation of the uterus; (**b**) ectopic pregnancy, a pregnancy that occurs outside the uterus; (**c**) miscarriage if pregnancy occurs; (**d**) abdominal pain; (**e**) backache (often a sign of infection); (**f**) heavy periods (common); (**g**) pelvic infection, which often causes infertility if left untreated. Expulsion of the IUD is also a possible problem; users should regularly check that the tail threads are in the vagina.

The pill
Oral contraception is the most reliable method of non-surgical birth control. By altering the body's natural hormone balance, the pill interferes with the woman's normal monthly cycle of ovulation and menstruation and suppresses fertility. The pill is easy to use and does not interfere with lovemaking, but is not recommended for forgetful people. Possible side-effects include: (**a**) headaches; (**b**) tiredness; (**c**) depression; (**d**) nausea; (**e**) sore breasts; (**f**) weight gain; (**g**) blood clotting and thrombosis in women who smoke, or who have diabetes or circulatory problems; (**h**) decreased sex drive.

Efficiency of methods
The diagram *above* shows the failure rates for various different types of contraception. The figures are based on a survey in the USA and refer to the number of pregnancies per 100 users during the first year of using the method. Theoretical rates are given first, which predict the rates if the method is used conscientiously as instructed; actual rates, which take into account human factors such as forgetfulness and irregularity of use, are given in parentheses where these are appropriate.

1 Tubal ligation 0.04
2 Vasectomy 0.15
3 IUD 1–3 (5)
4 Combined pill 0.34 (4–10)
5 Minipill 1–1.5 (5–10)
6 Condom 3 (10)
7 Cap+spermicide 3 (17)
8 Temperature method 7 (20)
9 Calendar method 13 (21)
10 Mucus method 2 (25)
11 Spermicide 4 (20–25)
12 Withdrawal 9 (20–25)

Sex problems 1

Sex problems are a source of great unhappiness, anxiety, and pain. In this section we look at different sorts of sexual problem – genital pain or dysfunction, problems with intercourse, problems associated with aging, fertility problems, and sexually transmitted infections. Some of these problems, such as those resulting from genital abnormality or an infection, are obviously physical in origin although there may be psychological implications. Many others, particularly those involving difficulties with intercourse, have a variety of psychological causes. Superficial causes often produce temporary difficulties, but where causes are deep-seated conditions are more difficult to alter. Such problems as impotence and premature ejaculation may be caused by current circumstances – the man is sexually inexperienced, nervous, worried about work, or unused to his sexual partner. When circumstances improve he is able to relax and his sexual performance is restored. If a woman fears intercourse as an invasion or worries that the man is merely using her she may fail to reach orgasm or may suffer from vaginismus. Unexpressed resentments or other problems in a couple's marriage may find expression in sexual difficulties. A superficial problem may become more lasting and serious if the people involved become preoccupied with it and develop a sense of failure. Psychotherapy has great value in clarifying underlying emotional causes or bringing hidden fears to the surface.

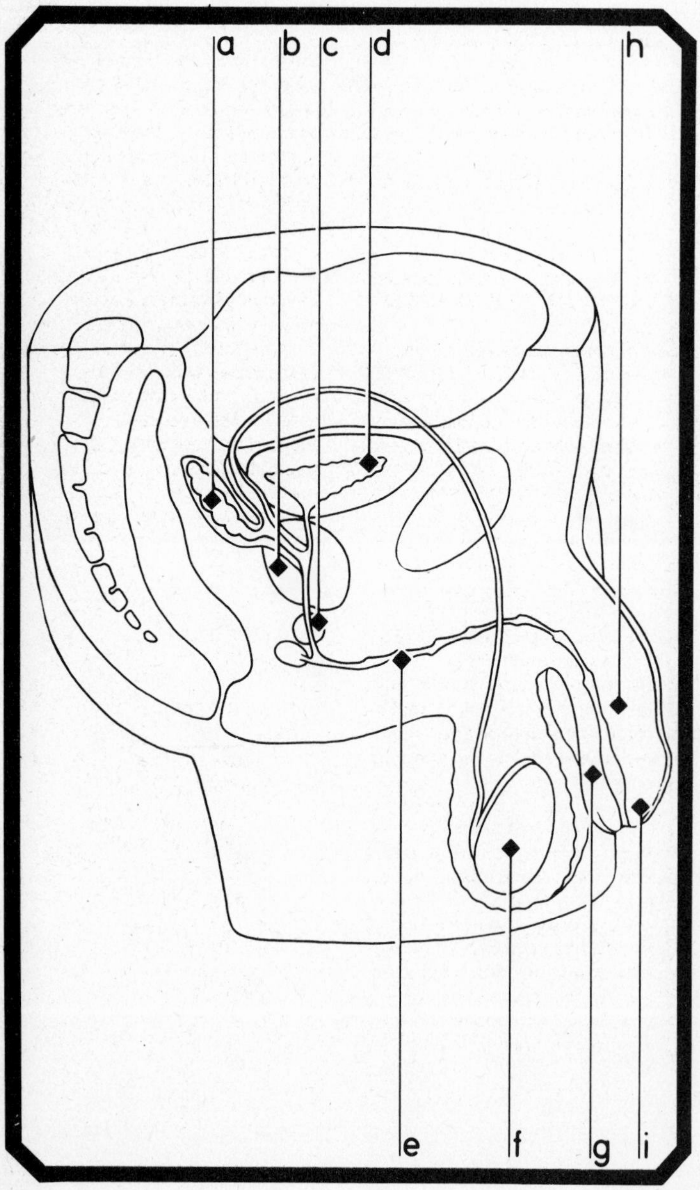

Male physical problems
The sites of some possible problems involving the male sex organs are located on the drawing *left*.

a Seminal vesicles: infection causes pain on intercourse; the production of too much or too little seminal fluid are causes of infertility.

b Prostate gland: infection, overenlargement, cancer and, in old men, spasmodic contractions are causes of pain during intercourse.

c Compressor muscles: failure of these muscles to relax at ejaculation causes seminal fluid to be discharged into the bladder instead of being discharged through the urethra. This problem – termed retrograde ejaculation – may result from prostate surgery or an accident.

d Bladder: infection causes pain on intercourse.

e Urethra: adhesions following gonorrheal infection cause pain on intercourse.

f Testes: failure of the testes to descend before puberty causes infertility, as does inadequate production of sperm; painful intercourse can result from unrelieved congestion of the testes following prolonged erection without ejaculation.

g Blood vessels: hardening of blood vessels leading to the erectile tissue of the penis means that older men take longer to obtain an erection.

h Shaft of the penis: pain on intercourse may be the result of badly performed circumcision, or may be caused by Peyronie's disease (in which the penis on erection is painfully bowed up and bent sideways) or by chordee (in which the erect penis is painfully bowed down).

i Glans penis: pain in the glans on intercourse may be caused by a build-up of smegma (see p.111) and bacteria, by adhesion of the glans to an overtight foreskin, by inflammation of the urethra or prostate, or by contact with germs, acid or a partner's contraceptive cream.

Other physical problems that interfere with a man's sexual performance include disorders of hormone production in the pituitary or the testes, and defects of the central nervous system.

Psychological origins
Guilt is one of the most common causes of deep-seated sexual problems, but it is not merely that the sexual act is thought to be bad or dirty in itself. Often a person has not fully broken away emotionally from a loved parent; intimacy may then take on an incestuous tone. Sometimes fear of sexual fantasies is so great that a person becomes sexually over-controlled. Common fantasies that worry many people concern promiscuity, homosexuality, anal sex, sado-masochism, prostitution and rape. The person often fears – usually unnecessarily – that he will act out the fantasies if they are not totally restrained.

Some serious sexual problems are rooted in a disturbance of the whole personality. Severe deprivation and disturbance in early childhood cause some people to develop an emotionally repressed personality. Fearing that their defenses against their own vulnerability and dependency needs will crumble, such people avoid close contact and emotional commitment. For some the sex act is divorced from emotion and is indulged in promiscuously or compulsively. Another serious problem occurs when the sexual personality does not develop clearly in childhood. The person becomes sexually confused, and often looks for security and affection rather than sex.

Types of therapy
Therapy for sexual problems may be physical or emotional. In sex therapy, for example, the therapist may give the couple exercises or sex-play routines; underlying problems are not dwelt on. In psychotherapy, by contrast, underlying emotional problems are brought to the surface. The client or patient talks in a free, unplanned way. The therapist listens for hints about the real nature of the problem. Gradually, with the therapist's help and clarification, the patient is able to experience consciously problems that had previously been ignored, rejected or repressed, and so deal with them.

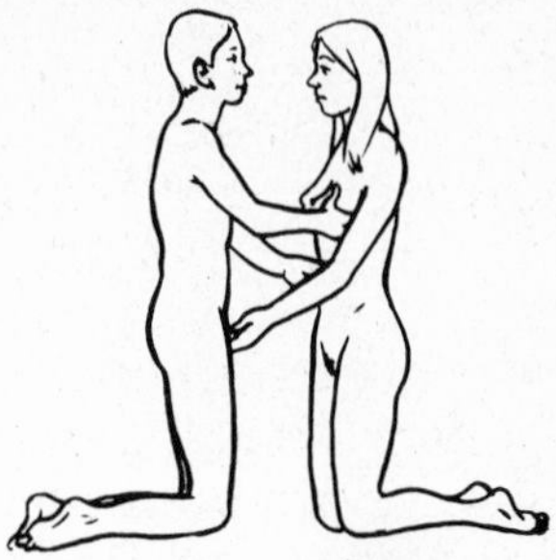

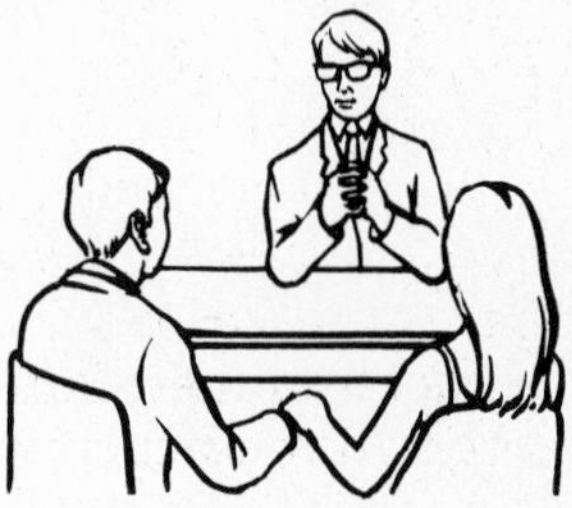

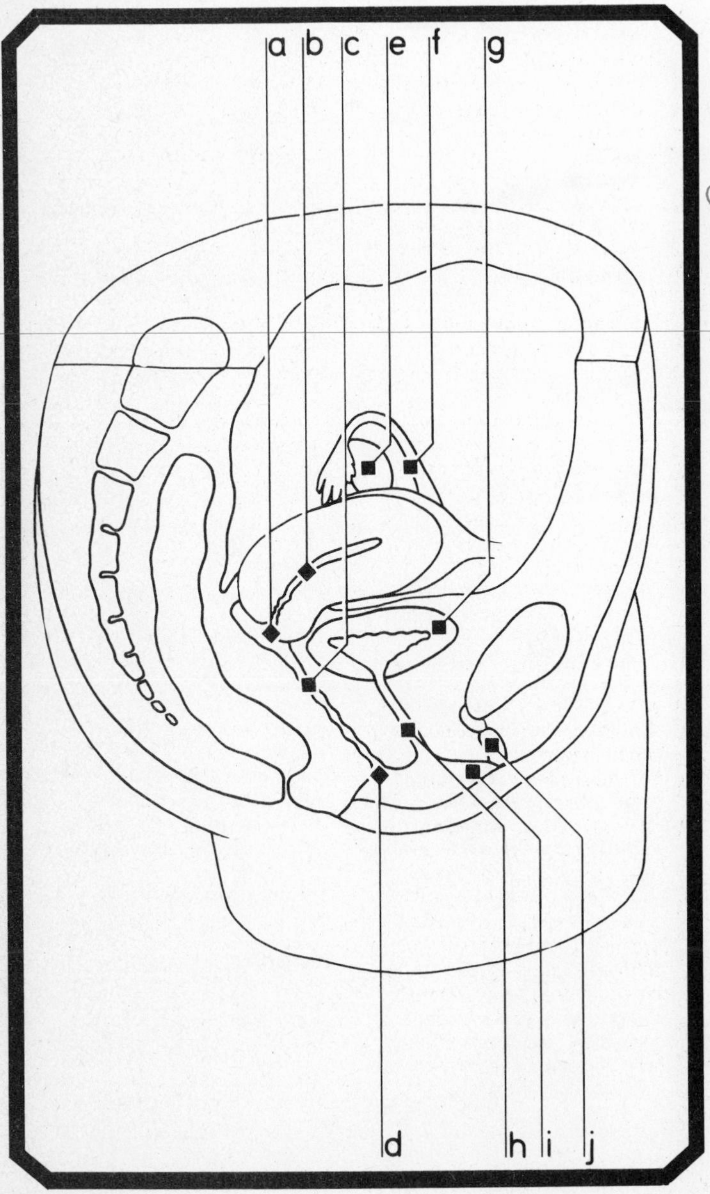

Female physical problems
As in men there may be hormone disorders and defects of the central nervous system. Other problem sites are shown *left*.

a Cervix: infection, injury or the presence of fibrous growths (endometriosis) cause pain.
b Uterus: there may be pain (as in **a**); fertility may be affected if the uterus is tilted, divided or double.
c Vagina: causes of pain on intercourse include infection, lack of lubrication, slackness or tightness of the vaginal walls, sensitivity to rubber devices, and vaginismus.
d Vaginal outlet: labia fused over the outlet prevent intercourse; pain may result from a very rigid hymen, from atrophy due to aging, or from injury associated with first intercourse, IUD strings, rape, abortion or childbirth.
e Ovaries: ovulatory problems are a cause of infertility; pain on intercourse may be due to inflammation, displacement or ovarian cysts.
f Fallopian tubes: infection may cause pain on intercourse; blocking of the tubes – often a result of infection – is a common cause of infertility.
g Bladder: infection is a cause of painful intercourse.
h Urethra: infection is a cause of painful intercourse.
i Vulva: atrophy in old age may make intercourse painful.
j Clitoris: smegma, infection and injury are causes of pain on intercourse.

Vaginismus
In this condition the muscles surrounding the vagina go into spasm so that the vagina and its opening are narrowed. If the contraction is very strong, perhaps lasting many hours, attempts at intercourse produce excruciating pain in the woman and the partner's penis will be quite unable to enter the vagina. Psychological causes of the problem include fear, guilt and memory of past pain on intercourse. Many sufferers respond well to psychotherapy. Some sex therapists recommend stretching the vaginal muscles by inserting progressively larger dilators into the vagina over a period of several days.

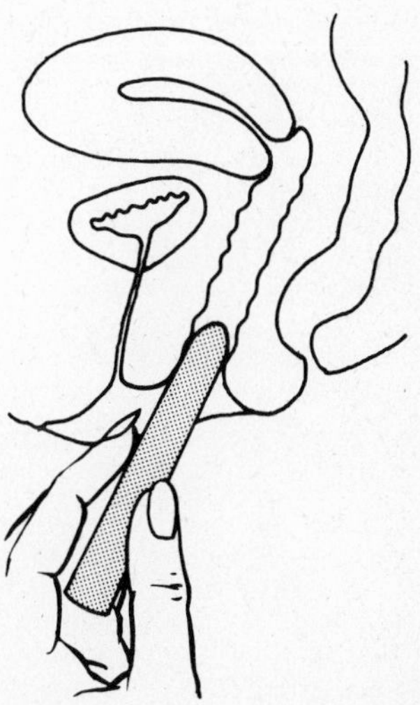

Sex problems 2

Lack of orgasm in women
This is the commonest form of sexual inadequacy in women. Sometimes there is a physical cause, such as a defect in the reproductive organs, hormonal imbalance, inflammation or injury. More commonly the cause is psychological. Possible psychological causes include rejection of the partner as a suitable mate, or being so eager to succeed that tension sets in and prevents orgasm. Deep-rooted psychological causes can be uncovered and treated by psychotherapy. The sex therapy techniques described briefly *right* were pioneered in the 1960s by the US sexologists W.H. Masters and V.E. Johnson.

Stimulation techniques
Treating lack of orgasm in women often involves the encouragement of considerate and stimulating sex play in an atmosphere of relaxation and mutual harmony. Some women find it helpful to look at erotic literature, to discuss sexually stimulating topics, or to concentrate on a sexual fantasy. Masturbation by vibrator or by hand, oral-genital contact, and deep penetration by the penis may be helpful to women who are capable of sexual arousal but who find orgasm elusive. Any method that brings orgasm once makes it easier to reach orgasm again in the future.

Orgasmic therapy for women
1 The couple sit nude in the position shown. She guides his hands briefly over her genitals, so controlling her own sexual sensations and preventing them from becoming too intense.
2 In later sessions the couple work up to a point where they adopt this new position and she enjoys keeping still with his penis in her vagina. Next she makes thrusting movements with her hips. Later he also thrusts his hips.
3 The final stage involves adopting this side-by-side intercourse position which, because it provides good opportunity for uncontrolled hip movements, is very conducive to female orgasm.

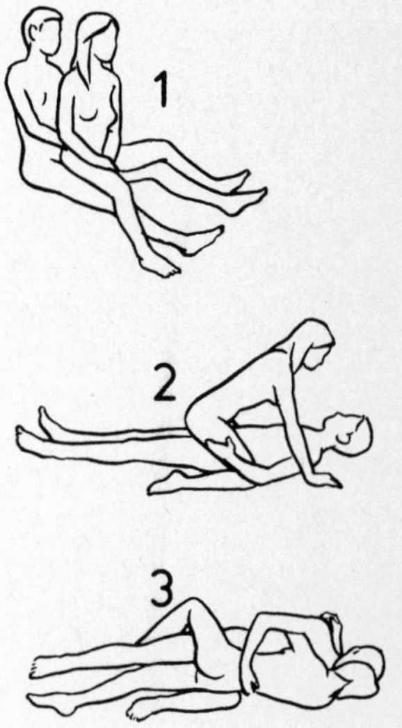

Impotence
This may be primary, meaning the man has never sustained an erection for intercourse, or secondary, meaning the man has lost previous coital capacity. Physical causes, such as a genital defect, hormonal imbalance, fatigue or too much alcohol, are thought to account for only about 10% of cases; the remainder result from a variety of psychological causes. Men who suffer from more than short-term impotence should seek professional help. The therapy summarized *right* is that of Masters and Johnson. By stressing aspects of lovemaking other than the gaining of an erection, it has the effect of making an erection more likely.

Incidence of impotence
A man is considered impotent if one in four sexual attempts fails to produce an erection. As the diagram *right* shows the incidence of impotence rises markedly from late middle age onward. Note that this picture is somewhat misleading: many very old men continue to enjoy intercourse occasionally.

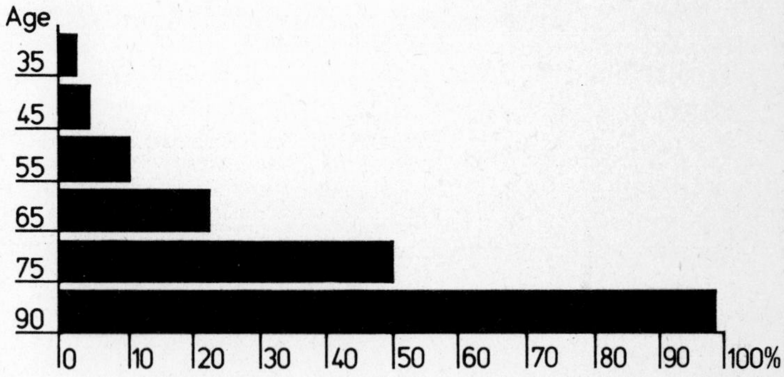

Impotence therapy
1 For about 10 days the couple limit sex to fondling breasts and genitals. When he has an erection he lets it subside.
2 The couple try intercourse as shown, recommencing if his penis goes limp. When he can keep an erection in her vagina, he thrusts his hips. If the couple can relax, orgasm follows.

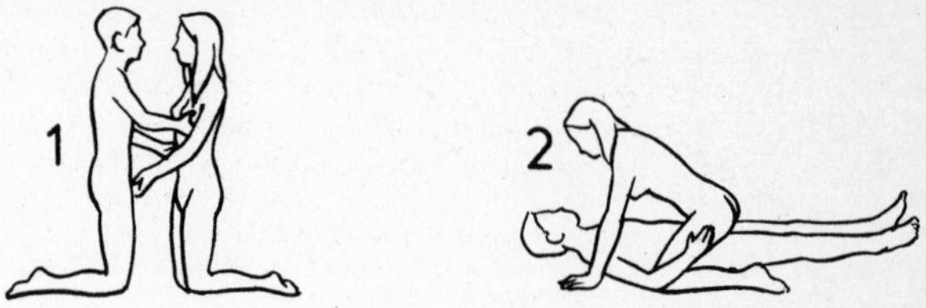

Ejaculatory incompetence
Failure to ejaculate during intercourse may stem from fears that are conscious, such as fear of disturbance, or subconscious. In the latter case, psychotheraphy may be needed. Masters and Johnson's sex therapy is summarized here.
1 The woman masturbates the man so that he ejaculates outside her vagina.
2 Later, adopting the position shown, she again masturbates him to ejaculate outside her vagina. Next, she masturbates him until he feels orgasm is inevitable and then she quickly places his penis in her vagina so at least some of his semen is ejaculated there. In the last stage the man ejaculates entirely within her vagina.

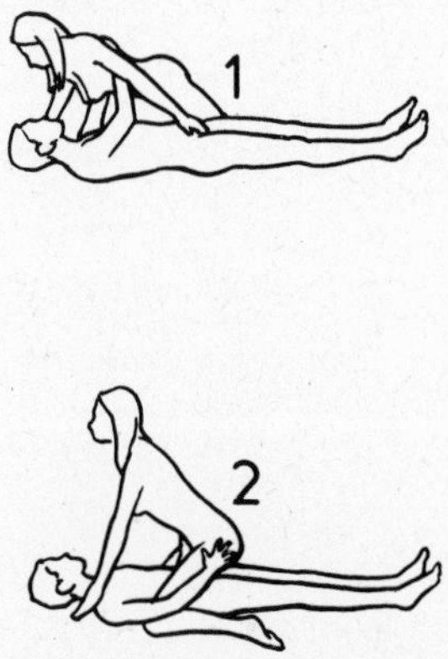

Premature ejaculation
This becomes a problem only when the man ejaculates too soon for the woman so often that the couple's emotional relationship suffers. Usually the problem is easily solved. It may be possible to fend off ejaculation by unsexy thoughts. Some men find that intercourse soon after orgasm delays ejaculation. In a few cases premature ejaculation is due to a physical problem that needs medical treatment. More often the problem is due to sexual inexperience, to making love in cramped or hurried conditions, or to anxiety about premature ejaculation in the past. Persistent sufferers are likely to benefit from some form of therapy.

Delaying ejaculation
Masters and Johnson recommend this therapy for premature ejaculation. She masturbates him until just before he feels ejaculation is inevitable. Then she squeezes the head of his penis quite hard for 3–4 seconds until his urge to ejaculate goes. Alternating stimulation and squeezing is continued for 15–20 minutes. Later she kneels over him for intercourse; he plays a fairly inactive role and withdraws his penis for squeezing if he feels he is going to ejaculate too soon.

Sex and special needs
Certain conditions, which may or may not be problems in themselves, have implications for a couple's sex life. In some cases the condition necessitating changes in sexual activity is of limited duration, as for example during pregnancy or following an accident. In other cases there may need to be a more long-term adaptation of sexual practices. Physical handicap, for example, may permanently affect a couple's options in the selection of positions for intercourse. In old age, couples may well find that new sexual techniques are invaluable in encouraging a continuing and fulfilling enjoyment of sexual activity.

Intercourse in pregnancy
Early in pregnancy a couple can generally have intercourse as usual, except when it is banned by the doctor because of previous miscarriage. A couple should also take their own doctor's advice about how late in pregnancy to continue having sex. As pregnancy proceeds couples are advised to use positions that keep direct pressure off the woman's abdomen. It is also important that the man should not thrust too deeply. Four recommended positions are shown *right*.
a Rear entry, kneeling.
b Rear entry, side-by-side.
c On the edge of a bed, with her legs supported.
d Sitting on a chair.

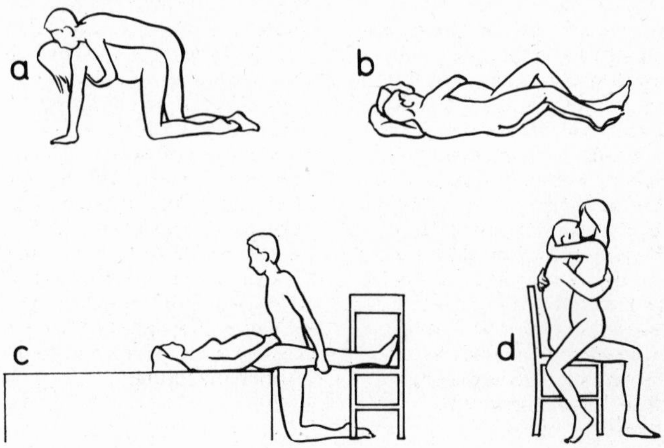

Intercourse and handicap
Even in cases of severe physical handicap it is often possible for a couple to enjoy sexual intercourse. Specialist counseling and literature are becoming increasingly widely available and handicapped persons are recommended to seek them. The sex act is possible in many different positions and there is a good chance that at least one will prove possible. Good use can sometimes be made of sex aids, some of which are designed specially for the physically handicapped. If intercourse is impossible, many couples can find considerable sexual satisfaction in developing other forms of lovemaking.

Intercourse with back pain
Four positions that may be suitable if you or your partner has back pain are illustrated *right*, but seek medical advice first. In each case the partner who does not have the back pain should do the thrusting. (In positions **1** to **3** the man is the back pain sufferer. In position **4** it is the woman.)
1 He stands for rear entry as she kneels near the bed edge.
2 He sits on a chair; she sits facing him on his lap.
3 He lies on his back on the bed; she sits astride him and leans forward.
4 She lies on her back on the bed; he leans forward between her legs.

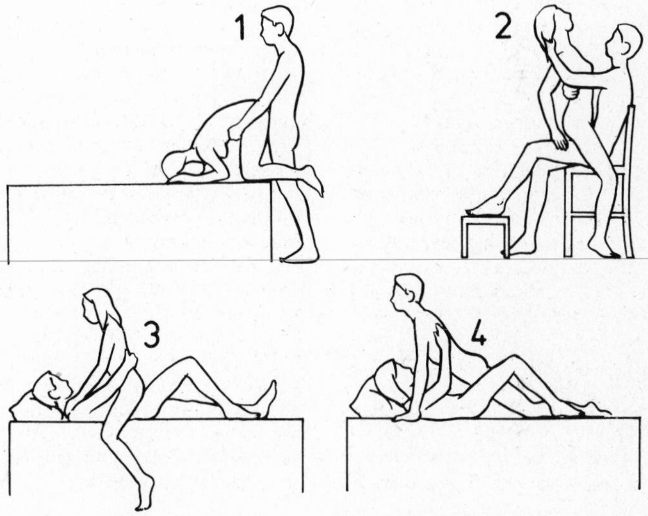

Sex and aging
Although the sex drive declines with age, this decline is often exaggerated. Ability to enjoy sexual activity often continues into extreme old age, particularly if an effort is made to respond to changes in the pattern of sexual response. Older couples must generally allow longer for sexual arousal. Once an older man obtains an erection, however, he has the advantage of being able to maintain it longer and may use his greater ejaculatory control to prolong intercourse almost indefinitely if he withdraws temporarily whenever orgasm is imminent. By avoiding orgasm an older man can also reduce the time needed between erections.

The aging male
Most old men remain physically capable of sexual activity. Impotence does increase with age, but in most cases this is due to psychological causes. By about age 60, however, aging will have brought the following physical changes.
a Hardening of blood vessels affects erectile capacity.
b Scrotal tissue sags and wrinkles.
c Testes shrink, lose firmness, and are less elevated on arousal.
d Thickening and degeneration of the seminiferous tubules inhibit sperm production.
e The prostate gland may be enlarged and its contractions during orgasm are weaker.
f Seminal fluid is thinner and reduced in quantity.

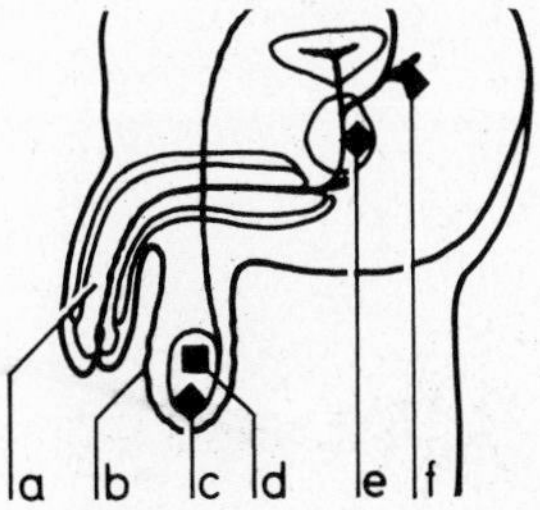

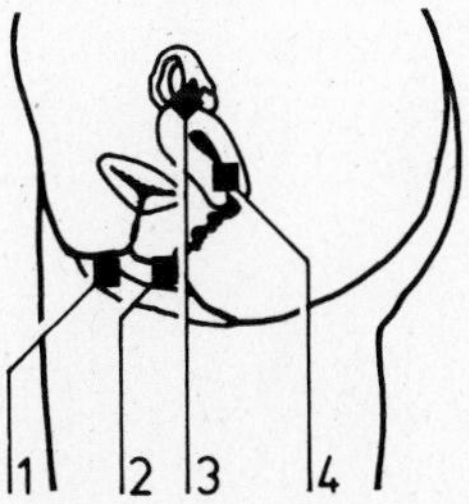

The aging female
Although the menopause ends a woman's reproductive potential, any loss of sex drive at this time is usually temporary. In fact women usually find that their cycle of sexual response is less affected by age than is that of their partner. The postmenopausal changes listed here may make intercourse uncomfortable for some women, but hormone pills and local applications are available to alleviate their effects.
1 The vulva atrophies.
2 The vaginal walls get thinner; reduced lubrication may lead to vaginal irritation.
3 Ovaries shrink.
4 The uterus shrinks; uterine muscle becomes fibrous but is probably still contractile.

Sex problems 3

Infertility
As a general guideline if a couple who want children have been having sex regularly without contraception for more than a year and conception has not occurred, they should seek medical advice. Causes of infertility (temporary inability to have children) or sterility (where the problem is permanent) are many and varied. Treatments for different infertility problems include:

- psychiatric help to deal with emotional problems;
- antibiotics for infections;
- surgery, for example to unblock the Fallopian tubes;
- use of fertility drugs;
- artificial insemination, with sperm from partner or donor.

Incidence of infertility
As shown in the top diagram *right,* an estimated 25% of all couples have some form of fertility problem. Out of every 100 couples:
a 75 can produce as many children as they want;
b 15 have fewer children than they want;
c 10 cannot have children.

Male and female infertility
When infertility occurs it may be the man, the woman or both who are infertile. As shown in the lower diagram *right:*
1 in 50–55% of cases it is the woman who is infertile;
2 in 30–35% of cases it is the man who is infertile;
3 in 15% of cases both partners are infertile.

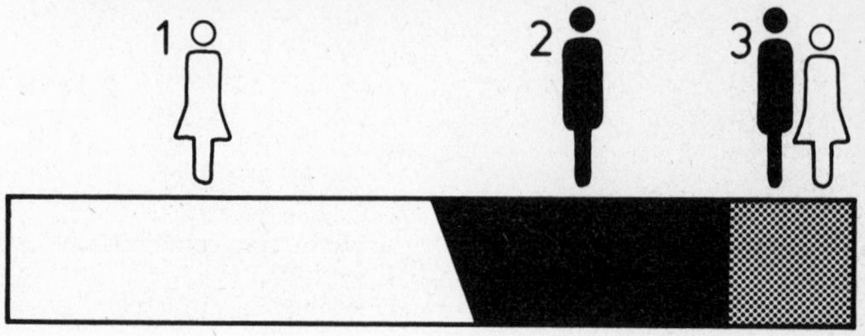

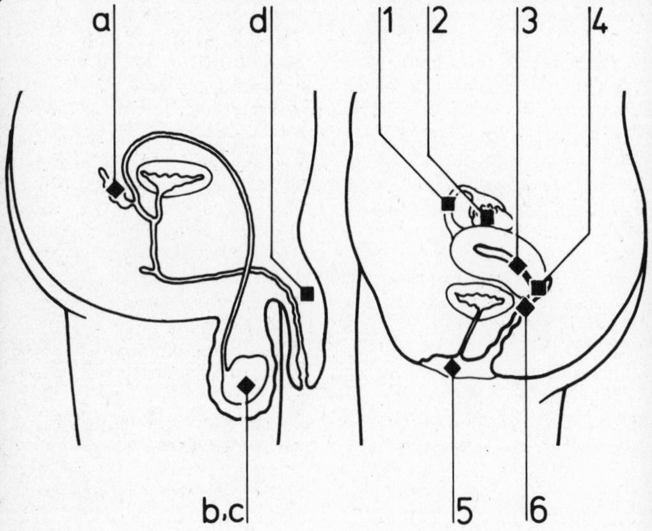

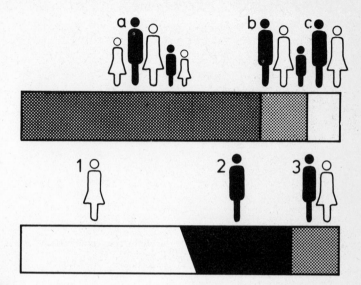

Infertility in men
The following problems, keyed *above,* may contribute to infertility in men.
a Too much or too little seminal fluid; both problems can hinder the sperm's journey to the Fallopian tubes.
b Failure of the testes to descend before puberty.
c Low sperm production caused by prolonged abstinence, overtight underwear, ill health, obesity or poor diet. Sperm can also be malformed or have a short life-span.
d Impotence, making complete intercourse impossible.
Infertility in men may also result from VD, exposure to radiation, and late contraction of some childhood illnesses.

Infertility in women
The following problems, keyed *above,* may contribute to infertility in women.
1 Blocked or malfunctioning Fallopian tubes.
2 Malfunctioning ovaries.
3 Divided or tilted uterus.
4 Disorders of the cervix, perhaps leading to persistent miscarriage, or cervical fluid that is hostile to sperm or the unfertilized egg.
5 Fused labia or strong hymen preventing intercourse.
6 Very narrow, tight or divided vagina.
Other causes of infertility include hormone disorders that affect the menstrual cycle, and nonconsummation because of pain when intercourse is tried.

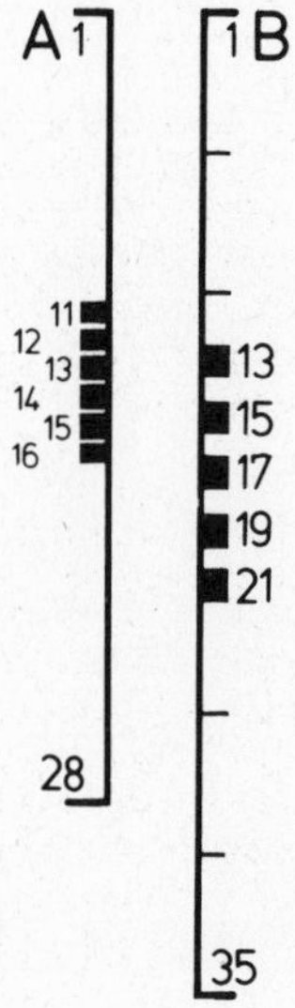

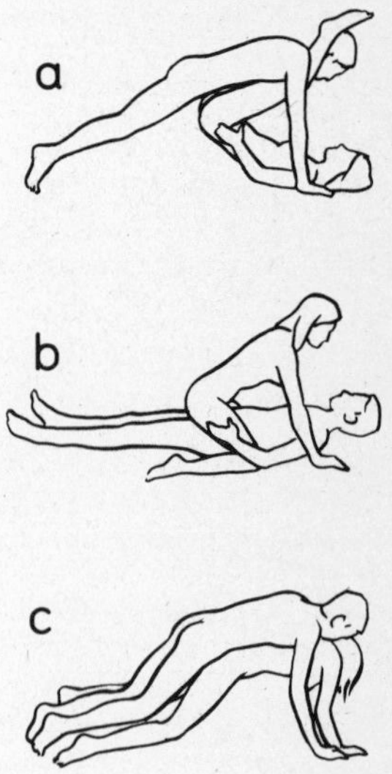

Timing of intercourse
By combining knowledge about the likely time of a woman's ovulation (12 to 16 days before the next menstruation) with information about the life-span of sperm inside a woman (up to 3 days), it becomes possible to predict those times of the month when a couple is most likely to conceive. Fertility counselors will make recommendations for individual couples. The diagram *above* indicates recommended days for intercourse for couples where the woman has a 28-day cycle (**A**) or a 35-day cycle (**B**).

Intercourse positions
Some couples can increase the likelihood of conception by using one of the intercourse positions shown *above.*
a This deep-penetration position brings semen close to the woman's cervix; conception chances further increase if she remains still for 10 minutes after he ejaculates.
b If vaginal tightness is a problem the woman may be advised to squat on top of the man's penis after first dilating the vagina by finger or with a glass dilator.
c Rear-entry positions with the woman kneeling or lying aid fertility in cases where a woman's fertility is being adversely affected by a retroverted (tilted) uterus.

Sexually transmitted diseases
Although modern medicine can cure most sexually transmitted diseases, annual numbers of cases remain alarmingly high. In the USA there are more than one million reported cases of gonorrhea each year, and very many more are believed to go unreported. Meanwhile US cases of syphilis exceed half a million and there may be more than five million Americans with genital herpes. Hindrances in the eradication of sexual diseases include increased promiscuity, more travel by the unattached, declining use of condoms, and the appearance of new disease strains that resist treatment and produce symptom-free carriers.

Sexual infections in the USA
The diagram *right* shows the relative prevalence of the 10 commonest sexually transmitted diseases among persons visiting US venereal clinics in the late 1970s. Listed are numbers of men (first) and women (second) diagnosed as having each disease for every 100 clinic visits by persons of each sex.

a Gonorrhea 24.0, 15.0
b NSGI 24.8, 11.3
c Trichomoniasis 10.4 (women)
d Genital warts 4.3, 3.0
e Candidosis 6.1 (women)
f Genital herpes 3.4, 1.5
g Crab lice 2.9, 1.6
h Molluscum contagiosum 1.0, 3.4
i Syphilis 1.7, 1.4
j Scabies 1.3, 0.4

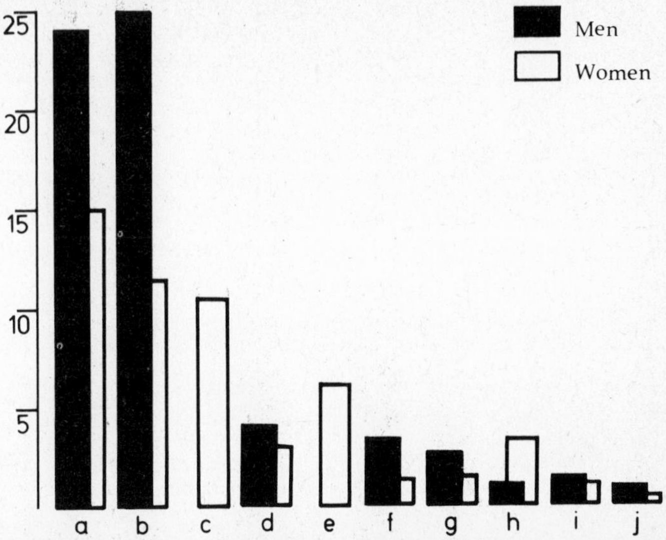

Symptoms and treatments
● NSGI (non-specific genital infections – usually urethritis in men, and vaginitis or cervicitis in women): 1–4 weeks after infection men may have some discharge from the penis and pain on urination; women may have increased vaginal discharge, pain on urination, and abdominal pain. All are treated with antibiotics.
● Gonorrhea: first symptoms in men, usually 2–10 days after infection, are a watery (later thicker, greenish-yellow) penile discharge, frequent urge to urinate and pain on urination; only 20% of females infected show early symptoms – a red, raw vulva, white, yellow or green vaginal discharge, and perhaps pain on urination. Complications can be serious if the disease goes untreated; treatment is with antibiotics.
● Trichomoniasis: symptoms in women are a foul-smelling, greenish, foamy vaginal discharge, and inflammation of the vagina and vulva; men usually have no symptoms but can transmit the disease. Treatment is by drugs.
● Genital warts: appearing 1–6 months after infection, these form a tiny "cauliflower" around genitals or anus. Caustic substances, freezing or cauterization remove them.
● Candidosis (thrush): women have an itchy, swollen vulva, curdy vaginal discharge, and pain on coitus and urination; men may have a red, spotty penis and inner foreskin, with a burning sensation. Treatment is with fungicide.
● Genital herpes: 4–5 days after infection itchy blisters appear on the genitals and then burst to produce shallow, painful ulcers. Sufferers may experience fever and other symptoms. All symptoms go in 2 weeks but milder attacks may recur. As yet there is no cure, but research is promising.
● Crab lice: these produce itching in areas covered by pubic or other body hair. Special lotions cure the problem.
● Molluscum contagiosum: small, painless pink spots with a white plug appear in the genital area up to 3 months after sexual contact. Caustic substances will remove them; otherwise they may last months.
● Syphilis: in stage one, 10–40 days after infection, a small painless sore appears on the part directly infected and persists 4–10 weeks; in stage two, 1½–3 months after infection and lasting up to a year, there is a skin rash, patchy hair loss and perhaps other symptoms; stage three is symptom-free; in stage four, as much as 30 years after infection, vital organs suffer serious, irreversible damage. Before serious damage has occurred, treatment is possible by injections of antibiotics.
● Scabies: shows as small itchy lumps and thin dark lines where mites burrow into the skin. Special lotions effect a cure if meticulously applied.

VD prevention
The following precautions reduce the risk of genital infection.
● Wash genitals daily.
● Change underwear daily.
● Avoid underwear made of nylon as this tends to harbor germs.
● Avoid contact with chemicals that irritate the genitals.
● Wipe the bottom from front to back at toilet visits to avoid transferring germs from the anus to the urethra.
● Keep sexual contact to one infection-free partner.
● Leave 6 weeks between sexual partners in order to reduce your risk of unknowingly incubating a sexual infection that might be passed on.
● Look for discharge or sores on a new partner's genitals.
● Use a condom at intercourse — contraceptive creams and foams also help block infection.
● Wash genitals before and after intercourse.
● Urinate after intercourse.
Early treatment of venereal disease is essential. The following measures should prevent serious complications.
● If you suspect you have a sexually transmitted disease, have a confidential medical examination as soon as possible.
● Warn your partner to seek medical aid.
● Avoid sexual contact.
● Follow the treatment prescribed.
● Have a repeat test to make sure you are cured.
● Avoid reinfection.

VD warning signs
The following symptoms do not necessarily confirm venereal disease but they should be investigated by a doctor.
● A sore, ulcer or rash on the penis, vagina or vulval lips.
● A sore, ulcer or rash on or near the anus.
● Swollen glands in the groin.
● A burning sensation or pain on urination.
● An itchy or sore vagina or itchy penis tip.
● Pain on intercourse.
● Unusual discharge from the penis or vagina.
● A frequent urge to urinate.
● Patchy hair loss.
● Eye infection.
● A sore, ulcer or rash in the mouth or on the lips.
● Body rash.
● Sores in soft skin folds.
● A rash, sore or ulcer on the finger or hand.
● Nausea.
● Low-grade fever.
● Abdominal pain.
● Low backache.
● Excessive, painful periods.

CHAPTER 5

There are many symptoms in the human body that can indicate a variety of physical conditions. The same symptom may appear in conditions that are harmless and also in ones that are potentially fatal; for instance a headache may indicate lack of sleep or may be early warning of meningitis. The diagnosis of the condition will depend on the nature of the symptom; a headache may be a dull throbbing caused by muscle tension or it may be the stabbing pain behind the eyeballs that is symptomatic of glaucoma. Our summary of common symptoms is no substitute for expert diagnosis – a doctor must often take into account whole groups of signs and symptoms – but if you learn to recognize and describe any bodily dysfunctions accurately you will be helping your doctor in his task.

SYMPTOMS

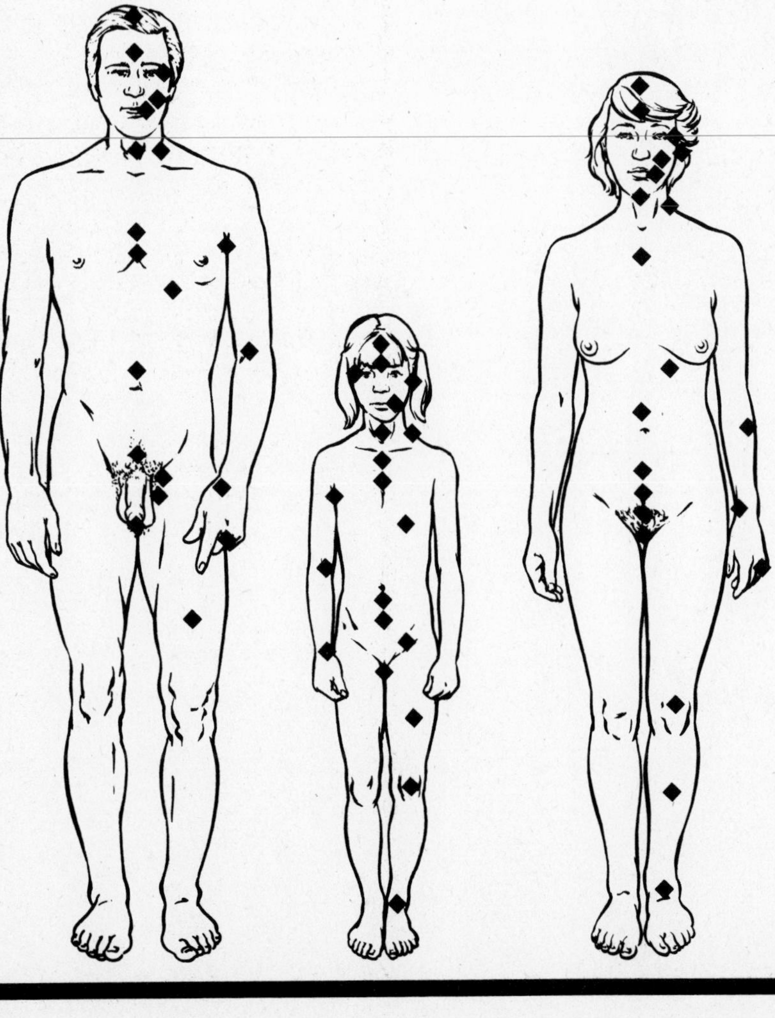

Symptoms in children

These pages list some of the commonest symptoms that infants and children are liable to suffer. Page references refer you to further information. Most illnesses comprise a battery of signs and symptoms, so individual ones are by no means infallible indicators of a particular disease. Children shrug off most troubles without medical help. But you should call your doctor if a baby seems discolored, listless, unconscious, convulsed, distressed; or suffers severe or persistent cough, diarrhea or vomiting; or bleeds from any orifice. Older children need medical help if they continue a high temperature; behave oddly; suffer a serious burn; bleed heavily; lose consciousness or appetite; or suffer from breathing difficulty.

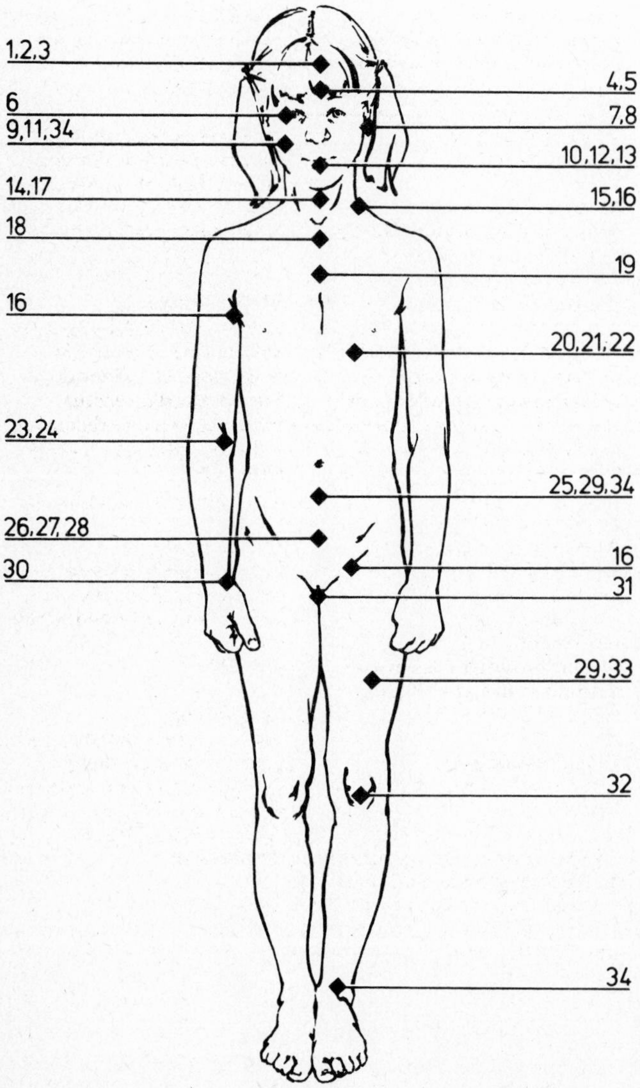

1 Headache
Headaches in children are usually toxic headaches caused by fever; they may sometimes be caused by anxiety.
(Pp. 126–127.)

2 Dizziness
This can be a symptom of infectious diseases and ear troubles, and also anemia.
(Pp. 60–61, 126–127.)

3 Fainting
This is very rare in children before puberty.
(Pp. 88–89.)

4 Fatigue
Emotional stress or influenza are common causes.
(Pp. 92–93, 147.)

5 High temperature
The height of a child's temperature during illness is not an indicator of the severity of the illness, since a high fever often indicates good bodily resistance to the disease. However, a doctor should be called if the fever is prolonged or if the child exhibits other symptoms that could be serious.
Appendicitis, blood-poisoning, bronchitis, chickenpox, croup, gastroenteritis, German measles, influenza, measles, mumps, roseola, sinusitis, tonsillitis and whooping cough may all be accompanied by a fever.
(Pp. 62–63, 92–93, 98–99, 126–127.)

6 Blurred vision
Nearsightedness makes distant objects seem blurred.
(Pp. 58.)

7 Earache
Earache is usually caused by an inflamed eardrum, and may be associated with tonsillitis.
(Pp. 60–63.)

8 Discharge
Ear discharge often indicates a perforated eardrum. Common cold, hay fever and sinusitis yield nasal discharge.
(Pp. 60–63, 90–93.)

9 Pallor
This may follow a knock on the head or accompany stomach ache and motion sickness. It may also be a reaction to cold or emotional shock.
(Pp. 96–97, 126–127.)

10 Crying
Crying babies may be hungry, too cold or hot, uncomfortable from a dirty diaper, or suffering pain from teething, colic, or more severe problems. An experienced mother will usually notice anything unusual in her child's cry.
(Pp. 60–61, 96–97.)

11 Discoloration
Heart or lung troubles may turn skin and lips bluish; liver ailments turn skin and whites of eyes yellow. Bruising may cause livid discoloration that slowly fades.
(Pp. 80–81, 106–107.)

12 Thirst
Excessive thirst may mean dehydration or diabetes; if the thirst is insatiable, seek a doctor's advice quickly.
(Pp. 106–107.)

13 Toothache
This is usually due to tooth decay or injury.
(Pp. 64–67.)

14 Sore throat
This may be due to common cold, pharyngitis, laryngitis, tonsillitis or the onset of a childhood illness.
(Pp. 62–63, 90–91, 126–127.)

15 Stiff neck
Common causes are sleeping awkwardly, exposure to cold, and tonsillitis.
(Pp. 62–63.)

16 Swollen glands
Swollen glands in neck, armpits, or groin may indicate spread of infection (rarely, cancer).
(Pp. 60–63, 126–127.)

17 Hoarseness
Shouting and laryngitis are often to blame for this.
(Pp. 62–63, 126–127.)

18 Cough
Colds, croup, whooping cough and other respiratory irritants produce coughs.
(Pp. 62–63, 90–93, 126–127.)

19 Breathlessness
This can be due to croup, whooping cough, cystic fibrosis or heart or lung troubles.
(Pp. 80–81, 92–93.)

20 Indigestion
Indigestion may be caused by an upset stomach, anxiety, hurried meals or ingesting gas-producing foods. Prolonged indigestion in children over 5 may indicate appendicitis.
(Pp. 94, 96–99.)

21 Nausea and vomiting
Overfed or underfed infants are liable to vomit. Any child with an infection or a cough may be sick. Motion sickness or excessive excitement are other causes.
(Pp. 90–91, 94–99.)

22 Loss of appetite
Intestinal infections, whooping cough, pinworms, obstructive adenoids and emotional stress are common causes.
(Pp. 29, 92, 94–95, 100–101, 126–127, 147.)

23 Itching
Chicken pox, scabies, pinworms and allergy are common causes of itching.
(Pp. 62–63, 76–77, 100–101, 126–127.)

24 Rashes
Infants may suffer diaper rash, prickly heat, roseola (a virus infection). Many children get impetigo, measles, chickenpox, or rashes caused by eczema.
(Pp. 76–79, 102–103, 126–127.)

25 Stomach ache
Abdominal pain in infants may mean feeding wrongly, emotional distress or infection. Some children often suffer gastroenteritis. Severe pain may indicate poisoning, or a surgical condition.
(Pp. 20–21, 94–99, 147.)

26 Constipation
This may affect underfed bottle-fed babies, newly weaned babies, and children dehydrated by fever.
(Pp. 96–97, 100–101, 126–127.)

27 Diarrhea
Bowel infections produce loose green, foul movements in babies and watery movements in older children. Digestive upsets from eating too much fruit, and even respiratory infections commonly produce diarrhea.
(Pp. 100–101.)

28 Flatulence
Air-swallowing by greedy feeders produces intestinal discomfort in some babies.
(Pp. 96–97, 126–127.)

29 Aches and pains
Colicky pain suggests spasm or inflammation of an internal organ; nerve pain may be a diffuse, burning feeling; skin pain burns or pricks; and bone or muscle pain is diffuse and aching.
(Pp. 70–71.)

30 Pulse changes
Most fevers raise the pulse rate by 10 beats per minute for each Fahrenheit degree rise in body temperature.
(Pp. 126–127.)

31 Enuresis (bedwetting)
This can mean late development of the brain's bladder-control center, worry, physical illness or emotional disturbance.
(Pp. 102–103.)

32 Stiff joints
Active children rarely get stiff joints under normal circumstances; if they do occur they may indicate virus infection, juvenile rheumatoid arthritis, rheumatic fever or leukemia.
(Pp. 68–69, 72–73, 167.)

33 Aching legs
Leg pain can be a lesser symptom in infections including measles and scarlet fever.
(Pp. 127.)

34 Swelling
Swelling of the face may occur in response to an allergen; swelling of the face, abdomen and ankles may indicate kidney disease or heart failure.
(Pp. 104–105.)

Symptoms in men

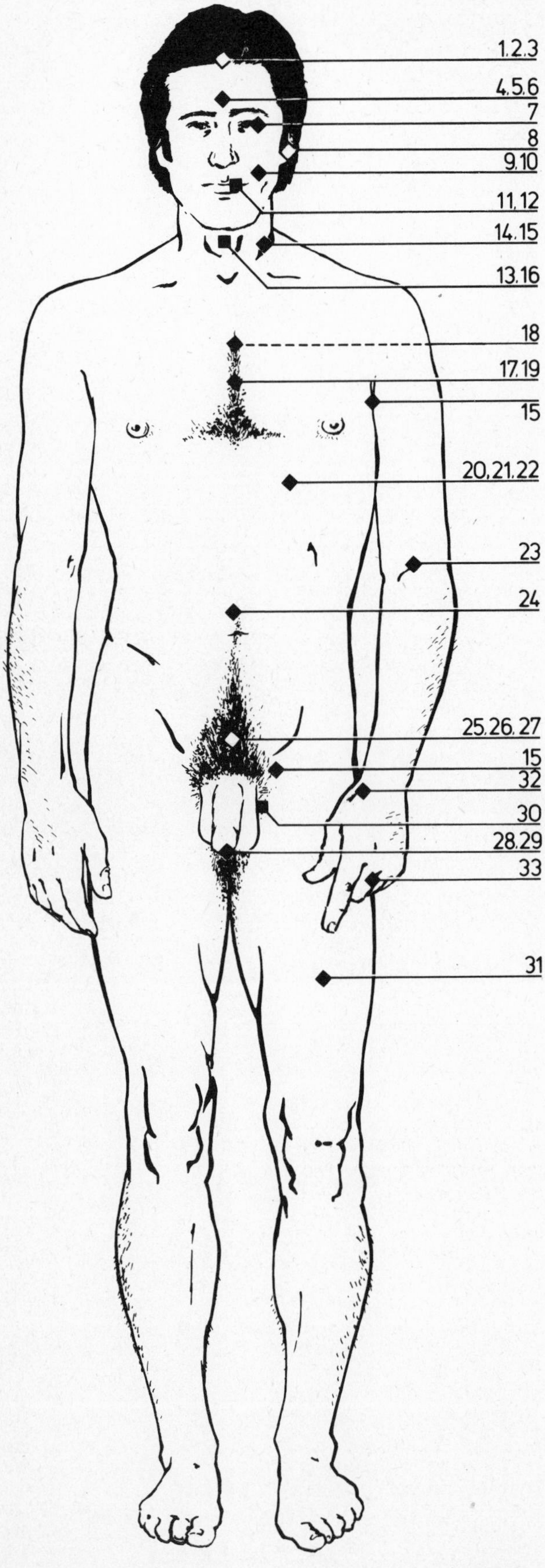

Some of the symptoms on these pages arise from ailments peculiar to males, particularly adults. Because men are more muscular than women and perform more heavy work, they are more liable to injure ligaments and muscles. Moreover diseases including stomach cancer and peptic ulcers occur more frequently in men than women, and under age 45 or so men are more liable to heart attacks. However, many symptoms spring from diseases that both men and women suffer (see pages 184–185). Space restricts us to listing a few, mainly common symptoms and causal conditions. Our pointers offer no substitute for thorough medical diagnosis.

1 Headaches
Most headaches have minor significance, but new or severe types should be investigated. (Pp. 160–161.)

2 Dizziness
Rising after kneeling can make you dizzy. Dizziness can mean ear, heart or circulation problems, brain injury or heat exhaustion. (Pp. 60–61.)

3 Fainting
Causes include long standing (as in troops on parade), strangulated inguinal hernia, a sudden blow to the testes or internal bleeding, such as a bleeding peptic ulcer. (Pp. 88–89, 98–99.)

4 Fatigue
Emotional stress or various diseases may be responsible. (Pp. 129, 160–161.)

5 Depression
Job loss, marriage breakdown, bereavement, or organic disease (such as chronic gastritis) may produce depression. (Pp. 82–83, 98–99, 146–147, 172–175.)

6 High temperature
Many infectious diseases cause a fever in either sex. (See children's symptoms.)

7 Blurred vision
Various disorders of eye, kidney or pancreas can blur vision. (Pp. 58–59, 104–107.)

8 Earache
Ear, nose or throat infection or injury to the eardrum (perhaps the result of an explosion, deep diving or a sudden blow) can cause earache. (Pp. 60–63,.)

9 Pallor
Shock, heart attack, hiatus hernia, anemia, motion sickness and blood loss may all produce pallor. (Pp. 88–89, 96–99.)

10 Discoloration
Causes of discoloration are similar to those for women. (Pp. 106–107.)

11 Thirst
Diabetes, anemia, fluid loss and certain poisons are among factors that produce excessive thirst. (Pp. 88–89, 106–107.)

12 Toothache
Tooth decay, impacted wisdom teeth or injury are usually responsible; severe throat and nose infections may also produce pain that seems to be located in the jaw. (Pp. 64–65.)

13 Sore throat
Possible causes are as for children, also (more rarely) quinsy, syphilis and cancer. (Pp. 62.)

14 Stiff neck
This may be due to arthritis, back injury or slipped disk; see also children's symptoms. (Pp. 68–69.)

15 Swollen glands
Swollen glands in the neck, armpits or groin indicate infection (rarely, cancer). Swollen testes and scrotum can occur during mumps.
(Pp. 60–63.)

16 Hoarseness
Causes are as listed under women's symptoms; hoarseness persisting for two weeks should be investigated.
(Pp. 62.)

17 Cough
Causes are similar to those listed for women. A persistent cough starting in middle age sometimes means lung cancer.
(Pp. 90–93, 152–155, 166.)

18 Backache
Strained muscles, a slipped disk, and fatigue commonly cause backache. So may depression, stress and other emotional problems.
(Pp. 68–69, 72–73, 146–147.)

19 Breathlessness
Obesity, heart trouble, asthma, lung disease, anxiety, chronic bronchitis, pneumonia, perforated ulcer and high altitudes may all cause breathlessness.
(Pp. 29, 39, 92–93, 99.)

20 Indigestion
Emotional stress, overindulgence in food or alcohol, hasty eating, bad teeth, hiatus hernia, constipation, appendicitis and other factors, most trivial, can produce this.
(Pp. 64–65, 96–101, 146–147.)

21 Nausea and vomiting
Food poisoning, dyspepsia, infections and alcohol abuse are likely to produce nausea and vomiting.
(Pp. 62, 96–99.)

22 Loss of appetite
Possible causes include stress, intestinal infection, and diseases of the stomach.
(Pp. 82–83, 94–99, 146–147.)

23 Rashes
These range from skin infections and allergies to rashes of systemic origin.
(Pp. 76–79.)

24 Stomach ache
Gastrointestinal inflammation and salt deficiency are possible causes.
(Pp. 98–99.)

25 Constipation
Lack of exercise or of roughage in the diet are common causes of constipation; rarely the problem may be a bowel obstruction.
(Pp. 100–101.)

26 Diarrhea
This may be caused by infection, certain drugs, eating foods that disagree with you, or a gastrointestinal disease.
(Pp. 18–19, 96–101.)

27 Flatulence
Air-swallowing or disease of the esophagus, stomach, small or large intestine, or gallbladder may make men belch or pass wind.
(Pp. 96–99, 106–107.)

28 Discharge
Discharge from the penis suggests a genital infection.
(Pp. 110–111, 176–177.)

29 Painful urination
This may reflect infection of the urinary tract or an enlarged prostate gland.
(Pp. 103–105, 110–111.)

30 Itching
Itchy genitals may mean crab lice, nonspecific urethritis, fungus infection or scabies.
(Pp. 76–77, 110–111, 176–177.)

31 Aches and pains
These range from strained or sprained muscles or ligaments and arthritis in joints to male problems like prostatitis, urethritis and an infected glans and foreskin.
(Pp. 34, 40, 68–69, 72–73, 102, 111.)

32 Pulse changes
Normal pulse rate is 65–72 in men, slower in old age. High blood pressure and fever may raise the rate. Extra beats, missed beats and a slow pulse seldom indicate disease.
(Pp. 81, 88–89.)

33 Trembling
Violent physical exertion can produce a temporary tremor; see also women's symptoms.
(Pp. 117.)

Symptoms in women

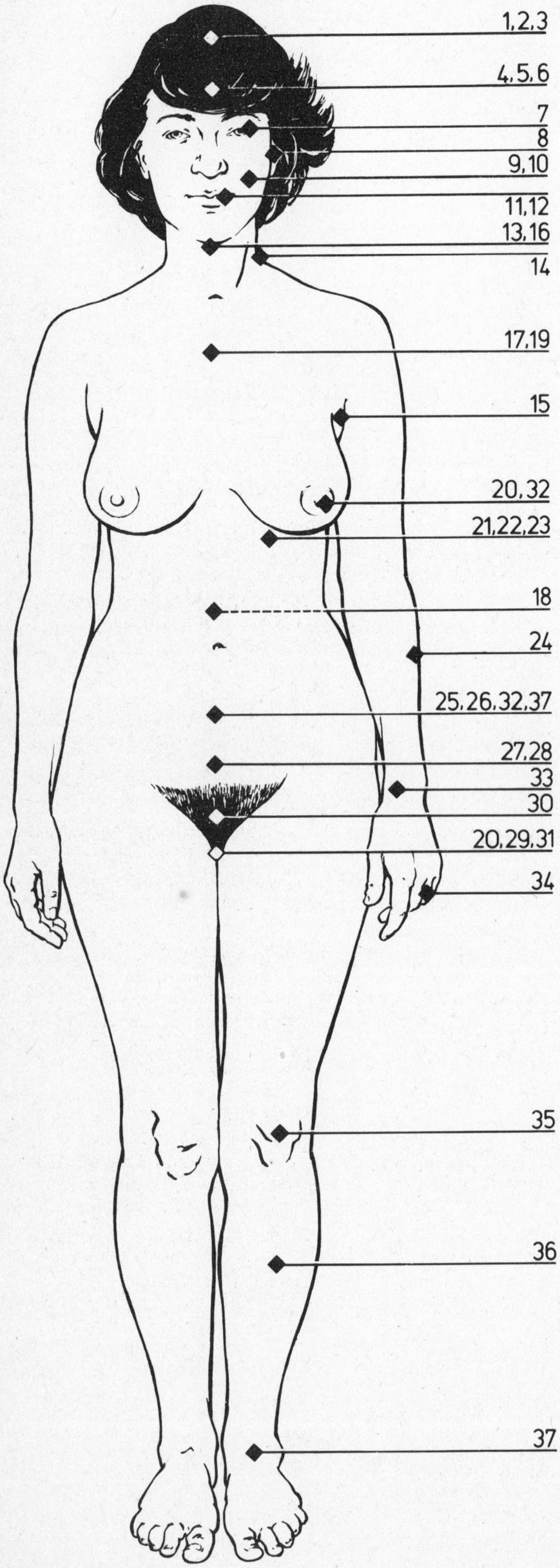

Periodic changes brought about by female sex hormones and the extensive body area taken up in women by the breasts and reproductive tract help to give rise to many (mostly minor) symptoms suffered only by females after puberty. The hormonal changes that usher in the menopause can cause further problems. For various reasons, women also suffer more than men from migraine, gallbladder troubles and some other problems such as fainting and varicose veins. These pages stress symptoms related to female problems, but include symptoms caused by ailments also found in men or children. So for further possible causes see also pages 180–183.

1 Headache
Women may suffer premenstrual, menstrual, or tension headaches, or migraine. See also men's symptoms.
(Pp. 114–115, 136–137, 160–161.)

2 Dizziness
Migraine, the contraceptive pill, toxemia of pregnancy, the menopause and anemia may produce dizzy spells. See also men's symptoms.
(Pp. 60–61, 132–133, 136–137, 170–171.)

3 Fainting
Women faint more easily than men, for instance in stuffy rooms, in early pregnancy, or when suffering from emotional stress or anemia.
(Pp. 17, 88–89, 130–131, 146–147.)

4 Fatigue
Premenstrual tension, emotional disturbances, the menopause, infections, diabetes, anemia and hypothyroidism all produce fatigue.
(Pp. 88–89, 114–115, 129, 136–137, 160–161.)

5 Depression
Childbirth, marriage problems or the menopause may be to blame. See also men's symptoms.
(Pp. 82–83, 136–137, 146–147, 172–173.)

6 High temperature
Many infectious diseases and chest and kidney infections produce high temperatures. See also children's symptoms.

7 Blurred vision
Nearsightedness, farsightedness, migraine, and toxemia of pregnancy can all blur vision. See also men's symptoms.
(Pp. 58–59, 132–133.)

8 Earache
Ear, nose or throat infection is usually the cause.
(Pp. 60–63.)

9 Pallor
Blood loss due to piles or menstrual flow can cause pallor. Shock and heart attack are other possible causes.
(Pp. 114–115.)

10 Discoloration
Liver and gallbladder diseases produce jaundice; bruising produces skin discoloration. Addison's disease browns skin on the knees, elbows, knuckles; heart or lung disease may tinge the lips and face blue.
(Pp. 106–107.)

11 Thirst
Anemia, dehydration and diabetes provoke excessive thirst.
(Pp. 88–89, 106–107.)

12 Toothache
Impacted wisdom teeth and tooth decay (a risk in pregnancy) make teeth ache.
(Pp. 64–65.)

13 Sore throat
See children's symptoms and men's symptoms for causes.

14 Stiff neck
This may be due to arthritis, neck injury or slipped disk. See also children's symptoms. (Pp. 68–69.)

15 Swollen glands
Swollen glands in neck, armpits, or groin indicate infection; mononucleosis (glandular fever) causes swollen glands in many parts of the body. Some cancers may cause swollen glands nearby. (Pp. 108–109, 164–167.)

16 Hoarseness
Laryngitis, upper respiratory tract infections, benign tumors and cancer of the larynx or esophagus can all make someone hoarse. (Pp. 62.)

17 Cough
Colds, smoking, asthma, bronchitis, pneumonia and other respiratory conditions or irritants make people cough. (Pp. 90–93, 152–155, 166.)

18 Backache
This is sometimes linked with menstruation, pregnancy, menopause or prolapsed uterus; other causes may be as for men. (Pp. 72–73, 112–115, 130–131, 136–137.)

19 Breathlessness
Early pregnancy, obesity, and various heart and lung troubles cause breathlessness. See also men's symptoms. (Pp. 29, 39, 130–133.)

20 Discharge
Benign cysts and breast cancer may produce nipple discharge. Unusual vaginal discharge suggests infection or possibly a cervical or uterine tumor. See also children's symptoms. (Pp. 78, 108–109, 114–115.)

21 Indigestion
Gallbladder trouble, pregnancy, and the menopause can cause indigestion. See also men's symptoms. (Pp. 96–97, 106–107, 130–131, 136–137.)

22 Nausea and vomiting
Migraine, early pregnancy and some infections cause these. (Pp. 62, 96–99, 130–131.)

23 Loss of appetite
Anorexia nervosa, depressive illness, menopause or intestinal infection may be to blame. (Pp. 28, 94–95, 98–99, 136–137, 146–147.)

24 Rashes
Rashes of special significance to women include those produced by rosacea and German measles. (Pp. 76–79.)

25 Stomach ache
This may accompany menstruation or be due to disease inside the genital tract. Agonizing cramps radiating to back and shoulder may mean gallstone trouble. (Pp. 106–107, 112–115.)

26 Painful periods
Hormonal changes in the uterus, and sometimes diseased reproductive organs, cause these. (Pp. 113–115.)

27 Constipation
This often coincides with painful periods, pregnancy and childbirth. (Pp. 28, 100–101, 114–115, 130–131.)

28 Diarrhea
This may be caused by infection, certain drugs, eating foods that disagree with you, or some gastrointestinal disease. (Pp. 18–19, 96–101.)

29 Flatulence
Belching or passing wind may indicate air-swallowing or disease of the digestive tract. (Pp. 97–99.)

30 Itching
Itchy genitals may mean genital infection or pubic infestation. (Pp. 76–77, 176–177.)

31 Painful urination
This may mean urinary tract infection, kidney stones, or inflammation of the vagina or vulva. (Pp. 103–105.)

32 Aches and pains
These range from minor muscle problems to arthritis. Women are liable to pains in the breasts, lower back and abdomen. (Pp. 34, 40, 68–69, 72–73, 108–109, 114–115.)

33 Pulse changes
Normal heartbeat for women is 70–80, slower in old age. Rapid heartbeat (tachycardia) often occurs in menstruation, pregnancy and menopause. (Pp. 81, 114–115, 131, 136–137.)

34 Trembling
Anxiety, cold, fear, drugs and old age may produce trembling. (P. 117.)

35 Stiff joints
Stiff knees and hips may signal osteoarthritis. Rheumatoid arthritis affects many joints. (Pp. 68–69.)

36 Aching legs
Obesity makes legs ache. Cramping leg pains may be caused by painful periods or varicose veins. (Pp. 29, 40, 120–121.)

37 Swelling
Premenstrual tension, the contraceptive pill, toxemia of pregnancy and kidney trouble cause general edema; pregnancy and ovarian cysts produce abdominal swelling. See also men's symptoms. (Pp. 104–105, 114–115, 132–133.)

Index

Index

Index